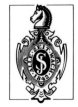

J. A. Young · P. Y. D. Wong (Eds)

Epithelial Secretion of Water and Electrolytes

With 24 Tables and 94 Illustrations

Springer-Verlag Berlin Heidelberg New York
London Paris Tokyo Hong Kong

J. A. Young, DSc MD (Qld) FAA FRACP
Department of Physiology, University of Sydney, Sydney, NSW 2006, Australia

P. Y. D. Wong, MA PhD (Cantab) DSc (Lond) FRSC FIBiol
Department of Physiology, Faculty of Medicine, University of Hong Kong, Li Shu Fan Building, Sassoon Road, Hong Kong

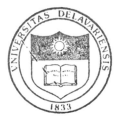

ISBN 3-540-51627-1 Springer-Verlag Berlin Heidelberg New York
ISBN 0-387-51627-1 Springer-Verlag New York Berlin Heidelberg

List of Contributors

Argent, B.E.
Department of Physiological Sciences, University Medical School, Framlington Place, Newcastle upon Tyne NE2 4HH, UK

Bijman, J.
Department of Cell Biology and Genetics, Faculty of Medicine, Erasmus University Rotterdam, Dr. Molewaterplein 50, 3000 DR Rotterdam, The Netherlands

Brown, P.D.
Department of Physiological Sciences, University of Manchester, Stopford Building, Oxford Road, Manchester M13 9PT, UK

Case, R.M.
Department of Physiological Sciences, University of Manchester, Stopford Building, Oxford Road, Manchester M13 9PT, UK

Cook, D.I.
Department of Physiology, University of Sydney, Sydney, NSW 2006, Australia

Curci, S.
Istituto di Fisiologia Generale, Università degli Studi, Via Amendaola 165A, 70126 Bari, Italy

Cuthbert, A.W.
Department of Pharmacology, University of Cambridge, Hills Road, Cambridge CB2 2QD, UK

Dunne, M.J.
The M.R.C. Secretory Control Research Group, The Physiological Laboratory, University of Liverpool, Brownlow Hill, P.O. Box 147, Liverpool L69 3BX, UK

Elliott, A.C.
Department of Physiological Sciences, University of Manchester, Stopford Building, Oxford Road, Manchester M13 9PT, UK

Frömter, E.
Zentrum der Physiologie, Klinikum der J.W.-Goethe-Universität, Theodor-Stern-Kai 7, 6000 Frankfurt/Main 70, FRG

Giaume, C.
Laboratoire de Neurobiologie, Ecole Normale Supérieure, 46, rue d'Ulm, 75230 Paris Cedex 05, France

Gitter, A.H.
Hals-Nasen-Ohren-Klinik der Universität Tübingen, Silcherstraße 5, 7400 Tübingen 1, FRG

Gögelein, H.
Max-Planck-Institut für Biophysik, Kennedyallee 70, 6000 Frankfurt/Main 70, FRG

Graf, J.
Institut für Allgemeine und Experimentelle Pathologie der Universität Wien, Währinger Straße 13, 1090 Wien, Austria

Gray, M.A.
Department of Physiological Sciences, University Medical School, Framlington Place, Newcastle upon Tyne NE2 4HH, UK

Greenwell, J.R.
Department of Physiological Sciences, University Medical School, Framlington Place, Newcastle upon Tyne NE2 4HH, UK

Greger, R.
Physiologisches Institut der Universität Freiburg, Hermann-Herder-Straße 7, 7800 Freiburg, FRG

Hayashi, H.
Department of Physiology, Tohoku University School of Medicine, 2–1 Seiryo-cho, Sendai 980, Japan

Hoogeveen, A.M.
Department of Cell Biology and Genetics, Faculty of Medicine, Erasmus University Rotterdam, Dr. Molewaterplein 50, 3000 DR Rotterdam, The Netherlands

Imai, Y.
Department of Physiology, Osaka Medical College, 2–7 Daigaku-machi, Takatsuki City, Osaka 569, Japan

De Jonge, H.R.
Department of Biochemistry I, Faculty of Medicine, Erasmus University Rotterdam, Dr. Molewaterplein 50, 3000 DR Rotterdam, The Netherlands

Van der Kamp, A.W.M.
Department of Cell Biology and Genetics, Faculty of Medicine, Erasmus University Rotterdam, Dr. Molewaterplein 50, 3000 DR Rotterdam, The Netherlands

Kanno T.
Department of Physiology, Faculty of Veterinary Medicine, Hokkaido University, Sapporo 060, Japan

Kansen, M.
Department of Cell Biology and Genetics, Faculty of Medicine, Erasmus University Rotterdam, Dr. Molewaterplein 50, 3000 DR Rotterdam, The Netherlands

Kemmer, T.P.
Max-Planck-Institut für Biophysik, Kennedyallee 70, 6000 Frankfurt/Main 70, FRG

Kunzelmann, K.
Physiologisches Institut der Universität Freiburg, Hermann-Herder-Straße 7, 7800 Freiburg, FRG

Lau, K.R.
Department of Physiological Sciences, University of Manchester, Stopford Building, Oxford Road, Manchester M13 9PT, UK

Marshall, A. T.
Department of Zoology, La Trobe University, Bundoora, Victoria 3083, Australia

Martinez, J. R.
Biomedical Research Division, Lovelace Medical Foundation, 2425 Ridgecrest Boulevard, S.E. Albuquerque, NM 87108, USA

Maruyama, Y.
Department of Physiology, Jichi Medical School, Minamikawachi-machi, Tochigi-ken 329-04, Japan

Murakami, M.
Department of Molecular Physiology, National Institute for Physiological Sciences, Okazaki, Japan

Nauntofte, B.
Institute of Oral Function, The Panum Institute, The Royal Dental College, 2200 Copenhagen, Denmark

Nishiyama, A.
Department of Physiology, Tohoku University School of Medicine, 2–1 Seiryo-cho, Sendai, Miyagi 980, Japan

Novak, I.
Physiologisches Institut, Albert-Ludwigs-Universität, Hermann-Herder-Straße 7, 7800 Freiburg, FRG

Ozawa, T.
Department of Physiology, Tohoku University School of Medicine, 2–1 Seiryo-cho, Sendai, Miyagi 980, Japan

Petersen, O. H.
The M.R.C. Secretory Control Research Group, The Physiological Laboratory, University of Liverpool, Brownlow Hill, P.O. Box 147, Liverpool L69 3BX, UK

Poulsen, J. H.
Department of General Physiology and Biophysics, The Panum Institute, University of Copenhagen, Blegdamsvej 3, 2200 Copenhagen, Denmark

Quissell, D. O.
Oral Sciences Research Center, University of Colorado Health Science Center, 1300 South Potomac Street, Suite 110, Aurora, CO 80012, USA

Randriamampita, C.
Laboratoire de Neurobiologie, Ecole Normale Supérieure, 46, rue d'Ulm, 75230 Paris Cedex 05, France

Reid, A. M.
Department of Veterinary Physiology, University of Sydney, Sydney, NSW 2006, Australia

Roberts, M. L.
Department of Physiology, University of Adelaide, G.P.O. Box 498, Adelaide, SA 5001, Australia

Saito, Y.
Department of Physiology, Tohoku University School of Medicine, 2–1 Seiryo-cho, Sendai, Miyagi 980, Japan

Schmid, A.
Max-Planck-Institut für Biophysik, Kennedyallee 70, 6000 Frankfurt/Main 70, FRG

Scholte, B.J.
Department of Cell Biology and Genetics, Faculty of Medicine, Erasmus University Rotterdam, Dr. Molewaterplein 50, 3000 DR Rotterdam, The Netherlands

Schulz, I.
Max-Planck-Institut für Biophysik, Kennedyallee 70, 6000 Frankfurt/Main 70, FRG

Seo, Y.
Department of Molecular Physiology, National Institute for Physiological Sciences, Okazaki, Japan

Steward, M.C.
Department of Physiological Sciences, University of Manchester, School of Medicine, Manchester M13 9PT, UK

Takahashi, H.
Department of Physiology, Tohoku University School of Medicine, 2–1 Seiryo-cho, Sendai 980, Japan

Titchen, D.A,
Department of Veterinary Physiology, University of Sydney, Sydney, NSW 2006, Australia

Trautmann, A.
Laboratoire de Neurobiologie, Ecole Normale Supérieure, 46, rue d'Ulm, 75230 Paris Cedex 05, France

Watari, H.
Department of Molecular Physiology, National Institute for Physiological Sciences, Okazaki, Japan

Wong, P.Y.D.
Department of Physiology, University of Hong Kong, Li Shu Fan Building, Sassoon Road, Hong Kong

Young, J.A.
Department of Physiology, University of Sydney, Sydney, NSW 2006, Australia

Preface

In 1976, when Springer-Verlag commissioned Professors Giebisch, Tosteson, and Ussing to edit what was destined to become a monumental five-volume *Handbuch* ("Membrane Transport in Biology", 1978 [Vols I, II, III] and 1979 [Vols IV A, B]), the subject of transepithelial secretion was still in its infancy. Not surprisingly, therefore, their *Handbuch* concentrated mainly on transepithelial absorption, although substantial chapters dealing with some secretory organs were included, viz. "Ion Transport Across the Choroid Plexus" (by E. M. Wright), "Sweat Glands" (by J. H. Thaysen), "Lacrimal Gland" (by J. H. Thaysen) and "Transport Across Insect Excretory Epithelia" (by J. P. H. Maddrell) in Volume III and "Transport in Salivary and Salt Glands" (by J. A. Young and E. W. Van Lennep), "Gastric Secretion" (by T. E. Machen and J. G. Forte), "Transport Processes in the Exocrine Pancreas" (by I. Schulz and K. J. Ullrich), and "Transport of Ions in Liver Cells" (by M. Claret) in Volume IV B. The publication in 1977 of the seminal paper of Silva and his colleagues on the mechanism of secretion of salt and water in the salt excreting gland of the dogfish (American Journal of Physiology 233, F298–F306, 1977) provided physiologists with their first real insight into the mechanisms underlying transepithelial fluid secretion, however, and, in the ensuing years, interest in the topic has exploded as is evidenced by the numerous international symposia on exocrine secretion held since that date.

It was the most recent of these symposia, organized by Dr. P. Y. D. Wong and myself in Hong Kong in February 1988, that provided the inspiration for the present volume. When we planned that conference, we were agreed that the conference proceedings should be published in time to be of use at the conference; this was achieved with the publication in January 1988 of "Exocrine Secretion" (Hong Kong University Press, edited by P. Y. D. Wong and J. A. Young). Nevertheless it was also apparent that the time was ripe for publication of a review volume on exocrine secretion that would put the advances in our knowledge of the subject since 1977 in perspective. Since most of those whom we would have wished to contribute to such a book were present at the conference, we took the opportunity to approach each for an article and we entered into arrangements with Springer-Verlag to publish the volume. Rapid publication was clearly essential if the book was to be of more than archival value, so we set a deadline of eight months for preparation of the manuscripts, three months for the editors to do their part, and six months for Springer to produce the volume. This, too, has been achieved.

In some respects the coverage of the volume is wider in its scope than we originally intended although in other respects it is narrower. The scope is wider, in that, in addition to chapters on the mechanism of secretion of salt and water, we have included chapters on the control of secretion and on the secretion of exportable protein. These additions need no apology since the broadened coverage clearly helps put the topic of fluid transport into better perspective. Coverage is narrower than originally planned in that we have not included chapters on all the major secreting organs, the intestine, sweat glands, and the choroid plexus being notable omissions. Although such omissions will doubtless distress those with specialist interests, we feel that the information available about secretion by the seven exocrine organs that are included will provide an amply broad perspective for the more general reader.

The coverage of this volume falls into two sections. In the first, entitled General Aspects of Secretion, we have included chapters on the role in secretion of cation and anion channels in the plasma membranes, as well as the role of gap junctions and ion channels in intracellular organelles. We have also included a chapter on signal transduction and, in addition, several chapters on some new techniques that are helping to increase our knowledge of secretion: capacitance measurements, nuclear magnetic resonance, use of mutant cell lines, and use of network thermodynamic analysis. In the second section, entitled "Secretion in Individual Tissues", we have included six chapters on various aspects of salivary secretion as well as chapters on lacrimal glands, the pancreas, the gastric mucosa, the liver, the epididymis, and vertebrate salt glands. Finally, we have included a chapter specifically dealing with cystic fibrosis, a disease predominantly affecting secretory epithelia.

My own interest in exocrine secretion dates back to 1964 when I had the good fortune to take up an Australian Government scholarship to study in Berlin in the laboratories of Professor K.J. Ullrich. I had gone there hoping to study urea transport in the loop of Henle, but Professor Ullrich persuaded me instead to undertake a project involving the micropuncture of rat salivary glands, initiated in Berlin in the previous year by Professor J.R. Martinez. A quarter of a century later, I know I will never get around to studying urea transport in Henle's loop but I also know that I owe a great debt of gratitude to Professor Ullrich for introducing me to the fascinating field of secretion, a field that has become my life's work. Looking over the list of papers in this volume, I see that no less than 10 of the 25 chapters in it come from the laboratories of past or present collaborators of Professor Ullrich, from which it will be clear that the topic of secretion owes a great deal to him even though he himself remains firmly committed to absorption and the kidney. At the Hong Kong conference we were greatly honored to have Professor Ullrich attend and present a paper on secretion (in the kidney proximal tubule). Now, as I write this preface, I should like to pay tribute to his eminence by dedicating this volume to him.

Sydney, May 1989   *John Atherton Young*

Contents

3 Exocrine Pancreas

4 Endocrine Pancreas

5 Gastric Mucosa

6 Liver

7 Epididymis

8 Salt Glands

9 Cystic Fibrotic Epithelia

A General Aspects of Secretion

Epithelial Chloride Channels *

R. Greger and K. Kunzelmann

Introduction

The present short overview summarizes the role of chloride channels in epithelial transport. At present, we are aware of a general concept in which chloride uptake is carrier mediated and driven by the electrochemical gradient for chloride and the cotransported or countertransported ions, and in which chloride exit occurs via chloride channels. Basically, two concepts have been suggested to account for hormonal upregulation of chloride transport. The first involves primary stimulation of potassium pathways (Petersen 1987), resulting in cell hyperpolarization and a consequent increase in the driving force for conductive chloride exit from the cell. The other involves a primary increase in chloride conductance and, thus, depolarization of the cell. This results in an increased driving force for conductive potassium exit from the cell (Greger et al. 1986). In the many different chloride-secreting epithelia that exist, it may turn out that the models described above may only be extremes and that intermediate constellations may also occur (Marty et al. 1984; Young et al. 1988). The currently known mechanisms of channel activation make it seem likely that we will have to deal with more than one or two general mechanisms of channel regulation.

Chloride Channels

The chloride channels observed in epithelia are currently subdivided into three categories: small, intermediate, and large channels. Table 1 attempts to utilize such a formalistic subdivision to classify the different epithelia. It is apparent that the large chloride channels, with a conductance greater than 100 pS, have been found in only a few cultured epithelia. The most frequently encountered chloride channels are of 5–100 pS conductance. There is, however, substantial evidence making it appear very likely that chloride channels with a conductance of less than 5 pS occur in a variety of chloride-secreting epithelia.

---

* The work from the authors' laboratory cited in this review has been supported by DFG 480/9 and by a grant from the EC: ST 2 y-0095-2-D (CD).

Table 1. Epithelial chloride channels

Tissue	Membrane	Conductance (pS)	Reference
Small channels:			
Lacrimal gland	Apical	1–2	Marty et al. 1984
Salivary gland	Apical	1–2	Young et al. 1988
Pancreas duct	Apical	4.5	Argent et al. 1987
Intermediate channels:			
Thick ascending limb	Basolateral	20–30	Greger and Kunzelmann 1988
Urinary bladder	Basolateral	64	Hanrahan et al. 1985 (cf. also large channel)
Malpighian tubule	Apical	25	Summarized in Gögelein 1988
Choroid plexus	Apical	31	Zeuthen et al. 1987
Sweat gland	Apical	25, 50	Gögelein 1988; Welsh et al. 1987
Rectal gland	Apical	11, 45	Gögelein et al. 1987b; Greger et al. 1987a
Trachea and respiratory epithelial cells	Apical	10–80	Kunzelmann et al. 1987b; Frizzell 1987; Frömter and Disser 1988; Welsh 1987a
Colon crypt cell	Apical	15–50	Halm et al. 1988; Hayslett et al. 1987
Cornea	Apical	70	Koniarek and Leibovitch 1985
Large channels:			
Urinary bladder	Basolateral	360	Hanrahan et al. 1985
A6 cells	Apical	360	Nelson et al. 1984
Alveolar cell	Apical	380	Krouse et al. 1986; Schneider et al. 1985
Amphiuma diluting segment	Basolateral	150–200	Kawahara and Giebisch 1987
Collecting duct principal cell	Apical	120	Christine et al. 1987
MDCK cells	Apical	460	Kolb et al. 1985

The very large conductance channels are difficult to categorize as their role in secretion or reabsorbtion of chloride is quite uncertain. The small conductance chloride channels appear to play an important role in various glands such as the lacrimal gland (Marty et al. 1984), mandibular gland (Young et al. 1988), and pancreas (Petersen 1986). In these glands, the chloride channel activation is apparently parallel or secondary to the initial activation of K^+ channels (Petersen 1986). It is worth noting at this point that these small chloride channels have not been resolved by single channel analysis, and their existence has been deduced exclusively from whole-cell current recordings (Marty et al. 1984; Young et al. 1988) and from microelectrode potential measurements (Petersen 1986). In these whole-cell preparations no larger conductance chloride channels have been identified. It is somehow disturbing that single channel analysis has not been performed in these preparations, and that, conversely, whole-cell current measurements have been attempted only very rarely in the preparations exposing clearly defined single channel chloride currents. The dilemma presents two aspects. One is due to the fact that the amplitude resolution of the single channel analysis is limited to rather less than 1 pA, i.e., channels with a conductance of less than $1-2$ pS can hardly be detected at reasonable driving forces. The other dilemma has to do with the biological preparation. In many secretory acinar cells the luminal membrane is very small when compared with the basolateral membrane surface. Thus, it is very likely that the patch pipette will record from the basolateral surface, and very unlikely that the properties of the apical membrane will be recorded. This, however, is the membrane in which chloride channels are to be expected. The present review will focus mostly on the chloride channels of intermediate conductance.

Chloride Channels with Intermediate Conductance

Intermediate-conductance chloride channels have now been found in several chloride reabsorbing and secreting epithelia. Examples include the thick ascending limb of Henle's loop (Greger 1986), the rectal gland tubule of the dogfish (*Squalus acanthias*; Gögelein et al. 1987; Greger et al. 1987a), colonic carcinoma cells (Halm et al. 1988; Hayslett et al. 1987) which appear to resemble the chloride-secreting cells of the colonic crypts, and respiratory epithelial cells in primary culture as they are derived from human nasal polyps (Frizzell 1987; Kunzelmann et al. 1988a; Welsh and Liedtke 1986). The chloride channels in these preparations have many properties in common. Some of these are summarized in Table 2. The conductance is close to 50 pS. In several of these channel types it has been noted that the conductance for outward currents, i.e., the anion current flowing into the cell, is $1.5-2$ times larger then the conductance for the inward current (Frizzell 1987; Hayslett et al. 1987; Welsh and Liedtke 1986). It has also been noted in most preparations that the probability for the channel to be open is increased with depolarization of the cytosolic side of the membrane (Frizzell 1987; Greger et al. 1987a; Hayslett et al. 1987; Kunzelmann et al. 1988). In terms of macroscopic currents these two properties contribute to the outward rectification of chloride currents. This is apparent from the following simple formula:

$$I_{Cl} = i_{Cl} \cdot p_0 \cdot n.$$

In this equation I_{Cl}, and i_{Cl} are the macroscopic and microsopic chloride current, respectively, p_0 is the open-state probability, and n is the number of chloride channels per unit area. The total extent of rectification may be by a factor of $2-10$ if one varies the driving force from $+50$ to -50 mV (Hayslett et al. 1987). It should be noted that no potential dependence of i_{Cl} has been noted in the rectal gland chloride channel (Greger et al. 1987a), and that the potential dependence of p_0 for the respiratory epithelium chloride channel was found to be large in two (Frizzell 1987; Kunzelmann et al. 1988) but very small in a third laboratory (Welsh and Liedtke 1986). The reason for this seeming discrepancy is not clear.

Table 2 Properties of epithelial chloride channels of intermediate conductance

Tissue	Conductance	Function	Selectivity	Regulation	Inhibitor	Reference
TAL	20–50	Cl reabsorbing	$Cl \gg Na$	cAMP	DPC, NPPB	Greger 1986; Greger and Kunzelmann 1988
RGT	45	Cl secreting	$Cl > Br > I > Gluc > Na$	cAMP, PD	DPC, NPPB	Greger et al. 1987a
Colon rat	50	Cl secreting	$I > Br > Cl > F = HCO_3 > SO_4$	PD	DIDS	Reinhardt et al. 1987
T_{84}	30–50	Cl secreting	$ClO_4 > I > NO_3 > Cl \gg F$	PD		Halm et al. 1988
			$Cl = Br = I \gg Na$	PD	NPPB	Unpublished, from the authors' laboratory
HT_{29}	50	Cl secreting	$Cl = Br = I \gg Gluc = Na = 0$	PD	NPPB	Hayslett et al. 1987
Trachea	20–50	Cl secreting	$Cl > Na$	PD	DPC	Welsh 1987a
Respiratory epithelial cells	30–80	Cl secreting	$Cl = Br = I \gg Glu = Na = 0$	PD	NPPB	Kunzelmann et al. 1988b

TAL, thick ascending limb of Henle's loop; DPC, diphenylamino-2-carboxylate; NPPB, 5-nitro-2-(3-phenylpropylamino)-benzoate; PD, voltage dependence, in the case of the present chloride channels this implies outward rectification; RGT, rectal gland tubule; T_{84} and HT_{29} are colonic carcinoma cell lines representing the function of the crypt cell; Gluc, gluconate

The chloride channels in all of the epithelia mentioned above are highly selective for chloride over sodium and potassium (Greger et al. 1987a; Hayslett et al. 1987; Kunzelmann et al. 1987b; Welsh and Liedke 1986). This has been shown by a shift in the zero current potential when the solution on one side is diluted. In addition, something all of these chloride channels have in common is that they are impermeable to large anions such as sulfate, gluconate, cyclamate, etc. (Frizzell 1987; Greger et al. 1987a; Hayslett et al. 1987; Kunzelmann et al. 1988b; Welsh and Liedtke 1986) although they are permeable to nitrate and other halides (Frizzell 1987; Kunzelmann et al. 1988b; Welsh and Liedtke 1986). Certain sequences have been deduced from the shifts obtained in zero current potentials although we do not believe that these sequences can be determined with sufficient accuracy. Two problems have to be taken into account: (1) the shift of the zero current potential is frequently only a few mV, and this is very little in view of rather large liquid junction potentials, and (2) the Goldman formula is not appropriate for most of the above chloride channels. Nevertheless, it seems fair to conclude that small halides can permeate these channels to some extent, that large anions are excluded from the channel, and that the discrimination among the different halides is rather poor.

A kinetic analysis of these chloride channels has been attempted in several reports (Dreinhöfer et al. 1988; Greger et al. 1987a; Hayslett et al. 1987; Kunzelmann et al. 1988b; Welsh and Liedtke 1986). In general, two open states and two closed states have been identified. These four states have time constants of about $1-20$ ms. A reaction scheme of the channel opening has been deduced in one report on the basis of an inhibitor study (Dreinhöfer et al. 1988). It was noted in this report, and it should be kept in mind, that the currently used methodology will always underestimate the number of different states of the channel. For instance, if the chloride channel had a closed state of very long duration, one would hardly detect it because the number of such events accumulating over the limited period of the recording would be too small. Conversely, if the chloride channel possessed very short-lived states, one would hardly detect them since the required filtering would have a cutoff at some 0.5 ms. With this in mind, it should be evident that the four states of the channel that have been described so far must necessarily be an underestimate.

The chloride channels in all of the epithelia mentioned above can be blocked by a new class of chloride channel blockers (Dreinhöfer et al. 1988; Greger et al. 1987a; Hayslett et al. 1987; Kunzelmann et al. 1988b; Wangemann et al. 1987; Wittner et al. 1987) all of which belong to the aryl-amino-benzoate type. Inhibition occurs at $10^{-8}-10^{-4}$ mol/l depending on the blocker used and the preparation. It is important to note that the inhibition appears to occur from the outside of the channel, which explains at least one part of the large span of required inhibitory concentrations. In the thick ascending limb of Henle's loop the blockers have been added to the peritubular side, and very small concentrations were sufficient to block the chloride channels (Wangemann et al. 1987). In patch-clamp studies in the rectal gland tubule (Greger et al. 1987a), in colonic carcinoma cells (HT_{29} and T_{84}) (Hayslett et al. 1987; and unpublished observations from the authors' laboratory), and in respiratory epithelium chloride channels (Kunzelmann et al. 1988b) the concentrations required for complete inhibition were of the order $10^{-6}-10^{-5}$ mol/l. This is not surprising since the membrane patches are usually of inside-out configuration, i.e., the blocker has to penetrate the membrane before it can reach its binding site. In fact, we have also used these blockers in outside-out patches of the same preparations and made two important observations: (1) the blocking effect occurred immediately, i.e., with the speed of the fluid exchange, and (2) fairly low concentrations were sufficient to exert this inhibitory effect.

Chloride channel blockers have a characteristic effect on the kinetic appearance of the above chloride channels. At low concentrations they reduce the occurrence of the long open state and induce flickering. The time constant of this flickering may be so short that the full current amplitude is not reached (Dreinhöfer et al. 1988). Very similar observations of blocker-induced flickering have been reported for the effect of amiloride on the Na^+ channel (Gögelein and Greger 1986; Li and Lindemann 1983; Palmer 1985) and for quinidine and quinine on the K^+ channel (Gögelein et al. 1987a). It has also been claimed that the stilbene derivatives, 4-acetamino-4'-isothiocyanatostilbene-2,2'-disulfonic acid (SITS) and DIDS, block these chloride channels (Frizzell et al. 1988). We cannot confirm this, but we point to the fact that fairly high doses had to be used by Frizzell et al. (1988) to obtain this effect. Nevertheless, we are well aware of such cross reactivity of blockers. It is known, for instance, that band-3 inhibitors block certain chloride channels (Gögelein 1988). Conversely, chloride channel blockers inhibit exchange by the band-3 protein (Cousin and Motais 1982; Passow 1986) and the $Na^+-K^+-2Cl^-$-cotransporter (Greger et al. 1987c, 1987d; Wangemann et al. 1986; Wittner et al. 1986, 1987). This may simply reflect the fact that all these chloride transporters belong to one family of transport proteins and have some molecular homology. Apart from this consideration it should be noted that interaction of loop diuretics such as furosemide with chloride channels has been postulated (Evans et al. 1986; Patarca et al. 1983). We propose that this effect of furosemide is indirect: the fall in cytosolic chloride concentration after furosemide (Greger et al. 1983; Greger and Schlatter 1984) leads to a marked reduction in chloride conductance (Greger and Schlatter 1984).

Hormonal Regulation of Chloride Channels

Again we shall restrict ourselves to the regulation of the chloride channel with intermediate conductance. It is well known that chloride transport across the respective epithelia can be increased by certain hormones: antidiuretic hormone increases NaCl reabsorption in the thick ascending limb of Henle's loop via V2 receptors (Greger 1985), prostaglandin E_2 increases NaCl secretion in colonic krypt cells as well as in colonic carcinoma cells (Heintze et al. 1983; Weymer et al. 1985), rectin and vasointestinal peptide (VIP) increase NaCl secretion in the rectal gland (Greger et al. 1986), and adrenaline increases NaCl secretion in respiratory epithelial cells (Welsh 1987a). All these regulatory pathways use cyclic AMP as a second messenger. From macroscopic measurements in the intact cells of these epithelia it has been suggested that the first effect of hormonal stimulation is an increase in the chloride conductance (Greger et al. 1984). The increase in chloride conductance then leads to increased coupled uptake of Na^+, Cl^-, and K^+ via the $Na^+-K^+-2Cl^-$-cotransporter which in turn increases cytosolic Na^+ concentration. This latter change may then augment the rate of the Na^+-, K^+-ATPase. The required increase in K^+ recycling may have two causes. First, the driving force for K^+ exit increases at least in some of the above epithelia as the cells depolarize. Second, it has been shown for some preparations that K^+ conductance is upregulated with some delay (Welsh 1987a). It has been claimed that this upregulation of K^+ conductance may be due to an increase in cytosolic Ca^{2+} concentration (Welsh 1987a).

More recently the patch-clamp technique has been used to examine the mechanisms of hormone-induced increase in transcellular chloride transport. In several studies it has been shown that the respective hormone or the membrane permeable second messenger, dibutyryl-cyclic AMP, increases the density of operating chloride channels in cell-attached membrane patches (Greger et al. 1985; Welsh 1987a). These findings prove unequivocally that the primary effect of stimulation is the activation of chloride channels. Conversely, it has been shown that potassium channels can operate with and without any stimulating agent. From these data it appears attractive to postulate that chloride channels are activated directly by phosporylation via a cyclic AMP-dependent protein kinase A. This hypothesis was examined in cell-free patches with ATP and the catalytic subunit of protein kinase A added to the cytosolic side. It was found that under these conditions chloride channels could be activated in previously silent membrane patches (Greger et al. 1988; Li et al. 1988; Schoumacher et al. 1987). Nevertheless, these experiments are probably not as conclusive as one would wish them to be. (1) These experiments have to be compared to time controls, and these time controls in which no agent is added are necessarily unpaired observations. (2) Only a large series of control experiments can exclude the possibility that channel activation can also occur spontaneously, for instance, simply because a vesicle ruptures. (3) It cannot be excluded a priori that the excision leaves part of the activation machinery intact so that ATP alone would be sufficient to produce channel activation. The above experiments would be more conclusive if channel activation generated in this fashion could be abolished by dephosphorylation, i.e., after addition of phosphatase. This has not yet been reported.

For some of the K^+ channels it has been shown that they are regulated by cytosolic Ca^{2+}. This is the case for respiratory epithelial cells (Kunzelmann et al. 1988b; Welsh and Liedtke 1986), but not for the rectal gland (Greger et al. 1987b) and the thick ascending limb of Henle's loop (unpublished from the authors' laboratory). On the other hand, experiments in intact cells have suggested that increases in cytosolic Ca^{2+} do not only increase the K^+ conductance, but also increase chloride secretion and chloride conductance (Marty et al. 1984; Welsh 1987a; Weymer et al. 1985; Young et al. 1988). This might suggest that the chloride channels are regulated by cytosolic Ca^{2+}. In fact it has been claimed that chloride channels in excised patches can be activated by high Ca^{2+} concentrations (Frizzell et al. 1986). Re-examination of this issue in several laboratories uniformly leads to the conclusion that chloride channels in excised patches cannot be activated by elevated Ca^{2+} concentrations (Greger and Kunzelmann 1988; Kunzelmann et al. 1988a, 1988b; Welsh 1987a). It is highly likely that the current concept of stimulation of transcellular chloride transport is incomplete. It is probably true that chloride channel activation is the first step and that it is induced by cyclic AMP, and it is also true that some potassium channels are activated by elevated cytosolic Ca^{2+}, but it is equally likely that chloride channel phosphorylation by an A kinase is one, but not the only mechanism of stimulation in several epithelia. Several new experimental findings point to more complex regulatory systems. First, it has been reported recently in respiratory epithelial cells that phorbol esters acutely increase NaCl secretion, but that they also reduce the activation induced by adrenaline (Welsh 1987b). Furthermore, the finding that excision of cell membranes of cystic fibrosis respiratory cells leads to spontaneous chloride channel activation in these previously silent patches is hardly compatible with chloride channel phosphorylation. This latter finding has generated a few new hypotheses. One is that the excision of these channel-"free" patches leads to channel activation because the medium into which the patch is moved contains high Ca^{2+} concentrations (Frizzell et al. 1986). This hypothesis has found no experimental support (Greger and Kunzelmann 1988; Kunzelmann et al. 1988b; Welsh 1987a). Another hypothesis claimed that depolarization of the excised patch caused irreversible channel activation (Frömter and Disser 1988; Schoumacher et al. 1987; Welsh 1987a). We have examined this hypothesis and are unable to confirm it (Kunzelmann et al. 1988a). We find that spontaneous chloride channel activation occurs immediately whether the patch is excised at positive or negative clamp voltages. We argue that the delayed channel activation observed in other studies at positive clamp voltages has some other cause. From our experience it is very probable that the excision led to vesicle formation. These vesicles can be ruptured with long-lasting depolarization, and this may have unmasked chloride channels in the other membrane. Further studies will be needed to clarify this point. At present, it appears very attractive to assume that chloride-channel activation may be caused differently in the various epithelia discussed in this review. It may involve direct phosphorylation in some epithelia (Greger et al. 1988), but it may involve disinhibition in others. In these latter epithelia a cytosolic inhibitor may keep the channels closed until this inhibitor is modified, e.g., by phosphorylation, and only then can the chloride channels be opened (Kunzelmann et al. 1988a). We believe that clarification of this issue will also be the key to the understanding of the underlying pathology of cystic fibrosis.

Conclusion

The present short overview discussed the properties of chloride channels in epithelia. We have only focused on those chloride channels for which we possess single-channel data. It became evident that these channels recorded in various epithelia have several properties in common. They all are of medium conductance (20–80 pS). They are outwardly rectifying, i.e., they favor inward movement of chloride over outward movement. This may seem paradoxical because, physiologically, these channels conduct chloride currents from cell to medium. On the other hand the rectification may limit, or downregulate, the stimulated chloride current in a negative feedback loop. All of these channels are inhibited by chloride-channel blockers. The regulation of the channels plays a predominant role in the hormonal regulation of NaCl transport. Current concepts of chloride-channel regulation are insufficient to account for all of the experimental observations. It appears likely that chloride-channel regulation is very complex and involves several regulatory loops. Overstimulation, as occurs in diarrhea, probably leads to uncontrolled stimulation of chloride currents, and tonic inhibition of chloride channels is probably responsible for cystic fibrosis.

References

Argent BE, Gray MA, Greenwell JR (1987) Secretin- regulated anion channel in the apical membrane of rat pancreatic duct cells in vitro. J Physiol 391:33P

Christine CW, Laskowski FH, Gitter AH, Gross P, Frömter E (1987) Chloride-selective single ion channels in the apical membrane of cultured collecting duct principal cells. Pflügers Arch 408:R32

Cousin JL, Motais R (1982) Inhibition of anion red blood cell by anionic amphiphilic compounds. I. Determination of the flufenamate-binding site by proteolytic dissection of the band-3 protein. Biochim Biophys Acta 687:147–155

Dreinhöfer J, Gögelein H, Greger R (1988) Blocking kinetics of Cl⁻ channels in colonic carcinoma cells (HT_{29}) as revealed by 5-nitro-2-(3-phenylpropylamino)-benzoic acid (NPPB). Biochim Biophys Acta 956:135–142

Evans MG, Marty A, Tan YP, Trautmann A (1986) Blockage of Ca-activated Cl conductance by furosemide in rat lacrimal glands, Pflügers Arch 406:65–68

Frizzell RA (1987) Cystic fibrosis: a disease of ion channels? Trends Neurosci 10:190–193

Frizzell RA, Halm DR, Rechkemmer GR, Shoemaker RL (1986) Chloride channel regulation in secretory epithelia. Fed Proc 45:2727–2731

Frizzell RA, Schoumacher RA, Shoemaker RL, Bridges RL, Halm DR (1988) Disorders of chloride channel regulation in cystic fibrosis (CF) and secretory diarrhea (SD). Symposium: Disorders of chloride channel regulation: cystic fibrosis and secretory diarrhea, May 1988, Amsterdam

Frömter E, Disser J (1988) Properties of Na⁺ channels and Cl⁻ channels in sweat duct and nasal polyp epithelia. Symposium: Disorders of chloride channel regulation: cystic fibrosis and secretory diarrhea, May 1988, Amsterdam

Gögelein H (1988) Chloride channels in epithelia. Biochim Biophys Acta 947:521–547

Gögelein H, Greger R (1986) Na⁺ selective channels in the apical membrane of rabbit late proximal tubule (pars recta). Pflügers Arch 406:198–203

Gögelein H, Greger R, Schlatter E (1987a) Potassium channels in the basolateral membrane of the rectal gland of Squalus acanthias. Regulation and inhibitors. Pflügers Arch 409:107–113

Gögelein H, Schlatter E, Greger R (1987b) The "small" conductance chloride channel in the luminal membrane of the rectal gland of the dogfish (Squalus acanthias). Pflügers Arch 409:122–125

Greger R (1985) Ion transport mechanisms in thick ascending limb of Henle's loop of mammalian nephron. Physiol Rev 65:760–797

Greger R (1986) Chlorid transportierende Epithelien. In: Bromm B (ed) Hauptvorträge der Tagungen der Deutschen Physiologischen Gesellschaft. Fischer, Stuttgart, pp 19–28

Greger R, Kunzelmann K (1988) Chloride channels. Symposium: Disorders of chloride channel regulation: cystic fibrosis and secretory diarrhea, May 1988, Amsterdam

Greger R, Schlatter E (1984) Mechanism of NaCl secretion in rectal gland tubules of spiny dogfish (Squalus acanthias). II. Effects of inhibitors. Pflügers Arch 402:364–375

Greger R, Oberleithner H, Schlatter E, Cassola AC, Weidtke C (1983) Chloride activity in cells of isolated perfused cortical thick ascending limbs of rabbit kidney. Pflügers Arch 399:29–34

Greger R, Schlatter E, Wang F, Forrest Jr (1984) Mechanism of NaCl secretion in rectal gland tubules of spiny dogfish (Squalus acanthias) III. Effects of stimulation of secretion by cyclic AMP. Pflügers Arch 402:376–384

Greger R, Schlatter E, Gögelein H (1985) Cl^- channels in the apical cell membrane of the rectal gland "induced" by cAMP. Pflügers Arch 403:446–448

Greger R, Schlatter E, Gögelein H (1986) Sodium chloride secretion in rectal gland of dogfish, Squalus acanthias. NIPS 1:134–136

Greger R, Schlatter E, Gögelein H (1987a) Chloride channels in the luminal membrane of the rectal gland of the dogfish (Squalus acanthias). Properties of the "larger" conductance channel. Pflügers Arch 409:114–121

Greger R, Gögelein H, Schlatter E (1987b) Potassium channels in the basolateral membrane of the rectal gland of the dogfish (Squalus acanthias). Pflügers Arch 409:100–106

Greger R, Lang HJ, Englert HC, Wangemann P (1987c) Blockers of the $Na^+-K^+-2Cl^-$-carrier and of chloride channels in the thick ascending limb of the loop of Henle. In: Puschett J (ed) Diuretics. Elsevier, Amsterdam, pp 33–38

Greger R, Wangemann P, Wittner M, Di Stefano A, Lang HJ, Englert HC (1987d) Blockers of active transport in the thick ascending limb of the loop of Henle. In: Andreucci VE, Dal Canton (eds) Diuretics: basic, pharmacological, and clinical aspects. Martinus Nijhoff, Boston, pp 33–38

Greger R, Gögelein H, Schlatter E (1988) Stimulation of NaCl secretion in the rectal gland of the dogfish Squalus acanthias. Comp Biochem Physiol [A] 90 (4): 733–737

Halm DR, Rechkemmer GR, Schoumacher RA, Frizzell RA (1988) Apical membrane chloride channels in a colonic cell line activated by secretory agonists. Am J Physiol 254:C505–C511

Hanrahan JW, Alles WP, Lewis SA (1985) Single anion-selective channels in basolateral membrane of a mammalian tight epithelium. Proc Natl Acad Sci USA 82:7791–7795

Hayslett JP, Gögelein H, Kunzelmann K, Greger R (1987) Characteristics of apical chloride channels in human colon cells (HT_{29}). Pflügers Arch 410:487–494

Heintze K, Stewart CP, Frizzell RA (1983) Sodium dependent chloride secretion across rabbit descending colon. Am J Physiol 244:G357–G365

Kawahara K, Giebisch G (1987) Single K and Cl channels in basal membrane of Amphiuma diluting segment. 10th International congress of nephrology, 26.–31. July 1987, London

Kolb HA, Brown CDA, Murer H (1985) Identification of a voltage-dependent anion channel in an apical membrane of a Cl^--secretory epithelium (MDCK). Pflügers Arch 403:262–265

Koniarek JP, Leibovitch LS (1985) Patch-clamp studies of in vitro rabbit corneal epithelial cells. J Gen Physiol 86:20a–21a

Krouse ME, Schneider GT, Gage PW (1986) A large anion-selective channel has seven conductance levels. Nature 319:58–60

Kunzelmann K, Ünal Ö, Beck C, Emmrich P, Arndt HJ, Greger R (1988a) Regulation of ion channels in respiratory cells of cystic fibrosis patients and normal individuals. Pflügers Arch 412:R10 (Abstract)

Kunzelmann K, Ünal Ö, Beck C, Emmrich P, Arndt HJ, Greger R (1988b) Ion channels of cultured respiratory epithelial cells of patients with cystic fibrosis. Pflügers Arch 411:R68 (Abstract)

Li JHY, Lindemann B (1983) Competitive blocking of epithelial sodium channels by organic cations: the relationship between macroscopic and microscopic inhibition constants. J Membr Biol 76:235–251

Li M, McCann JD, Liedtke CM, Nairn AC, Greengard P, Welsh MJ (1988) Cyclic AMP-dependent protein kinase opens chloride channels in normal but not cystic fibrosis airway epithelium. Nature 331:358–360

Marty A, Tan YP, Trautmann A (1984) Three types of calcium-dependent channel in rat lacrimal glands. J Physiol 357:293–325

Nelson DJ, Tang JM, Palmer LG (1984) Single-channel recordings of apical membrane chloride conductance in A6 epithelial cells. J Membr Biol 80:81–89

Palmer LG (1985) Modulation of apical Na permeability of toad urinary bladder by intracellular Na, Ca, and H. J Membr Biol 83:57–69

Passow H (1986) Molecular aspects of band 3 protein-mediated anion transport across the red blood cell membrane. Rev Physiol Biochem Pharmacol 103:62–123

Patarca R, Candia OA, Reinach PS (1983) Mode of inhibition of active chloride transport in the frog cornea by furosemide. Am J Physiol 245:F660–F669

Petersen OH (1986) Calcium-activated potassium channels and fluid secretion by exocrine glands. Am J Physiol 251:G1–G13

Petersen OH (1987) Potassium channels and fluid secretion. NIPS 1:92–95

Reinhardt R, Bridges RJ, Rummel W, Lindemann B (1987) Properties of an anion-selective channel from rat colonic enterocyte plasma membranes reconstituted into planar phospholipid bilayers. J Membr Biol 95:47–54

Schneider GT, Cook DI, Gage PW, Young JA (1985) Voltage sensitive, high-conductance chloride channels in the luminal membrane of cultured pulmonary alveolar (type II) cells. Pflügers Arch 404:354–357

Schoumacher RA, Shoemaker RL, Halm DR, Tallant EA, Wallace RW, Frizzell RA (1987) Phosphorylation fails to activate chloride channels from cystic fibrosis airway cells. Nature 330:752–754

Wangemann P, Di Stefano A, Wittner M, Englert HC, Lang HJ, Schlatter E, Greger R (1986) Cl⁻-channel blockers in the thick ascending limb of the loop of Henle. Structure activity relationship. Pflügers Arch 407:128–141

Welsh MJ (1987a) Electrolyte transport by airway epithelia. Physiol Rev 67:1143–1184

Welsh MJ (1987b) Effect of phorbol ester and calcium ionophore on chloride secretion in canine tracheal epithelium. Am J Physiol 253:C828–C834

Welsh MJ, Liedtke CM (1986) Chloride and potassium channels in cystic fibrosis airway epithelia. Nature 322:467–470

Welsh MJ, McCann JD, Dearborn DG (1987) Chloride and sodium channel currents in normal and cystic fibrosis sweat duct epithelium. Fed Proc 46:5567

Weymer A, Huott P, Liu W, McRoberts JA, Dharmsathaphorn K (1985) Chloride secretory mechanism induced by prostaglandin E_1 in a colonic epithelial cell line. J Clin Invest 76:1828–1836

Wittner M, Di Stefano A, Schlatter E, Delarge J, Greger R (1986) Torasemide inhibits NaCl reabsorption in the thick ascending limb of the loop of Henle. Pflügers Arch 407:611–614

Wittner M, Di Stefano A, Wangemann P, Delarge J, Greger R (1987) Analogues of torasemide – structure function relationships – experiments in the thick ascending limbs of the loop of Henle of rabbit nephron. Pflügers Arch 408:54–62

Young JA, Gard GB, Champion MP, Cook DJ (1988) Patch clamp studies on muscarinic stimulus-secretion coupling in rat mandibular gland endpiece cells. In: Wong PYD, Young JA (eds) Exocrine secretion. Hong Kong University Press, Hong Kong, pp 219–222

Zeuthen T, Christensen O, Cherksey B (1987) Electrodiffusion of Cl⁻ and K⁺ in epithelial membranes reconstituted into planar lipid bilayers. Pflügers Arch 408:275–281

Cation Channels and Secretion*

D. I. Cook and J. A. Young

Introduction

Soon after two cation-selective channels, a Ca^{2+}-activated K^+ channel and a non-selective cation channel, were first demonstrated in a secretory epithelium by single-channel recording techniques (Maruyama and Petersen 1982a, b; Maruyama et al. 1983a), it became apparent that they were very widely distributed among the secretory epithelia. The present review will first deal with the possible roles of these and other cation-selective channels in epithelial secretion and then with their distribution and characteristics.

The Role of Cation Channels in Secretion

Models Relying on Secondary Active Cl^- Transport

The Importance of K^+ Channels

Any discussion of the mechanism of epithelial secretion must begin with the model first proposed by Silva et al. (1977) to explain secretion by the shark rectal gland. This model, which is based on the secondary active transport of Cl^-, utilises a basolateral $Na^+-K^+-2Cl^-$ cotransporter to maintain the concentration of Cl^- in the cytosol above electrochemical equilibrium. The details of its operation are provided in other chapters in this volume.

Basolateral K^+ channels are critical for the operation of this model for several reasons. (a) They keep the apical (as well as the basolateral) cell membrane potential more negative than the Nernst potential for Cl^-, thereby providing a driving force for the sustained electrogenic efflux of Cl^- across the apical membrane. Were the K^+ channels not present, the cell potential would move towards the Nernst potential for Cl^-, so reducing the driving force for Cl^- exit. (b) The $Na^+-K^+-2Cl^-$ cotransporter and the

---

*The authors' experimental work reported in this paper was supported by the National Health and Medical Research Council of Australia.

Young · Wong, Epithelial Secretion of Water and Electrolytes
© Springer-Verlag Berlin · Heidelberg 1990

Na^+-, K^+-ATPase together pump five K^+ ions into the cell for each six Cl^- ions secreted. If these K^+ ions remained in the cytosol, the cytosolic K^+ concentration would increase, leading to inhibition of the $Na^+-K^+-2Cl^-$ cotransporter and the Na^+-, K^+-ATPase, and/or cell swelling and eventual lysis would occur. The K^+ channels prevent this by providing an exit pathway for K^+. (c) The K^+ channels may also play a role in the regulation of the $Na^+-K^+-2Cl^-$ cotransporter by controlling the K^+ gradient across the basolateral membrane (Petersen and Maruyama 1984). This is because opening the K^+ channels reduces the cytosolic K^+ concentration and locally increases the interstitial K^+ concentration, leading to a reduction in the energy gradient for K^+ ions against which the $Na^+-K^+-2Cl^-$ cotransporter has to operate. Since interstitial K^+ activities rise to as high as 19 mmol/l during the initial stages of secretion (Poulsen and Bledsoe 1978), and cytosolic K^+ activities fall to about 80 mmol/l (Poulsen and Oakley 1979; Murakami et al. 1988), the change in the Nernst potential for K^+ is sufficiently large that it might conceivably provide a means of control over the $Na^+-K^+-2Cl^-$ cotransporter. Although the case for a role for such a mechanism in the control of secretion rate is strengthened by the observation that the $Na^+-K^+-2Cl^-$ cotransporter (in the rabbit parotid) has a low affinity for K^+ ($K_{0.5}=30$ mmol/l: Turner et al. 1986), it is nevertheless unlikely to be the predominant control mechanism since a reduction in the Nernst potential for K^+ would also reduce the driving force for Cl^- secretion, as has been demonstrated experimentally in the canine tracheal mucosa (Welsh 1983).[1]

The importance of basolateral K^+ channels in epithelial electrolyte secretion has been well demonstrated by the experiments of Evans et al. (1986) in which in vitro gland perfusion was used to demonstrate that K^+ channel blockers such as tetraethylammonium and decamethonium, which have been shown by whole-cell patch-clamp studies to block all the K^+ channels in secretory cells (Llano et al. 1987), cause a rapid and reversible inhibition of fluid and electrolyte secretion when added to the perfusion medium. Similar results have been obtained in canine tracheal mucosa (Welsh 1983; Smith and Frizzell 1984) and in rat intestine (Hardcastle and Hardcastle 1986).

---

[1] Let us take an extreme example to illustrate the difficulties that would arise with this method of control. Suppose that the cytosolic K^+ concentration is 145 mmol/l and the interstitial K^+ is 5 mmol/l and that during stimulation the cytosolic K^+ concentration falls to 110 mmol/l and the interstitial K^+ concentration rises to 20 mmol/l. The Nernst potential for K^+ will thus be -89 mV at rest and -45 mV during stimulation. In other words, the Nernst potential for K^+ will be reduced by $+44$ mV during stimulation. Consequently, if the driving force for Cl^- exit is to increase during stimulation, the Nernst potential for Cl^- must increase by more than $+44$ mV. In many epithelia, the resting Cl^- concentration is approximately 40 mmol/l with a Cl^- Nernst potential of -35 mV (Cook and Young 1989a). Consequently, if decreasing the K^+ gradient is to stimulate secretion, it would have to increase the cytosolic Cl^- concentration to greater than the interstitial level.

Desirable Properties of the Cation Channels

We can predict what properties cation channels should have in order to fulfil the above mentioned functions effectively. (a) They should be strongly K^+ selective since any movement of Na^+ through them into the cytosol would reduce the efficiency of the secretory mechanism by shunting out the Na^+ gradient and by reducing the cation efflux that balances the Cl^- current across the apical membrane. (b) They should be activated by depolarisation since their function is to oppose a fall in cell potential. (c) Their activity should be under neurohumoral control since secretion itself is under autonomic control, and, in the secondary active Cl^- transport model, the activity of the K^+ channels is one of the major determinants of the secretion rate.

Basolateral Versus Apical Placement of K^+ Channels

The secondary active Cl^- transport model postulates that secretory cells have K^+ channels in their basolateral membranes. The question therefore arises as to whether it is essential that the K^+ channels be located solely in the basolateral membrane. Our recent model studies show that placing K^+ channels in the apical membrane has one effect that promotes and another that impedes the movement of Cl^- into the lumen (Cook and Young 1989b). Thus, insertion of K^+ channels in the apical membrane tends to increase secretion rate because the current loop now only passes across the apical Cl^- and apical K^+ channels, whereas the current loop in the usual model passes also across the tight junctional resistance; at the same time, however, it tends to reduce secretion rate because the accumulation of K^+ in the lumen leads to a reduction in the Nernst potential for K^+ across the apical membrane, so reducing the driving force for Cl^- exit. Whether or not apical K^+ channels will increase the efficiency of secretion depends on the balance between these opposing factors. For an epithelium with properties similar to those of the canine tracheal mucosa (Welsh 1987), our model studies (Cook and Young 1989b) show that an increase in secretory rate occurs when a part of the total cell K^+ conductance is placed in the apical membrane, provided the proportion does not exceed 60%. When the proportion does exceed 60%, there is a reduction in the secretory rate, with almost total inhibition when it is 100%. Maximum stimulation (of about 10%) is obtained when approximately 20% of the total cell K^+ conductance is placed in the apical membrane. The ability of apical K^+ channels to increase the rate of secretion is enhanced by increasing the resistance of the paracellular pathway relative to the transcellular pathway. Another important conclusion of our study (Cook and Young 1989b) is that the efficiency of paracellular exchange of Na^+ for K^+ is sufficiently great in an epithelium like canine tracheal mucosa that regardless of the proportion of the total K^+ conductance placed in the apical membrane, the primary secretion produced by secondary active Cl^- transport will be Na^+ rich.

Models Relying on Direct Active K^+ Transport

There is an alternative model for epithelial secretion that is not based on secondary active Cl^- transport but, rather, on direct active secretion of K^+ ions (Cook and Young 1989a). In this model, K^+ is pumped into the cell across the basolateral membrane by the Na^+-, K^+-ATPase and then flows down its electrochemical gradient into the lumen. Charge balance is maintained by movement of Cl^- into the lumen from the interstitium, either transcellularly, via Cl^- channels in the apical and basolateral membranes, or paracellularly, via the tight junctions. Subsequent exchange of K^+ for Na^+ through the tight junctions would be necessary for the formation of a Na^+-rich primary secretion. In this model, non-selective cation channels in the basolateral membrane can be used to balance the current due to K^+ efflux across the apical membrane by permitting an inward Na^+ current across the basolateral membrane, whilst simultaneously providing the cytosolic Na^+ required to maintain the activity of the Na^+-, K^+-ATPase. This model has been proposed as an explanation for electrolyte secretion by the rat lacrimal gland (Marty et al. 1984), although direct proof of its validity has not been obtained. The model has several interesting characteristics. (a) Its maximum efficiency for secretion is only two Cl^- ions per ATP molecule (cf. six Cl^- ions per ATP molecule in the secondary active Cl^- transport model), and even this is attained only when the intercellular junctions are made completely impermeable to cations. If paracellular cation permeabilities comparable in size to those reported for the canine tracheal mucosa are present (Welsh 1987), the efficiency of the model falls to as little as 0.04 Cl^- ions per molecule of ATP. (This contrasts with the model based on secondary active Cl^- transport in which the tight junctions can be made quite leaky to cations without noticeable impairment of transport efficiency.) (b) Since the primary driving force for secretion in this model is the movement of K^+ ions into the lumen, the luminal potential must be positive. Furthermore, the influx of Na^+ across the basolateral membrane will depolarise the cell potential, and, when the mechanism is operating at high transport rates, might even cause it to become positive if the Gibbs-Donnan effect is not very large. (c) The primary fluid must remain K^+ rich if the epithelium is to secrete efficiently.

Although these are not properties that accord well with our current knowledge of most secretory epithelia, there are some to which the model may be applicable since it predicts an electrogenic Na^+ entry pathway in the basolateral membrane as well as K^+ channels in the apical membrane and Cl^- channels in both membranes. Consequently, it might operate in those secretory cells, such as in mouse pancreatic acini (Maruyama and Petersen 1982a, b), in which only a non-selective cation channel has been observed in the basolateral membrane.

Cation Channels Types in Secretory Epithelia

The BK Channel

Distribution in Secretory and Non-secretory Tissues

Ca^{2+}-activated K^+ channels are very widely distributed and can be categorised on the basis of differences in single-channel conductance, sensitivity to changes in cytoplasmic Ca^{2+} and differential sensitivity to blockers such as tetraethylammonium, charybdotoxin and apamin (Blatz and Magleby 1987; Farley and Rudy 1988). The first such channel to be described in patch-clamp studies was the high-conductance Ca^{2+} and voltage-activated K^+ channel (the so-called BK channel; see Fig. 1) of bovine adrenal chromaffin cells (Marty 1981), cultured rat skeletal muscle (Pallotta et al. 1981), rabbit muscle t tubules (Latorre et al. 1982), frog sympathetic neurones (Adams et al. 1982) and clonal rat pituitary cells (Wong et al. 1982). The channel is characterised by a high single-channel

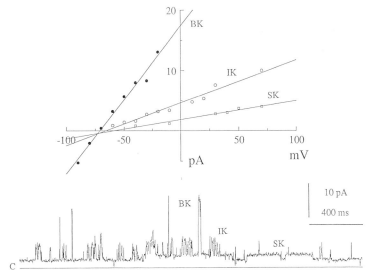

Fig. 1. The three different channel types (SK, IK and BK) seen in the plasma membrane of a secretory cell from a sheep parotid gland. *Below* is a record of the current flowing across a cell-attached patch clamped at a holding potential of $-10\,mV$ (relative to the bath) when the pipette contained an isotonic KCl solution. The *horizontal line* labelled C indicates the zero current level. There are three SK channels visible, at least one of which is open throughout almost all of the recording period, as well as two IK channels, opening periodically in short bursts, and one BK channel, opening only occasionally for brief periods. *Above* are shown the current–voltage relations of the three channel types depicted: the slope conductances were 29 pS (SK), 75 pS (IK) and 250 pS (BK); (E.A. Wegmen, unpublished data)

conductance (160–330 pS), high selectivity for K^+ over Na^+, and activation by cytosolic Ca^{2+} and by depolarisation (Blatz and Magleby 1987) – all properties appropriate for an epithelial secretory process driven by the secondary active transport of Cl^-.

The first report of the BK channel in a secretory epithelium was in basolateral membranes of rat and mouse mandibular and parotid glands (Maruyama et al. 1983a), but subsequently it has been found in a wide range of secretory epithelia (Table 1). The statement that the channels are located

Table 1. Conductances (pS) of putative BK channels bathed in symmetrical isotonic KCl solutions.

Species	Tissue	pS	Reference
Human	Submandibular gland	250	Morris et al. 1987b
	Parotid gland[a]	160	Maruyama et al. 1986b
	Pancreatic acini	250	Petersen et al. 1985
Monkey	JTC-12 renal cells	215	Kolb et al. 1986
Dog	MDCK	221	Bolivar and Ceriejido 1987
	Tracheal smooth muscle	266	McCann and Welsh 1986
Rat	Mandibular gland	200	Cook et al. 1988b
	Pancreatic ducts	237	Gray et al. 1988
	Enterocytes	256	Morris et al. 1986
	Skeletal muscle	218	Barrett et al. 1982
	Sympathetic neurones	200	Smart 1987
	Pituitary	208	Wong et al. 1982
	Pancreatic islet	250	Findlay et al. 1985
	Brain synaptosomes	250	Farley and Rudy 1988
Mouse	Lacrimal gland	200	Findlay 1984
	Parotid gland	250	Maruyama et al. 1983a
	Mandibular gland	245	Gallacher and Morris 1986
	Dorsal root ganglion	259	Simonneau et al. 1987
Guinea pig	Pancreatic acini	215	Suzuki and Petersen 1988
	Arterial smooth muscle	183	Benham et al. 1986
Rabbit	Collecting duct	180	Gitter et al. 1987
	Jejunal smooth muscle	198	Benham et al. 1986
	Proximal tubule	200	Merot et al. 1989
	Muscle t tubules	226	Latorre et al. 1982
Pig	Pancreatic acini	200	Maruyama et al. 1983b
Sheep	Parotid	229	Wegman et al. 1988
Cow	Adrenal chromaffin	180	Marty 1981
	Adrenal chromaffin	265	Yellen 1984a, b
Chick	Lens epithelium	230	Rae 1985
	Osteoblast cultures	247	Ypey et al. 1988
Necturus	Enterocytes[a]	167	Sheppard et al. 1988
	Choroid plexus	227	Christensen and Zeuthen 1987
Frog	Choroid plexus	227	Christensen and Zeuthen 1987

[a] More detailed studies may show that these smaller-conductance channels are really IK channels as seen in the sheep parotid gland (Wegman et al. 1988).

in the basolateral membrane should not, however, be taken as indicating that they are not also in the apical membrane. There is no theoretical reason why they should be absent from the apical membrane (Cook and Young 1989b), and, to date, there are only a few secretory epithelia in which it has proved technically possible to study the apical membranes with patch-clamp techniques. Among those few that have been so investigated, it is clear, however, that K^+ channels are not demonstrable in the apical membranes of secretory cells of shark rectal gland (Greger et al. 1987) and rat pancreatic ducts (Gray et al. 1988). The BK channel is also found in some absorptive epithelia (Table 1).

The BK channels of secretory epithelia appear to be similar to those described in non-secretory tissues. When bathed in symmetrical 150 mmol/l KCl solutions, they have a conductance in the range of 160–310 pS (Table 1) and their current–voltage relations appear to be linear in the range ± 50 mV. [Studies over a wider range in non-secretory tissues show that the relation may really be sublinear (Yellen 1984a; Eisenman et al. 1986), presumably because of the existence of multiple ion-binding sites within the channel.] Variability of up to 20% in the single-channel conductance among the channels from a single cell type is one of the most striking properties of the BK channel (Methfessel and Boheim 1982), and another common feature is the existence of a subconductance state with approximately 50% of the fully open conductance.

The Permeability Properties of the BK Channel

The dependence of single-channel conductance on the K^+ concentration has been found to follow a Michaelis-Menten relation in skeletal muscle t tubules (Latorre and Miller 1983) and in cultured rat skeletal muscle cells (Blatz and Magleby 1984), with a maximum conductance (V_{max}) of 500 pS and a dissociation constant (K_m) for K^+ of 140 mmol/l. The conductance is temperature dependent, increasing linearly from 100 pS at 1 °C to 300 pS at 36 °C (Barrett et al. 1982) and is diffusion limited (Yellen 1984a). The BK channel is highly selective for K^+ over Na^+ (Gallacher and Morris 1986; Gallacher et al. 1984; Trautmann and Marty 1984; Blatz and Magleby 1987; Cook et al. 1988b) and impermeable to Li^+ and Cs^+ (Marty et al. 1984; Cook et al. 1988b; Gallacher et al. 1984). The position with respect to Rb^+ is more complicated. In excised patch experiments in which 150 mmol/l K^+ is present on one side of the patch and 150 mmol/l Rb^+ on the other, the current–voltage relation reverses at 0 mV, indicating that Rb^+ has a similar permeability to K^+; however, no current appears to flow through the channel from the Rb^+ to the K^+ side, indicating that the channel has a very low conductance for Rb^+ (Gallacher et al. 1984). This discrepancy between permeability and conductance is readily explained in terms of electrodiffusion theory (Barry and Gage 1984) in which permeability is defined as the product of the ionic mobility through the channel and the affinity of the ion for the channel, whereas conductance is defined solely in terms of mobility.

Rb^+ evidently has a high affinity for the BK channel, but a low mobility through it. It is implicit in this analysis that the channel has multiple binding sites for K^+ (Barry and Gage 1984).

These findings on the cation selectivity of the BK channel in glandular tissues are in agreement with more extensive studies on the analogous channel in skeletal muscle, chromaffin cells and smooth muscle (Yellen 1984a, 1987; Blatz and Magleby 1984; Eisenman et al. 1986; Benham et al. 1986). In the BK channel from rat skeletal muscle the order of cation permeabilities is $Tl^+ > K^+ > Rb^+ > NH_4^+$, and the rank order of conductances at $0 mV$ is $K^+ > Tl^+ > NH_4^+ > Rb^+$ (Blatz and Magleby 1984; Eisenman et al. 1986). In contrast to secretory epithelia, in these tissues there is a measurable Rb^+ conductance (Benham et al. 1986; Yellen 1984a; Eisenman et al. 1986). Recent experiments in muscle cells confirm that the BK channel has more than one ion-binding site within its pore (Eisenman et al. 1986; Yellen 1987; Cecchi et al. 1987).

Blockers of the BK Channel

There is extensive literature on the sensitivity of BK channels to various blockers. Millimolar concentrations of Na^+ on the cytosolic side of the channel reduce open-channel currents and induce a rapid flickering blockade accompanied by a reduction in open probability (Marty 1983; Yellen 1984a; Cook et al. 1988b; Gitter et al. 1987). Na^+ blockade is competitive with internal K^+ and is enhanced by positive membrane potentials. External K^+, Cs^+ and Rb^+ relieve Na^+ blockade by enhancing the rate of Na^+ exit from the channel (Yellen 1984b). In low concentrations in the external solution, Rb^+ reduces the K^+ conductance of the BK channel in non-epithelial tissues (Eisenman et al. 1986), but not in mouse mandibular secretory cells (Gallacher et al. 1984).

Cs^+ also is an effective blocker of BK channels. Although Cs^+ in the pipette solution has been used to block whole-cell K^+ currents in secretory epithelia (Marty et al. 1984; Cook et al. 1988b), most studies on the mechanism of Cs^+ blockade have been performed in non-epithelial tissues. In bovine chromaffin cells internal Cs^+ binds at 25% of the electrical distance across the membrane with a dissociation constant of 100 mmol/l (Yellen 1984a), but in rabbit intestinal smooth muscle it binds at 54% with a dissociation constant of 70 mmol/l (Cecchi et al. 1987), suggesting some difference in channel structure between the two tissues. External Cs^+ (0.1–5.0 mmol/l) produces a voltage-dependent blockade of the BK channel (Yellen 1984a; Cecchi et al. 1987), but when the channel kinetics are analysed in terms of Woodhull's (1973) model of voltage-dependent blockade, it is found that the Cs^+ binding site has an electrical distance through the membrane in excess of 100%, and that this distance depends on the external K^+ and Cs^+ concentrations. This anomalous behaviour is consistent with the BK channel being a multi-ion pore in which external Cs^+ can be pushed through the channel by K^+ (Yellen 1987; Cecchi et al. 1987).

Another ion that is commonly used to block BK channels is Ba^{2+}. When present in the external solution in concentrations of 0.5–5.0 mmol/l, it causes a slow, voltage-dependent block of the BK channel of pig pancreatic acinar cells (Iwatsuki and Petersen 1985a), and in whole-cell experiments in pig pancreatic and rat mandibular endpiece cells, it reduces, but does not abolish the resting K^+ conductance (Iwatsuki and Petersen 1985a; Cook et al. 1988b); complete blockade of the resting K^+ conductance requires a concentration of Ba^{2+} in excess of 22 mmol/l (Iwatsuki and Petersen 1985a). The relative ineffectiveness of Ba^{2+} as a blocker has also been seen in MDCK cells (Bolivar and Cereijido 1987). Ba^{2+} is effective in very much lower concentrations, however, when applied from the internal surface (Iwatsuki and Petersen 1985a), although its effects are complicated by the fact that Ba^{2+} also has a stimulatory effect on secretion at negative membrane potentials (Iwatsuki and Petersen 1985a). The features of Ba^{2+} blockade in secretory epithelia are similar to those found in rabbit skeletal muscle (Vergara and Latorre 1983) where they are believed to be due to the divalent ion becoming wedged in the channel pore. Consistent with this are the findings that increasing the K^+ concentration either *cis* or *trans* to the side on which the divalent ion is added can overcome Ba^{2+} blockade (Vergara and Latorre 1983), and that the Ba^{2+} ion can only reach its binding site when the channel is open (Miller et al. 1987). Ca^{2+} ions can also block in a manner similar to Ba^{2+} (Iwatsuki and Petersen 1985a; Vergara and Latorre 1983).

Tetraethylammonium (TEA) has been used to block BK channels in several secretory epithelia: rat lacrimal gland (Trautmann and Marty 1984), rat mandibular gland (Cook et al. 1988b), rat parotid gland (Maruyama et al. 1986a) and pig pancreatic acini (Iwatsuki and Petersen 1985b). The drug is of particular importance because the sensitivity and sidedness of its action are two of the major criteria used to distinguish between types of K^+ channel (Farley and Rudy 1988; Suzuki and Petersen 1988). When applied from the external surface, it causes a complete blockade of BK channels in concentrations as low as 1 or 2 mmol/l (Trautmann and Marty 1984; Iwatsuki and Petersen 1985b), and at 0.2 mmol/l it causes a voltage-dependent reduction in single-channel conductance and open probability (Iwatsuki and Petersen 1985b). Internal TEA is much less effective in blocking BK channels: for example, 10 mmol/l TEA added to the cytosolic side of inside-out patches from pig pancreatic acini reduces the single-channel conductance only slightly (Iwatsuki and Petersen 1985b). Studies on bovine chromaffin cells (Yellen 1984a) and rat skeletal muscle (Blatz and Magleby 1984) also show that internal TEA has only a low affinity for the BK channel, its dissociation constants being 27 mmol/l and 64 mmol/l, respectively, whereas the dissociation constants for external TEA are very much lower, being 0.2 mmol/l and 0.3 mmol/l, respectively. Corresponding to this difference in affinity, there is also a difference in the type of blockade produced. Internal TEA produces a 'fast' blockade that reduces the single channel currents, whereas external TEA produces a 'slower' blockade that reduces the channel open probability and induces rapid flickering (Iwatsuki and Petersen 1985b; Yellen 1984a). In each case, the binding site for TEA appears to sense only a small fraction of the transmembrane potential, presumably because it has a fairly superficial location (Yellen 1984a). It should be noted that there have been reports of large-conductance K^+ channels in pituitary cells (Wong and Adler 1986) and in rat brain synaptosomes (Farley and Rudy 1988) that are more sensitive to internal than external TEA.

Several other quaternary ammonium compounds have also been found to block BK channels (Yellen 1987). Decamethonium, for example, has been used to abolish K^+ currents in whole-cell experiments on rat lacrimal cells (Llano et al. 1987), and, like TEA, it is a potent inhibitor of fluid secretion by rat mandibular glands (Evans et al. 1986). As discussed by Yellen (1987), quaternary ammonium ions have been used to delineate the geometry of the antechambers of the BK channel.

Quinine and its stereo-isomer, quinidine, also block BK channels. The action of these compounds in pancreatic acinar cells has been studied extensively by Iwatsuki and Petersen (1985a) who found that they produce a flickering ('intermediate') blockade of BK channels in concentrations of $100-500$ μmol/l, regardless of whether the drugs are added to the external or the internal surface of excised patches. These drugs also reduce, but do not abolish the resting K^+ current of pig pancreatic acinar cells studied by the whole-cell technique (Iwatsuki and Petersen 1985a). Similarly, Rae et al. (1988) have found that quinidine also produces a flickering type of blockade in a BK channel from chick lens epithelium. Recent studies on blockade of BK channels from bovine chromaffin cells by internal quinine (Glavinovic and Trifaro 1988) have shown that the drug produces a voltage-dependent blockade of the open channel, but that it is a poor blocker in the sense that it does not reduce the average current flowing through the channels. Although this last finding conflicts with the report of Iwatsuki and Petersen (1985a) in pig pancreatic acinar cells, there is some common ground between the two studies since Iwatsuki and Petersen (1985a) showed that quinidine failed to cause complete blockade of the K^+ conductance of pig pancreatic acinar cells. Quinidine does reduce K^+ efflux from rat submandibular cells (Kurtzer and Roberts 1982).

Calmodulin blockers such as trifluoperazine have been shown to inhibit the activity of Ca^{2+}-activated K^+ channels in a number of tissues (Klaerke et al. 1987; Okada et al. 1987; McCann and Welsh 1987), although, as yet, the only evidence suggesting that the BK channel in secretory tissues may be influenced by calmodulin blockers is the finding that trifluoperazine inhibits K^+ efflux from rat mandibular cells (Kurtzer and Roberts 1982).

The scorpion toxin, charybdotoxin, blocks BK channels from the external side in skeletal muscle (Miller et al. 1985). It binds to the BK channel in both the open and closed states, but has its highest affinity for the open state. The dissociation rate is increased by depolarisation, and the binding rate is decreased by increasing ionic strength (Anderson et al. 1988). Interestingly, internal K^+ or Rb^+ relieves charybdotoxin blockade (MacKinnon and Miller 1988). The venoms of several other scorpions, such as noxiustoxin, have also been found to block BK channels (Moczydlowski et al. 1988; Valdiva et al. 1988). A more unusual blocker is externally applied d-tubocurarine (Smart 1987). Neither apamin (Romey and Lazdunski 1984; Smart 1987) nor 4-aminopyridine (Bolivar and Cereijido 1987; Smart 1987) blocks the BK channel.

Activation of the BK Channel

The BK channels in non-epithelial tissues are activated by membrane depolarisation and by increases in cytosolic Ca^{2+} concentration (see Blatz and Magleby 1987 for a review), and the analogous channels of secretory epithelia mostly conform to this general pattern. With the exception of human and guinea pig pancreatic acini (Petersen et al. 1985; Suzuki and Petersen 1988), the BK channels in secretory tissue appear to be more sensitive to Ca^{2+}. Some idea of the relative Ca^{2+} sensitivities of the BK channels in various glandular tissues can be gained by looking at their open probability in inside-out patches exposed to 10^{-8} mol/l free Ca^{2+} and a transmembrane potential of 20 mV. Under these conditions the BK channels of mouse mandibular glands (75% open; Gallacher and Morris 1986), mouse lacrimal glands (80% open; Findlay 1984), rat lacrimal gland (60% open; Marty et al. 1984) and pig pancreatic acini (98% open; Maruyama et al. 1983 b) all appear to have a similarly high sensitivity to cytosolic Ca^{2+}, whereas guinea pig pancreatic acini (1% open; Suzuki and Petersen 1988) and human pancreatic acini (2% open; Petersen et al. 1985) have their maximum sensitivities to Ca^{2+} in the micromolar range. In non-glandular tissues, the BK channels of rat enterocytes (Morris et al. 1986) and clonal pituitary cells (Wong et al. 1982) belong to the high affinity group, whilst those in *Necturus* enterocytes (Sheppard et al. 1988), rat chromaffin cells (Marty 1981), rabbit jejunal and guinea-pig arterial smooth muscle (Benham et al. 1986), cultured rat skeletal muscle (Barrett et al. 1982), cultured rat sympathetic neurones (Smart 1987), neonatal dorsal root ganglion cells (Simonneau et al. 1987) and canine tracheal smooth muscle cells (McCann and Welsh 1986) belong to the low affinity group.

It is noteworthy that the open probability of the BK channel in rat lacrimal glands actually decreases when the cytosolic Ca^{2+} increases to high levels (Marty et al. 1984). This blockade by Ca^{2+} is accentuated by membrane depolarisation. Although blockade is apparent at 10 μmol/l Ca^{2+} in rat lacrimal glands, it has been seen in smooth muscle BK channels at Ca^{2+} concentrations concentrations as low as 1 μmol/l (Benham et al. 1986). It is believed to arise from the slow channel-blocking action of Ca^{2+} described by Vergara and Latorre (1983).

Secretion in many exocrine glands is evoked not only by agonists such as acetylcholine, which utilise Ca^{2+} for signal transduction, but also by agonists such as isoproterenol, which utilise cyclic AMP for this purpose

(Cook and Young 1989a). It is therefore of interest to note in the rat mandibular gland that both isoproterenol and acetylcholine control K^+ channel activity by modulating cytosolic Ca^{2+} activity and that cyclic AMP alone does not activate the channels (Cook et al. 1988a; Horn et al. 1988). The same appears to be the case in the rat lacrimal gland, where BK channels are activated not only by acetylcholine but also by VIP, an agonist that, like isoproterenol, utilises cyclic AMP in other tissues for signal transduction (Lechleiter et al. 1988).[2]

The BK channel from rat skeletal muscle t-tubules is activated by divalent cations in the order $Ca^{2+} > Cd^{2+} > Sr^{2+} > Mn^{2+} > Fe^{2+} > Co^{2+}$. The Ca^{2+} sensitivity of BK channels is enhanced by the presence of other divalent cations such as Mg^{2+}: rat skeletal muscle t-tubules (Golowasch et al. 1986; Oberhauser et al. 1988) and mouse parotid gland (Squire and Petersen 1987). In the channel from rat t-tubules, this enhancement has been attributed to the binding of Mg^{2+} to a modulator, site, the affinity sequence of which is: $Cd^{2+} > Mn^{2+} > Co^{2+} > Ni^{2+} > Mg^{2+} \gg Sr^{2+} = Ca^{2+}$ (Oberhauser et al. 1988). In mouse parotid glands, the sensitivity to Ca^{2+} is enhanced by Mg^{2+} in the range 1–1000 μmol/l (Squire and Petersen 1987).

Kinetics

There have been few studies performed on the kinetics of the BK channel in secretory epithelia. Whole-cell studies in the rat parotid suggest that the BK channel in this tissue has at least two closed and one open state (Maruyama et al. 1986a) although more extensive studies in non-epithelial tissues indicate that the BK channel has rather more complicated kinetics, with four different kinetic modes, the predominant one making up 96% of the activity. Whilst in the predominant mode, the channel protein can enter at least three to four open and six to eight closed states (McManus and Magleby 1988) as well as an inactivated state accessible only from a short-lived open state (Pallotta 1985b). Early studies suggested that Ca^{2+} binding was an essential prelude to BK channel opening (Moczydlowski and Latorre 1983; Magleby and Pallotta 1983) although the observation that Ca^{2+} sensitivity is acquired by BK channels during the development of spinal neurones (Blair and Dionne 1985) and the discovery that N-bromoacetamide abolished the Ca^{2+}-sensitivity of BK channels in rat skeletal muscle whilst leaving the voltage sensitivity intact (Pallotta 1985a) indicate that this is not so. These findings also suggest that the Ca^{2+}-sensitive part of the channel molecule is not closely associated with the conduction mechanism. The number of Ca^{2+} binding sites on each BK channel molecule has been estimated on kinetic grounds to be two or three (Barrett et al. 1982; Magleby and Pallotta 1983;

---

[2] This is in contrast to the position in *Necturus* oxyntic cells, which lack BK channels but have two smaller K^+ channels, one activated by Ca^{2+} and the other by cyclic AMP (Ueda et al. 1987).

Moczydlowski and Latorre 1983) although more recent studies suggest that the channel kinetics are too complex to justify drawing such a conclusion (Benham et al. 1986).

The Number of BK Channels per Cell

Several studies have been performed in which the number of BK channels present in a single exocrine cell has been determined by ensemble noise analysis: rat lacrimal acinar cells (Trautmann and Marty 1984), rat parotid cells (Maruyama et al. 1986a) and rat mandibular cells (Day et al. 1988). From these, it has been concluded that there are 50–150 BK channels per cell. Maruyama et al. (1983b) combined whole-cell and cell-attached patch-recording techniques and deduced that a single pig pancreatic acinar cell contains 25–60 BK channels.

Other K^+ Channels in Secretory Epithelia

In view of the variety of Ca^{2+}-activated K^+ channels detected in non-secretory tissues, for instance in rat brain synaptosomes (Farley and Rudy 1988), it is not altogether surprising that several other K^+ selective channel types have been reported in secretory epithelia. The majority of these fulfil the requirements of the secondary active Cl^- transport model of epithelial secretion extremely well, being highly selective for K^+ over Na^+ and activated both by depolarisation and by increases in an appropriate second messenger for control of signal transduction.

The IK Channel

In rat mandibular glands (Cook et al. 1988b), cultured human nasal epithelium (Kunzelmann et al. 1988), *Necturus* oxyntic cells (Ueda et al. 1987) and sheep parotid glands (Wegman et al. 1988) there are K^+ channels of intermediate conductance (IK channels; see Fig. 1). The best characterised is that in nasal epithelium which has a single-channel conductance of 78 pS, is blocked by quinidine, Ba^{2+} and TEA, and is activated by cytosolic Ca^{2+} concentrations greater than 0.1 µmol/l (Kunzelmann et al. 1988). The larger of the two K^+ channels in the basolateral membrane of *Necturus* oxyntic cells is similar. It has a single-channel conductance of 72 pS and is activated by depolarisation and by 500 nmol/l free Ca^{2+} in the internal solution (Ueda et al. 1987). Some channels with conductances of about 160 pS that have been reported as BK channels (Table 1) may really be IK channels.

The IK channel in salivary glands may actually be a substate of the BK channel. Thus, although there appear to be differences in the kinetics of the BK and IK channels in rat mandibular gland (Cook et al. 1988b) and in sheep parotid gland (Wegman et al. 1988), the observation in the sheep parotid that IK channel activity in cell-attached patches is often replaced by

BK channel activity once a ripped-off inside-out patch is formed (E. A. Wegman, personal communication) suggests that the conductance of the BK channel is under the control of cytoplasmic or cytoskeletal elements. This has also been proposed for the BK channel in an insulin-secreting cell line (Ribalet et al. 1988).

The SK Channel

There are several low-conductance K^+ channels in secretory epithelia (SK channels; see Fig. 1). In guinea pig pancreatic acini, the predominant K^+ channel has a single-channel conductance of 32 pS (Suzuki and Petersen 1988). It is opened by 1 µmol/l Ca^{2+} and by depolarisation, and it is blocked by 10 (but not 5) mmol/l TEA in the external solution (Suzuki and Petersen 1988). In addition to the Ca^{2+}-sensitive IK channel described above, Necturus oxyntic cells have a 33 pS K^+ channel in their basolateral membranes that is activated by increases in cytosolic cyclic AMP and is little influenced by the size of the transmembrane potential (Ueda et al. 1987). In sheep parotid cells (Wegman et al. 1988) there is a small K^+-selective channel with a conductance of 37 pS, but too little information is as yet available about it to allow us to speculate on its relation to those found in the guinea pig pancreatic acini or oxyntic cells. Cultured canine tracheal epithelium has a small inwardly rectifying K^+ channel with a conductance at 0 mV of 19 pS, increasing to 30 pS when the membrane is hyperpolarised (Welsh and McCann 1985). This channel is activated by Ca^{2+} in the range 0.1–1.0 µmol/l (Welsh and McCann 1985; Welsh and Liedtke 1986).

K^+ channels of a slightly higher conductance (50 pS) have been reported in mouse mandibular (Maruyama et al. 1983a) and in human pancreatic acinar cells (Petersen et al. 1985). In human pancreatic acinar cells, the channel is activated by depolarisation and by Ca^{2+} in the concentration range 0.2–1.0 µmol/l (Petersen et al. 1985), but the channel in mouse mandibular cells has not been characterised.

Anomalous Cation Channel Types

There are only two cation channel types so far reported in secretory cells that do not conform to the requirements of the secondary active Cl^- transport model: the K^+ channel in the shark rectal gland, for which no cytosolic regulator has yet been identified, and the 25 pS non-selective cation channel, which is not selective against Na^+.

The K^+ Channel in Shark Rectal Gland

In the basolateral membrane of shark rectal gland, an intermediate conductance (123 pS) K^+ channel has been found that is blocked by internal Ba^{2+}, quinine, quinidine, lidocaine, TEA (10 mmol/l), Cs^+ and Rb^+ (Greger et al. 1987; Gögelein et al. 1987) and is outwardly rectifying (Greger et al. 1987). Unlike the BK channel seen in other secretory epithelia, this channel is not activated by cytosolic Ca^{2+} (Gögelein et al. 1987).

The Non-selective Cation Channel

The non-selective cation channel does not fit into the framework of the secondary active Cl^- transport model. Its lack of selectivity between Na^+ and K^+ suggests that the mechanism of secretion in those secretory epithelia in which it is the predominant basolateral cation channel is entirely unlike that proposed by Silva et al. (1977). It has been reported in thyroid follicular cells (Maruyama et al. 1985) and mouse pancreatic acinar cells (Maruyama and Petersen 1982b, 1984b), in both of which it was the only cation channel observed, as well as in rat pancreatic acinar cells (Gögelein and Pfannmüller 1988), rat and mouse mandibular and parotid secretory cells (Maruyama et al. 1983a; Cook et al. 1988b), the ST_{885} mouse mandibular cell line (Cook et al. 1986), rat pancreatic duct cells (Argent et al. 1987), rat lacrimal secretory cells (Marty et al. 1984), guinea pig pancreatic acinar cells (Suzuki and Petersen 1988) and human parotid and submandibular secretory cells (Maruyama et al. 1986b). It is also widely distributed outside the secretory epithelia, having been reported in Purkinje fibres, neuroblastoma cells, Schwann cells, neutrophils, rat insulinoma cells, the apical membrane of cells of the inner medullary collecting duct of rat kidney, brown fat cells, bursting neurones from *Helix*, mouse neonatal dorsal root ganglion cells, mouse multipotential embryonal carcinoma cells and guinea pig ventricular myocytes (see Cook et al. 1990 for references). These non-selective cation channels all have a linear current–voltage relation with a single-channel conductance of between 25 pS and 35 pS when bathed in symmetrical 150 mmol/l NaCl solutions at 20°C. The single channel conductance is strongly temperature dependent, with a Q_{10} of 1.4 (Yellen 1982; Siemen and Reuhl 1987) and, in symmetrical NaCl solutions, it shows a simple Michaelis-Menten dependence on bathing solution Na^+, with a $K_{0.5}$ of 440 mmol/l and a maximum single-channel conductance (V_{max}) of 125 pS (Shahidi et al. 1989). The channel is strongly cation selective, having a negligible Cl^- permeability, but its most striking feature is its lack of selectivity among monovalent cations: it has similar permeabilities to Na^+, K^+, Rb^+, Cs^+, Li^+ and NH_4^+ (Cook et al. 1990), suggesting that it behaves as a weak-field binding site. In epithelial cells, the channel has a permeability to Mg^{2+} that is one twentieth that of Na^+, but it has no detectable permeability to Ca^{2+} (Petersen and Maruyama 1983; Cook et al. 1989) and Ba^{2+} cannot carry current through it (Gögelein and Pfannmüller 1988). In neutrophils and Schwann cells, however, the channel has a measurable Ca^{2+} permeability (Von Tscharner et al. 1986; Bevan et al. 1984).

In the ST_{885} cell line, the channel also permits the passage of quite large organic cations (Cook et al. 1990). The channel permeabilities (relative to Na^+) to organic cations are: guanidine (2.14) > ethanolamine (0.87) >

4-aminopyridine(0.79) > diethylamine(0.43) > piperazine(0.33) > TRIS(0.075) > N-methylglucamine(0.062). Since the Renkin equation fits these data well (Cook et al. 1990), it has been concluded that the non-selective cation channel behaves like a cylindrical pore with a radius of 0.49 nm. There does, however, appear to be some inhomogeneity in the permeability to large organic cations among non-selective cation channels from different sources. Thus, the channel from the bursting cells of *Helix* appears to be as permeable to TEA and TRIS as it is to Na^+ (Partridge and Swandulla 1987), and those in mouse neonatal dorsal root ganglion cells (Simonneau et al. 1987) and in macrophages (Lipton 1986) appear to be as permeable to TEA as they are to Na^+.

These studies on the permeation of large organic cations have shown that the non-selective cation channel has several remarkable similarities to the channel of the nicotinic acetylcholine receptor. Thus, its permeabilities to both inorganic and organic monovalent cations are almost indistinguishable from those established for the nicotinic receptor channel (Adams et al. 1980; Dwyer et al. 1980). Furthermore, in both channel types, 4-aminopyridine acts as an 'intermediate' blocker, whilst being more permeant than would be expected from its molecular radius. One important difference between the non-selective cation channel and the nicotinic acetylcholine receptor channel is that the latter is approximately 20% as permeable to Ca^{2+} as it is to Na^+ (Adams et al. 1980).

There is also evidence of inhomogeneity in the responses of the open probability of the non-selective cation to transmembrane voltage. The channel in ST_{885} cells, in both ripped-off and cell-attached patches (Cook et al. 1990), and in rat insulinoma cells (Sturgess et al. 1987) is activated by depolarisation, whereas that in macrophages (Lipton 1986) and in pancreatic (Maruyama and Petersen 1982a), thyroid (Maruyama et al. 1985), cardiac (Ehara et al. 1988), neuroblastoma (Yellen 1982) and dorsal root ganglion cells (Simonneau et al. 1987) is not influenced by transmembrane potential. The kinetics are complex, with clusters of flickering openings being separated by long periods of quiescence. The channel-open-time histogram requires at least two exponentials to describe it as does the closed-time histogram (Cook et al. 1990), suggesting that it has at least two closed and two open states.

The activity of the channel is also influenced by cytosolicfree Ca^{2+} levels, although the sensitivity to cytosolic Ca^{2+} differs widely among cell types. In cultured mouse mandibular cells (Cook et al. 1990), rat insulinoma cells (Sturgess et al. 1987) and rat Schwann cells (Beven et al. 1984), the free Ca^{2+} in the solution bathing the cytosolic surface of a ripped-off inside-out patch must be greater than 0.1 mmol/l to activate the channel whereas in rat thyroid follicular cells (Maruyama et al. 1985), rat lacrimal cells (Marty et al. 1984), cardiac cells (Ehara et al. 1988), neuroblastoma cells (Yellen 1982) and neutrophils (von Tscharner et al. 1986) the channels are activated in the range 1–10 μmol/l. The channel in rat pancreatic ducts is known to be activated by Ca^{2+} (Argent et al. 1987), but the concentration required has not yet been determined. In cultured mouse mandibular cells the Ca^{2+} dose-response curve has a Hill coefficient of 1.2 (Cook et al. 1990), suggesting that the binding of one Ca^{2+} ion is sufficient to open the channel.

There are several lines of evidence to suggest that the relative insensitivity to Ca^{2+} of non-selective cation channels in ripped-off patches may be an artefact. First, the channels are found to be active in cell-attached patches (Maruyama and Petersen 1982b; Cook et al. 1990). Second, Maruyama and Petersen (1984b), working with cell-attached patches from cells in which the plasma membrane had been permeabilised with saponin, showed that increasing the extracellular Ca^{2+} to greater than 50 nmol/l caused activation of the channel. Third, stimulating mouse pancreatic acinar cells with cholecystokinin (Maruyama and Petersen 1982b), rat lacrimal cells with acetylcholine or ionophore A23187 (Marty et al. 1984) and cultured mouse mandibular cells with ionophore A23187 (Poronnik et al. 1988), all treatments that increase intracellular free Ca^{2+}, causes an increase in channel activity. Fourth, in rat pancreatic acinar cells, the channel, when initially excised, has a high sensitivity to Ca^{2+} although it is rapidly lost (Maruyama and Petersen 1984b). Furthermore, in their studies on the non-selective cation channel in the apical membrane of the medullary collecting duct of the rat kidney, Light et al. (1988) showed that some channels in ripped-off patches respond to changes in free Ca^{2+} from 1 µmol/l to 10 nmol/l, whereas others do not. The authors speculated that this may have been due to differences in the phosphorylation status of the channels at the time of excision. In two of the tissues in which the non-selective cation channel has been found to have a very low Ca^{2+} sensitivity, viz., insulinoma cells and mouse mandibular cells, there is no apparent change in Ca^{2+} sensitivity following patch excision, which may indicate that the form showing high Ca^{2+} sensitivity in these preparations is extremely labile.

The sensitivity of the non-selective cation channels to a number of blockers has been determined. Of particular importance are the adenine derivatives, which inhibit the channel when added to the cytosolic surface. In rat insulinoma cells, their order of potency is AMP > ADP > ATP > adenosine. AMP is very potent, causing a 94% reduction in channel activity in concentrations of 1 µmol/l (Sturgess et al. 1987). AMP and ATP have also been shown to inhibit the non-selective cation channel in cultured mouse mandibular cells (Cook et al. 1990), as does ATP in guinea pig pancreatic acini (Suzuki and Petersen 1988). GMP is without inhibitory activity (Sturgess et al. 1987). Quinine or quinidine (10–1000 µmol/l) on either the intracellular or extracellular sides of the channel induces numerous brief closures ('intermediate' blockade) in rat insulinoma cells (Sturgess et al. 1987), in cultured-mouse mandibular cells (Cook et al. 1990) and in rat pancreatic acini (Gögelein and Pfannmüller 1988). In inside-out patches, with quinine in the bath, the frequency of the closures and their duration is greatest when the patch is depolarised. Quinine does not alter the open-state probability, indicating that it only blocks the open channel. 4-Aminopyridine (2–10 mmol/l) blocks the channel when added to the cytosolic side of the patch (Sturgess et al. 1987; Cook et al. 1990). It induces a blockade characterised by prolongation of the intervals between openings and a reduction in the mean open probability. The blockade is not influenced by transmembrane potential. Gögelein and Pfannmüller (1988) have found that Cl^- channel blockers in concentrations of 100 µmol/l reversibly inhibit the non-selective cation channel from the cytosolic side. The potency order of these compounds in blocking the non-selective cation channel was 3',5-dichlorodiphenylamine-2-carboxylic acid (DCDPC) > diphenylamine-2-carboxylic acid (DPC) > 5-nitro-2-(3-phenylpropylamino)-benzoic acid (NPPB), which is not the same as that for blockade of cyclic AMP-dependent Cl^- channels (Gögelein and Pfannmüller 1988). DPC has also been found to block the non-selective cation channel in mouse mandibular cells although in that case it acts only from the external surface (Cook et al. 1990). The blockade produced by DPC is similar to that produced by 4-aminopyridine, i.e. it is 'slow' and not influenced by voltage (Gögelein and Pfannmüller 1988; Cook et al. 1990).

Interestingly, SITS, DIDS and DNDS, stilbene disulfonic acid derivatives that block $Cl^- - HCO_3^-$ exchange, cause irreversible activation of the channel when added to the cytosolic surface (Gögelein and Pfannmüller 1988; Cook et al. 1990). This action appears to be dependent on the presence of Ca^{2+} in the intracellular solution (Gögelein and Pfannmüller 1988). The ability of SITS to hold the channel locked into an open conformation has been exploited to determine that the binding site for quinine from the intracellular surface senses 40% of the transmembrane potential (D. I. Cook and P. Poronnik, unpublished results). In general, the non-selective cation channel is not blocked by tetrodotoxin (Sturgess et al. 1987), TEA (Gögelein and Pfannmüller 1988), Ba^{2+} (Gögelein and Pfannmüller 1988) or amiloride (Sturgess et al. 1987; Cook et al. 1989). The non-selective cation channel of the inner medullary collecting duct is distinguished by being blocked by amiloride from the cytosolic surface and not being blocked by DPC (Light et al. 1988).

Ca^{2+} Channels

As mentioned above, the activity of many secretory epithelia is under neurohumoral control. In the case of those epithelia in which that control is exercised via control of intracellular free Ca^{2+} levels, there is good evidence not only that Ca^{2+} is released from intracellular stores, but also that it enters the cytosol via Ca^{2+} channels in the plasma membrane (Gallacher and Morris 1987; Morris et al. 1987a; Llano et al. 1987; Petersen and Gallacher 1988) which, in mouse lacrimal cells, may be activated by the synergistic action of IP_3 and IP_4 (Morris et al. 1987c; Changya et al. 1988) although studies in rat mast cells suggest that IP_3 alone is sufficient (Penner et al. 1988). Recent studies in thrombin-stimulated platelets (Zschauer et al. 1988) have demonstrated a calcium channel with a conductance of 10 pS in

150 mmol/l Ba^{2+} that appears to be a strong candidate for the IP_3-activated Ca^{2+} channel. To date, however, no Ca^{2+} channel has been demonstrated in patch-clamp studies on secretory epithelia.

References

Adams DJ, Dwyer TM, Hille B (1980) The permeability of endplate channels to monovalent and divalent metal cations. J Gen Physiol 75:493–510

Adams PR, Constanti A, Brown DA, Clark RB (1982) Intracellular Ca^{2+} activates a fast voltage-sensitive K^+ current in vertebrate sympathetic neurones. Nature 296:746–749

Anderson CS, MacKinnon R, Smith C, Miller C (1988) Charybdotoxin block of single Ca^{2+}-activated K^+ channels. Effects of channel gating, voltage, and ionic strength. J Gen Physiol 91:317–333

Argent BE, Arkle S, Gray MA, Greenwell JR (1987) Two types of calcium-sensitive cation channels in isolated rat pancreatic duct cells. J Physiol (Lond) 386:82P

Barrett JN, Magleby KL, Pallotta BS (1982) Properties of single calcium-activated potassium channels in cultured rat muscle. J Physiol (Lond) 331:211–230

Barry PH, Gage PW (1984) Ionic selectivity of channels at the end plate. In: Stein WD (ed) Ion channels: molecular and physiological aspects. Academic, Orlando, pp 1–51 (Current topics in membranes and transport, Vol 21)

Benham CD, Bolton TB, Lang RJ, Takewaki T (1986) Calcium-activated potassium channels in single smooth muscle cells of rabbit jejunum and guinea-pig mesenteric artery. J Physiol (Lond) 371:45–67

Bevan S, Gray PTA, Ritchie JM (1984) A calcium-activated cation-selective channel in rat cultured Schwann cells. Proc R Soc Lond [Biol] 222:349–355

Blair LAC, Dionne VE (1985) Development acquisition of Ca^{2+}-sensitivity by K^+ channels in spinal neurones. Nature 315:329–330

Blatz AL, Magleby KL (1984) Ion conductance and selectivity of single calcium-activated potassium channels in cultured rat muscle. J Gen Physiol 84:1–23

Blatz AL, Magleby KL (1987) Calcium-activated potassium channels. Trends Neurosci 10:463–467

Bolivar JJ, Cereijido M (1987) Voltage and Ca^{2+}-activated K^+ channel in cultured epithelial cells (MDCK). J Membr Biol 97:43–52

Cecchi X, Wolff D, Alvarez O, Latorre R (1987) Mechanisms of Cs^+ blockade in a Ca^{2+}-activated K^+ channel from smooth muscle. Biophys J 52:707–716

Changya L, Gallacher DV, Irvine RF, Petersen OH (1988) Effects of inositol polyphosphates on the Ca^{2+}-activated K^+ current in single perfused mouse lacrimal acinar cells. Proc Physiol Soc Nov: 24P

Christensen O, Zeuthen T (1987) Maxi K^+ channels in leaky epithelia are regulated by intracellular Ca^{2+}, pH and membrane potential. Pflügers Arch 408:249–259

Cook DI, Young JA (1989a) Fluid and electrolyte secretion by salivary glands. In: Forte JG (ed) Handbook of physiology (Section 6, Vol III, Salivary, pancreatic, gastric and hepatobiliary secretion). American Physiological Society, Washington, pp 1–23

Cook DI, Young JA (1989b) The effect of K^+ channels in the apical plasma membrane on epithelial secretion based on secondary active Cl^--transport. J Membr Biol 110: 139–146

Cook DI, Towner SP, Young JA (1986) Patch-clamp studies of cultured salivary cells. Biomed Res 7 (Suppl 2):203–207

Cook DI, Day ML, Champion M, Young JA (1988a) Ca^{2+} not cyclic AMP mediates the fluid secretory response to isoproterenol in the rat mandibular salivary gland: whole-cell patch-clamp studies. Pflügers Arch 413:67–76

Cook DI, Gard GB, Champion M, Young JA (1988b) Patch-clamp studies of the electrolyte secretory mechanism of rat mandibular gland cells stimulated with acetylcholine or isoproterenol. In: Thorn NA, Treiman M, Petersen OH, Thaysen JH (eds) Molecular mechanisms in secretion (25th Alfred Benzon symposium 1987). Munksgaard, Copenhagen, pp 131–151

Cook DI, Poronnik P, Young JA (1990) Characterisation of a 25 pS non-selective cation channel in a cultured epithelial cell line. J Membr Biol (in press)

Day ML, Cook DI, Young JA (1988) The measurement of the number of potassium channels in single rat mandibular cells by ensemble noise analysis. Proc Aust Physiol Pharmacol Soc 19:135P

Dwyer TM, Adams DJ, Hille B (1980) The permeability of the endplate channel to organic cations in frog muscle. J Gen Physiol 75:469–492

Ehara T, Noma A, Ono K (1988) Calcium-activated non-selective cation channel in ventricular cells isolated from adult guinea-pig hearts. J Physiol (Lond) 403: 117–134

Eisenmann G, Latorre R, Miller C (1986) Multi-ion conduction and selectivity in the high conductance Ca^{++} activated K^+ channel from skeletal muscle. Biophys J 50: 1025–1034

Evans LAR, Pirani DP, Cook DI, Young JA (1986) Intraepithelial current flow in rat pancreatic secretory epithelia. Pflügers Arch 407 (Suppl 2): S107–S111

Farley J, Rudy B (1988) Multiple types of voltage-dependent Ca^{2+}-activated K^+ channels of large conductance in rat brain synaptosomal membranes. Biophys J 53: 919–934

Findlay I (1984) A patch-clamp study of potassium channels and whole-cell currents in acinar cells of the mouse lacrimal gland. J Physiol (Lond) 350: 179–195

Findlay I, Dunne MJ, Petersen OH (1985) High-conductance K^+ channel in pancreatic islet cells can be activated and inactivated by internal calcium. J Membr Biol 83: 169–175

Gallacher DV, Morris AP (1986) A patch-clamp study of potassium currents in resting and acetylcholine-stimulated mouse submandibular acinar cells. J Physiol (Lond) 373:379–395

Gallacher DV, Morris AP (1987) The receptor-regulated calcium influx in mouse submandibular acinar cells is sodium dependent: a patch-clamp study. J Physiol (Lond) 384: 119–130

Gallacher DV, Maruyama Y, Petersen OH (1984) Patch-clamp study of rubidium and potassium conductances in single cation channels from mammalian exocrine acini. Pflügers Arch 401: 361–367

Gitter AH, Beyenbach KW, Christine CW, Gross P, Minuth WW, Frömter E (1987) High-conductance K^+ channel in apical membranes of principal cells cultured from rabbit renal cortical collecting duct Anlagen. Pflügers Arch 408: 282–290

Glavinovic MI, Trifaro JM (1988) Quinine blockade of currents through Ca^{2+}-activated K^+ channels in bovine chromaffin cells. J Physiol (Lond) 399: 139–152

Gögelein H, Pfannmüller B (1988) The non-selective cation channel in the basolateral membrane of rat exocrine pancreas. Inhibition by 3′,5-dichlorodiphenylamine-2-carboxylic acid (DCDPC). Pflügers Arch 413: 287–298

Gögelein H, Greger R, Schlatter E (1987) Potassium channels in the basolateral membrane of the rectal gland of Squalus acanthias. Regulation and inhibitors. Pflügers Arch 409: 107–113

Golowasch J, Kirkwood A, Miller C (1986) Allosteric effects of Mg^{2+} on the gating of Ca^{2+}-activated K^+ channels from mammalian skeletal muscle. J Exp Biol 124: 5–13

Gray MA, Greenwell JR, Argent BE (1988) Ion channels in pancreatic duct cells and their role in bicarbonate secretion. In: Wong PYD, Young JA (eds) Exocrine secretion. Hong Kong University Press, Hong Kong, pp 77–80

Greger R, Gögelein H, Schlatter E (1987) Potassium channels in the basolateral membrane of the rectal gland of the dogfish (Squalus acanthias). Pflügers Arch 409: 100–106

Hardcastle J, Hardcastle PT (1986) The involvement of basolateral potassium channels in the intestinal response to secretagogues in the rat. J Physiol (Lond) 379: 331–346

Horn VJ, Baum BJ, Ambudkar IS (1988) β-Adrenergic receptor stimulation induces inositol trisphosphate production and Ca^{2+} mobilization in rat parotid acinar cells. J Biol Chem 263: 12454–12460

Iwatsuki N, Petersen OH (1985a) Inhibition of Ca^{2+}-activated K^+ channels in pig pancreatic acinar cells by Ba^{2+}, Ca^{2+}, quinine and quinidine. Biochim Biophys Acta 819: 249–257

Iwatsuki, N, Petersen OH (1985b) Action of tetraethylammonium on calcium-activated potassium channels in pig pancreatic acinar cells studied by patch-clamp single-channel and whole-cell current recording. J Membr Biol 86: 139–144

Klaerke DA, Karlish SJD, Jørgensen PL (1987) Reconstitution in phospholipid vesicles of calcium-activated potassium channel from outer renal medulla. J Membr Biol 95: 105–112

Kolb HA, Brown CDA, Murer H (1986) Characterization of a Ca-dependent maxi-K channel in the apical membrane of a cultured renal epithelium (JTC-12.P3). J Membr Biol 92: 207–215

Kunzelmann K, Üna Ö, Beck C, Emmrich P, Arndt H, Greger R (1988) Ion channels of cultured respiratory epithelial cells of patients with cystic fibrosis. Pflügers Arch 411: R68

Kurtzer RJ, Roberts ML (1982) Calcium-dependent K^+ efflux from rat submandibular gland. The effects of trifluoperazine and quinidine. Biochim Biophys Acta 693: 479–484

Latorre R, Miller C (1983) Conduction and selectivity in potassium channels. J Membr Biol 71: 11–30

Latorre R, Vergara C, Hidalgo C (1982) Reconstitution in planar lipid bilayers of a Ca^{2+}-dependent K^+ channel from transverse tubule membranes isolated from rabbit skeletal muscle. Proc Natl Acad Sci USA 79: 805–809

Lechleiter JD, Dartt DA, Brehm P (1988) Vasoactive intestinal peptide activates Ca^{2+} dependent K^+ channels through a cAMP pathway in mouse lacrimal cells. Neuron 1: 227–235

Light DB, McCann FV, Keller TM, Stanton BA (1988) Amiloride-sensitive cation channel in apical membrane of inner medullary collecting duct. Am J Physiol 255: F278–F286

Lipton SA (1986) Antibody activates cationic channels via second messenger Ca^{2+}. Biochim Biophys Acta 856: 56–67

Llano I, Marty A, Tanguy J (1987) Dependence of intracellular effects of $GTP\gamma S$ and inositoltrisphosphate on cell membrane potential and on external Ca ions. Pflügers Arch 409: 499–506

MacKinnon R, Miller C (1988) Mechanism of charybdotoxin block of the high-conductance, Ca^{2+}-activated K^+ channel. J Gen Physiol 91: 335–349

Magleby KL, Pallotta BS (1983) Calcium dependence of open and shut interval distributions from calcium-activated potassium channels in cultured rat muscle. J Physiol (Lond) 344: 585–604

Marty A (1981) Ca-dependent K channels with large unitary conductance in chromaffin cell membranes. Nature 291: 497–500

Marty A (1983) Blocking of large conductance unitary calcium-dependent potassium currents by internal sodium ions. Pflügers Arch 396: 179–181

Marty A, Tan YP, Trautmann A (1984) Three types of calcium-dependent channels in rat lacrimal glands. J Physiol (Lond) 357: 293–325

Maruyama Y, Petersen OH (1982a) Single-channel currents in isolated patches of plasma membrane from basal surface of pancreatic acini. Nature 299: 159–161

Maruyama Y, Petersen OH (1982b) Cholecystokinin activation of single-channel currents is mediated by internal messenger in pancreatic acinar cells. Nature 300: 61–63

Maruyama Y, Petersen OH (1984a) Control of K^+ conductance by cholecystokinin and Ca^{2+} in single pancreatic acinar cells studied by the patch-clamp technique. J Membr Biol 79: 293–300

Maruyama Y, Petersen OH (1984b) Single calcium-dependent cation channels in mouse pancreatic acinar cells. J Membr Biol 81: 83–87

Maruyama Y, Gallacher DV, Petersen OH (1983a) Voltage and Ca^{2+}-activated K^+ channel in basolateral acinar cell membranes in mammalian salivary glands. Nature 302: 827–829

Maruyama Y, Petersen OH, Flanagan P, Pearson GT (1983b) Quantification of Ca^{2+}-activated K^+ channels under hormonal control in pig pancreas acinar cells. Nature 305: 228–232

Maruyama Y, Moore D, Petersen OH (1985) Calcium-activated cation channel in rat thyroid follicular cells. Biochim Biophys Acta 821:229–232

Maruyama Y, Nishiyama A, Izumi T, Hoshimiya N, Petersen OH (1986a) Ensemble noise and current relaxation analysis of K^+ current in single isolated salivary acinar cells from rat. Pflügers Arch 406:69–72

Maruyama Y, Nishiyama A, Teshima T (1986b) Two types of cation channels in the basolateral cell membrane of human salivary gland acinar cells. Jpn J Physiol 36:219–223

McCann JD, Welsh MJ (1986) Calcium-activated potassium channels in canine airway smooth muscle. J Physiol (Lond) 372:113–127

McCann JD, Welsh MJ (1987) Neuroleptics antagonize a calcium-activated potassium channel in airway smooth muscle. J Gen Physiol 89:339–352

McManus OB, Magleby KL (1988) Kinetic states and modes of single large-conductance calcium-activated potassium channels in cultured rat skeletal muscle. J Physiol (Lond) 402:79–120

Merot J, Bidet M, Le Maout S, Tauc M, Poujeol P (1989) Two types of K^+ channels in the apical membrane of rabbit proximal tubule in primary culture. Biochim Biophys Acta 978:134–144

Methfessel C, Boheim G (1982) The gating of single calcium-dependent potassium channels is described by an activation/blockade mechanism. Biophys Struct Mech 9:35–60

Miller C, Moczydlowski E, Latorre R, Phillips M (1985) Charybdotoxin, a protein inhibitor of single Ca^{2+}-activated K^+ channels from mammalian skeletal muscle. Nature 313:316–318

Miller C, Latorre R, Reisin I (1987) Coupling of voltage-dependent gating and Ba^{++} block in the high-conductance, Ca^{2+}-activated K^+ channel. J Gen Physiol 90:427–449

Moczydlowski E, Latorre R (1983) Gating kinetics of Ca activated K channels from rat muscle incorporated into planar lipid bilayers. J Gen Physiol 82:511–542

Moczydlowski E, Lucchesi K, Ravindran A (1988) An emerging pharmacology of peptide toxins targeted against potassium channels. J Membr Biol 105:595–111

Morris AP, Gallacher DV, Lee JAC (1986) A large conductance, voltage- and calcium-activated K^+ channel in the basolateral membrane of rat enterocytes. FEBS Lett 206:87–92

Morris AP, Fuller CM, Gallacher DV (1987a) Cholinergic receptors regulate a voltage-insensitive but Na^+-dependent calcium influx pathway in salivary acinar cells. FEBS Lett 211:195–199

Morris AP, Gallacher DV, Fuller CM, Scott J (1987b) Cholinergic receptor-regulation of potassium channels and potassium transport in human submandibular acinar cells. J Dent Res 66:541–546

Morris AP, Gallacher DV, Irvine RF, Petersen OH (1987c) Synergism of inositol trisphosphate and tetrakisphosphate in activating Ca^{2+}-dependet K^+ channels. Nature 330:653–655

Murakami M, Suzuki E, Seo Y, Miyamoto S, Watari H (1988) Activation-inactivation of Na^+/K^+ ATPase in the isolated perfused rat mandibular gland measured by NMR. In: Wong PYD, Young JA (eds) Exocrine secretion. Hong Kong University Press, Hong Kong, pp 125–128

Oberhauser A, Alvarez O, Latorre R (1988) Activation by divalent cations of a Ca^{2+}-activated K^+ channel from skeletal muscle membrane. J Gen Physiol 92:67–86

Okada Y, Yada T, Ohno-Shosaku T, Oiki S (1987) Evidence for the involvement of calmodulin in the operation of Ca-activated K channels in mouse fibroblasts. J Membr Biol 96:121–128

Pallotta BS (1985a) N-bromoacetamide removes a calcium-dependent component of channel opening from calcium-activated potassium channels in rat skeletal muscle. J Gen Physiol 86:601–611

Pallotta BS (1985b) Calcium-activated potassium channels in rat muscle inactivate from a short-duration open state. J Physiol (Lond) 363:501–516

Pallotta BS, Magleby KL, Barrett JN (1981) Single channel recordings on Ca^{2+}-activated currents in rat muscle cell culture. Nature 293: 471–474

Partridge LD, Swandulla D (1987) Single Ca-activated cation channels in bursting neurone of *Helix*. Pflügers Arch 410:627–631

Penner R, Matthews G, Neher E (1988) Regulation of calcium influx by second messengers in rat mast cells. Nature 334:499–504

Petersen OH, Gallacher DV (1988) Electrophysiology of pancreatic and salivary acinar cells. Annu Rev Physiol 50:65–80

Petersen OH, Maruyama Y (1983) What is the mechanism of the calcium influx to pancreatic acinar cells evoked by secretagogues. Pflügers Arch 396:82–84

Petersen OH, Maruyama Y (1984) Calcium-activated potassium channels and their role in secretion. Nature 307:693–696

Petersen OH, Findlay I, Iwatsuki N, Singh J, Gallacher DV, Fuller CM, Pearson GD, Dunne MJ, Morris AP (1985) Human pancreatic acinar cells: studies of stimulus-secretion coupling. Gastroenterology 89:109–117

Poronnik P, Cook DI, Young JA (1988) The use of Cytodex® microcarrier beads in patch-clamp studies on cultured epithelial cells. Pflügers Arch 413:90–92

Poulsen JH, Bledsoe SW (1978) Salivary gland K^+ transport: in vivo studies with K^+-specific microelectrodes. Am J Physiol 234:E79–E83

Poulsen JH, Oakley B (1979) Intracellular potassium ion activity in resting and stimulated mouse pancreas and submandibular gland. Proc R Soc Lond [Biol] 204:99–104

Rae JL (1985) The application of patch clamp methods to ocular epithelia. Curr Eye Res 4: 409–420

Rae JL, Laevis RA, Eisenberg RS (1988) Ionic channels in ocular epithelia. In: Narahashi T (ed) Ion channels, vol 1. Plenum, New York, pp 283–327

Ribalet B, Eddlestone GT, Ciani S (1988) Metabolic regulation of the K (ATP) and a Maxi-K (V) channel in the insulin-secreting RINm5F cell. J Gen Physiol 92:219–237

Romey G, Lazdunski M (1984) The coexistence in rat muscle cells of two distinct classes of Ca^{2+}-dependent K^+ channels with different pharmacological properties and different physiological functions. Biochem Biophys Res Commun 118:669–674

Shahidi S, Poronnik, P, Cook DI, Young JA (1989) Studies on the permeation mechanism in the 25 pS non-selective cation channel from ST_{885} cells. Proc Aust Physiol Pharmacol Soc 20 148 P

Sheppard DN, Giraldez F, Sepulveda FV (1988) Kinetics of voltage and Ca^{2+} activation and Ba^{2+} blockade of a large-conductance K^+ channel from *Necturus* enterocytes. J Membr Biol 105:65–76

Siemen D, Reuhl T (1987) Non-selective cationic channel in primary cultured cells of brown adipose tissue. Pflügers Arch 408:534–536

Silva P, Stoff J, Field M, Fine L, Forrest JN, Epstein FH (1977) Mechanism of active chloride secretion by shark rectal gland: role of Na-K-ATPase in chloride transport. Am J Physiol 233:F298–F306

Simonneau M, Distasi C, Tauc L, Barbin G (1987) Potassium channels in mouse neonate dorsal root ganglion cells: a patch-clamp study. Brain Res 412:224–232

Smart TG (1987) Single calcium-activated potassium channels recorded from cultured rat sympathetic neurones. J Physiol (Lond) 389:337–360

Smith PL, Frizzell RA (1984) Chloride secretion by canine tracheal epithelium. IV. Basolateral membrane K permeability parallels secretion rate. J Membr Biol 77: 187–199

Squire LG, Petersen OH (1987) Modulation of Ca^{2+}- and voltage-activated K^+ channels by internal Mg^{2+} in salivary acinar cells. Biochim Biophys Acta 899:171–175

Sturgess NC, Hales CN, Ashford MLJ (1987) Calcium and ATP regulate the activity of a non-selective cation channel in a rat insulinoma cell line. Pflügers Arch 409:607–615

Suzuki K, Petersen OH (1988) Patch-clamp study of single channel and whole cell K^+ currents in guinea pig pancreatic acinar cells. Am J Physiol 255:G275–G285

Trautmann A, Marty A (1984) Activation of Ca-dependent K channels by carbamylcholine in rat lacrimal glands. Proc Natl Acad Sci USA 81:611–615

Turner RJ, George JN, Baum BJ (1986) Evidence for a $Na^+/K^+/Cl^-$ cotransport system in basolateral membrane vesicles from the rabbit parotid. J Membr Biol 94:143–152

Ueda S, Loo DDF, Sachs G (1987) Regulation of K^+ channels in the basolateral membrane of *Necturus* oxyntic cells. J Membr Biol 97:31–41

Valdiva HH, Smith JS, Martin BM, Coronado R, Possani LO (1988) Charybdotoxin and noxiustoxin, two homologous peptide inhibitors of the $K^+(Ca^{2+})$ channel. FEBS Lett 226:280–284

Vergara C, Latorre R (1983) Kinetics of Ca^{2+}-activated K^+ channels from rabbit muscle incorporated into planar bilayers. Evidence for a Ca^{2+} and Ba^{2+} blockade. J Gen Physiol 82:543–568

Von Tscharner V, Prod'hom B, Baggiolini B, Reuter H (1986) Ion channels in human neutrophils activated by a rise in cytosolic calcium concentration. Nature 324:369–372

Wegman EA, Reid AM, Cook DI, Titchen DA, Young JA (1988) Potassium channels in secretory cells of the sheep parotid and mandibular glands. Proc Aust Physiol Pharmacol Soc 19:177P

Welsh MJ (1983) Evidence for basolateral membrane potassium conductance in canine tracheal epithelium. Am J Physiol 244:C377–C384

Welsh MJ (1987) Electrolyte transport by airway epithelia. Physiol Rev 67:1143–1184

Welsh MJ, Liedtke CM (1986) Chloride and potassium channels in cystic fibrosis airway epithelia. Nature 322:467–470

Welsh MJ, McCann JD (1985) Intracellular calcium regulates basolateral potassium channels in a chloride-secreting epithelium. Proc Natl Acad Sci USA 82:8823–8826

Wong BS, Adler M (1986) Tetraethylammonium blockade of calcium-activated potassium channels in clonal anterior pituitary cells. Pflügers Arch 407:279–284

Wong BS, Lecar H, Adler M (1982) Single calcium-dependent potassium channels in clonal anterior pituitary cells. Biophys J 39:313–317

Woodhull AM (1973) Ionic blockage of sodium channels in nerve. J Gen Physiol 61:687–708

Yellen G (1982) Single Ca^{2+}-activated non-selective cation channels in neuroblastoma. Nature 296:357–359

Yellen G (1984a) Ionic permeation and blockade in Ca^{2+}-activated K^+ channels of bovine chromaffin cells. J Gen Physiol 84:157–186

Yellen G (1984b) Relief of Na^+ block of Ca^{2+}-activated K^+ channels by external cations. J Gen Physiol 84:187–199

Yellen G (1987) Permeation in potassium channels: implications for channel structure. Annu Rev Biophys Biophys Chem 16:227–246

Ypey DL, Ravesloot JH, Buisman HP, Nijweide PJ (1988) Voltage-activated ionic channels and conductances in embryonic chick osteoblast cultures. J Membr Biol 101:141–150

Zschauer A, Van Breeman C, Bühler FR, Nelson MT (1988) Calcium channels in thrombin-activated human platelet membrane. Nature 344:703–705

Gap Junctions in Exocrine Glands*

A. Trautmann, C. Randriamampita and C. Giaume

In exocrine glands, the different cells of an acinus are associated by junctional complexes including, in addition to gap junctions, tight junctions and zonulae adherentes. The membrane-differentiation characteristics of gap junctions have been observed in pancreatic acini (Friend and Gilula 1972; Meda et al. 1983) and salivary glands (Kater and Galvin 1978). The specific role of the gap junction is the control of direct cell-to-cell communication. The existence of this type of communication can be demonstrated by dye or electrical coupling. Fluorescein and Lucifer Yellow are two dyes that have been shown to permeate gap junctions in the exocrine pancreas (Kater and Galvin 1978; Findlay and Petersen 1983; Meda et al. 1986) and in salivary glands of invertebrates (Rose 1971) and mammals (Hammer and Sheridan 1978). Electrical coupling has also been observed in a large number of exocrine glands (see for a review, Petersen 1980). In the pancreas, all the cells from the same acinus are electrically coupled and in some cases, cells from different acini seem also to be coupled (Iwatsuki and Petersen 1978a).

In the present review, some properties of the gap junction channels in exocrine glands will be discussed. The structure of the channel, the characteristics of the single-channel current, the mode of action of secretomotor agonists on gap junction channels, and the possible involvement of gap junction closure during secretion will be examined in more detail.

Characteristics of the Gap Junction Protein

Some 30 years after the original discovery of the existence of direct intercellular communication between invertebrate neurons (Furshpan and Potter 1959), several properties of gap junctions have been unravelled. The basic unit of a gap junction, the intercellular channel, is composed of two hemichannels or connexons (Makowski 1985; Zampighi and Simon 1985). The walls of a connexon seem to be made of six transmembrane proteins. In

---

* This work was supported by grants from the C.N.R.S., the Ministère de la Recherche et de la Technologie, and by the Université Pierre et Marie Curie.

various organs these proteins have been purified; their molecular weights were mostly between 26 and 32 kDa, but proteins of higher molecular weights were also detected. Antibodies obtained against the purified livergap junction protein (the 27-kDa protein) have been tested in various organs and a cross reactivity was found in the exocrine pancreas (Dermietzel et al. 1984; Hertzberg and Skibbens 1984; Paul 1986a). This suggests that pancreatic and liver gap junctions present common epitopes and therefore have a certain homology.

More recently, the molecular biological approach has helped to clarify the position. The gene of the protein making up the gap junction in exocrine glands has not yet been cloned (as at the end of 1988), but those of the liver and heart have been cloned and sequenced (Kumar and Gilula 1986; Paul 1986b; Beyer et al. 1987). There is a large homology between the 43-kDa gap junction protein from the heart (connexin 43) and the 32-kDa protein from the liver (connexin 32). In the lens, several proteins have been considered as putative gap junction subunits. One, called MIP26 (Gorin et al. 1984), presents no homology with the connexins, whereas two other proteins (46 and 70 kDa) are homologous to the connexins in the amino terminal region (Dupont et al. 1988; Kistler et al. 1988). It is worth noting that the more conserved regions (N-terminal domain) are the transmembrane and the extracellular ones. Most of the differences are found in the C-terminal region, corresponding to the cytoplasmic part of the connexins, which is probably the target of the intracellular molecules modulating junctional permeability. Molecular cDNA probes have revealed the existence in various organs of proteins homologous to the connexins (Paul 1986b; Beyer et al. 1987).

One may summarize the causes of the discrepancies between various estimates of the size of the gap junction protein as follows: (a) The technical approaches may be sources of artefacts (e.g. degradation or aggregation of proteins on the gels). In addition, the migration of these proteins is very sensitive to the concentration of acrylamide in the gel (Green et al. 1988). (b) It is probable that a connexon is not only composed of six monomers, but also possesses an additional, minor protein (Nicholson et al. 1987). (c) It now seems clear that gap junction proteins are homologous, but not identical in different organs of the same species (Kistler et al. 1988).

The Double Patch-Clamp Method

A new method derived from the whole-cell recording variant of the patch-clamp method (Marty and Neher 1983) was devised in order to measure directly the conductance of single gap junction channels (Neyton and Trautmann 1985). For this type of measurement, pairs of coupled cells are prepared by enzymatic dissociation of the tissue. A simultaneous double whole-cell recording of the cells of a pair allows the measurement of the current flowing from one cell to the other through the gap junction and estimation of the corresponding conductance. This estimation requires a correction for the error introduced by the series resistance, which can be very large when the junctional conductance is high and has sometimes been overlooked. If the background noise of this signal (proportional at low frequencies to the capacitance of the two cells and, thus, to the square of their diameter) is low enough, and if a small number of gap junction channels is open, single-channel events can be measured (Neyton and Trautmann 1985).

Before the introduction of the double patch-clamp technique, the method of choice for the study of the gap junction conductance was the double voltage-clamp technique (Spray et al. 1981). One advantage of the double patch clamp over the double voltage clamp is an enormous improvement of the signal-to-noise ratio. A second advantage is the possibility of measuring gap junction currents in small cells, which are not suitable for the double voltage clamp and in which quantitative measurements of gap junction conductance was previously impossible. This applies to cells from exocrine glands in general. A third advantage of this technique is that the composition of the intracellular solution is under control. This feature has allowed the determination of the ionic selectivity of gap junction channels (Neyton and Trautmann 1985). As will be shown in more detail below, we have also taken advantage of the ability to control the intracellular solution to analyse the modulation of gap junction conductance by a secretomotor agonist.

The double patch-clamp method suffers from an important drawback, however. After a double whole-cell recording has been established in a pair of acinar cells, gap junction channels close progressively during the next 5–30 min (Neyton and Trautmann 1985; Somogyi and Kolb 1988). This closure is reminiscent of the washout of Ca^{2+} curents observed in excitable cells, which is probably due to a Ca^{2+}-dependent protease and to the dephosphorylation of proteins normally phosphorylated by a cyclic AMP-dependent protein kinase (PKA; Chad and Eckert 1986; Amstrong and Eckert 1987). In pancreatic cells, spontaneous closure of gap junction channels is almost completely avoided by including ATP and cyclic AMP in the pipette (Somogyi and Kolb 1988). This suggests that gap junction channels require the activity of PKA to remain open. In lacrimal cells, washout seems to be linked to complex regulations. The inclusion of cyclic AMP and ATP in the pipette solution retards the washout; the further addition of leupeptin (which inhibits Ca^{2+}-dependent proteases) retards it even more, but the washout is not completely blocked (C. Randriamampita, C. Giaume and A. Trautmann, unpublished results). In these cells, spontaneous uncoupling could thus be due to a lack of activity of PKA, to the stimulation of proteases and to an additional unknown factor.

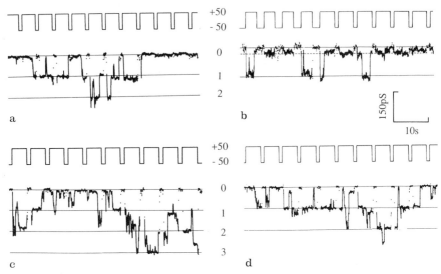

Fig. 1a–d. Single gap junction channel currents measured in lacrimal cells at the end of uncouplings **a** induced by 100 µmol/l arachidonic acid or **b** developing spontaneously, or **c** elicited by 1 µmol/l ACh or **d** 0.6 mmol/l octanol. The junctional conductance was derived from the current measured in cell 2 (at a constant holding potential of -50 mV), whilst stepping the voltage of cell 1 between -50 mV and $+50$ mV. *Dotted traces* show the current when the cells were isopotential. A subconductance state was observed in one recording (**b**), indicated by a *broken line*

Single-Channel Currents in Gap Junction

The first direct measurement of gap junction-channel conductance, obtained at the end of spontaneous uncouplings in rat lacrimal acinar cells, gave a value of 120 pS (Neyton and Trautmann 1985). This figure has to be treated with caution since the spontaneous uncoupling process could affect not only the number of open channels, but also their elementary conductance. Since then, we have observed that single-channel currents observed during uncoupling elicited by acetylcholine, arachidonic acid (see below) or octanol, had a similar amplitude, as shown in Fig. 1. This indicates that the initial measurements were not biased by washout.

A value of 120 pS fits quite well with indirect estimates made previously, based on the maximum size of molecules permeant through gap junction channels and on structural evidence, suggesting that this channel could be equivalent to a tube, 15–18 nm long with a diameter of 1.0–1.4 nm (Simpson et al. 1977). If ions were freely diffusing in such a structure, the expected conductance should be around 100 pS (Loewenstein 1975; Simpson et al. 1977).

Could it be that the conductance measured in patch-clamp experiments corresponds either to a substate of a larger channel or to the simultaneous opening of several smaller channels? Neither of these possibilities can be completely discarded, but the good agreement observed with indirect estimates does not argue in favour of either. In addition, at least in lacrimal glands, sudden conductance changes of larger amplitude were very rarely observed and were more likely to correspond to the occasional cooperative behaviour of a group of channels (Neyton and Trautmann 1985). On the other hand, smaller conductance changes were indeed observed although their amplitude was very variable, so that the only conductance change that showed quantal behaviour was the one around 100 pS.

Since then, other estimates of single-channel conductance have been obtained using the double patch-clamp technique. They gave consistent values for single-channel conductances ranging between 100 and 160 pS with frequent additional subconductance states. The conductance (respectively, subconductance) values were 130 (respectively, 27 pS) in pancreatic acinar cells (Somogyi and Kolb 1988), 120 pS (respectively, 22 to 70 pS) in Chinese hamster ovary cells (Somogyi and Kolb 1988), 166 pS (respectively, 60 and 80 pS) in adult mammalian heart cells (Veenstra and De Haan 1986, 1988) and 100 pS in embryonic muscle cells, measured with a slightly different method (Chow and Young 1987). By contrast, lower unitary conductances of 53 pS (Burt and Spray 1988) and 35–50 pS (Jongsma et al. 1986) have been measured in neonatal heart cells.

Modulation of Gap Junction Conductance in Exocrine Glands

Neurotransmitters, hormones and other regulatory molecules inducing secretion by exocrine glands belong to two main groups. The action of the first group is mediated by the dual pathway activated by the hydrolysis of polyphosphoinositides which results in an increase of intracellular Ca^{2+} and in the activation of protein kinease C (PKC). As summarized in the review of Williams (1987), secretomotor agonists increasing intracellular Ca^{2+} include: acetylcholine (ACh), noradrenaline (acting on α_1-adrenergic receptors; but see the exception presented by Cook et al. 1988), cholecystokinin, gastrin, bombesin and substance P. It was recently shown by Northern blot analysis with probes derived from subtype specific sequences that in the pancreas, muscarinic receptors are of the HM4 subtype (Peralta et al. 1987). The implication of PKC in the secretory process has also been documented recently (see Schulz et al. 1987 for a review). The action of the second group of secretomotor agonists is mediated by a rise in intracellular cyclic AMP. Agonists stimulating adenylate cyclase include: noradrenaline acting on β receptors, vasoactive intestinal peptide (VIP) and secretin (Williams 1987).

The action of the first series of secretomotor agonists on gap junctions has been studied initially by Petersen's group, who worked on fragments of pancreas, salivary and lacrimal glands (see Petersen 1980 for a review). These agonists elicit an increase in the cell membrane conductance and a decrease in gap junction conductance (Iwatsuki and Petersen 1978 a, b). The sequential order of these two events and the magnitude of the uncoupling could not be determined at that time because cell-to-cell coupling was measured with methods by which changes in junctional and non-junctional resistances could not be properly resolved (see below).

Up to the early 1980s, the two main condidates for the control of gap junction conductance were intracellular Ca^{2+} (Ca_i^{2+}) and intracellular protons (Loewenstein 1981; Spray and Bennett 1985). Iwatsuki and Petersen (1979) have shown that exposure of pancreatic acini to 100% CO_2 provoked an uncoupling presumably due to an intracellular acidification. Could it be that the uncoupling elicited by secretomotor agonists is due to such an acidification? Recent evidence suggests that this is not the case. ACh application causes a slight alkalinization of lacrimal cells (Saito et al. 1988), which could be due to the stimulation of the $Na^+ - H^+$ exchanger by PKC (Vigne et al. 1985), but an alkalinization of this magnitude does not cause closure of the gap junctions (J. Neyton and A. Trautmann, unpublished results). It seemed more likely, therefore, to suppose that the rise in Ca_i^{2+} induced by agonists like ACh, caerulein or bombesin (Iwatsuki and Petersen 1978 a) mediated their uncoupling effect. The Ca^{2+} concentration required to close gap junctions in exocrine glands was unknown, however, and a causal relation linking the Ca^{2+} increase to the gap junction closure has never been demonstrated.

In the past few years, several reports have shown that gap junction channels, like other ionic channels, may be modulated by various kinases. The effects of cyclic AMP on junctional communication include slow increases of coupling over periods of hours or days (see Loewenstein 1985 for a review), fast increases of coupling (De Mello 1984; Saez et al. 1986) or fast decreases of coupling (Teranishi et al. 1983; Piccolino et al. 1984). These effects are mediated in most cases, if not all, by PKA. In the liver, it has been shown that activation of PKA by glucagon results in an enhanced phosphorylation of the gap junction protein (Saez et al. 1986). In different cell lines, junctional permeability may be reduced by the activation of a tyrosine kinase. This phenomenon could play a role in the action of some transforming viruses (Loewenstein 1985). Finally, phorbol esters and diacylglycerol also reduce cell-to-cell communication in several cell lines, presumably by activating protein kinase C (e.g. see Enomoto et al. 1981; Yada et al. 1985).

Intracellular Messengers Involved in the ACh-Induced Uncoupling

The mechanism of gap junction regulation by ACh has been studied in detail in the rat lacrimal gland (Neyton and Trautmann 1986; Randriamampita et al. 1988a; Trautmann et al. 1988; Giaume et al. 1989). We first showed that a rise in Ca_i^{2+} could indeed induce a closure of gap junctions at a concentration between 1 and 10 µmol/l (Neyton and Trautmann 1986). However, Ca_i^{2+} does not seem to be the main molecule mediating the effect of ACh on gap junction for the following reasons: (a) The ACh-induced closure of gap junctions was unaffected by preloading the cells with a concentration of ethylene glycol tetraacetic acid (EGTA) large enough to block all the Ca^{2+}-dependent currents (Neyton and Trautmann 1986; see also Fig. 3). (b) The reduction in gap junction conductance caused by the Ca^{2+} ionophore, A23187, was smaller and more transient than that induced by ACh even though the former stimulus led to larger rises of Ca_i^{2+} than the latter (Trautmann et al. 1988). (c) The correlation between the increase in Ca_i^{2+} and the decrease in gap junction conductance was far from perfect. The peak of Ca_i^{2+} (and the corresponding increase of Ca^{2+}-dependent conductance) always took place well before maximum uncoupling was reached. Indeed, occasionally, ACh-induced uncouplings could be observed without any detectable increases in Ca_i^{2+} as indicated by the absence of Ca^{2+}-dependent currents (Neyton and Trautmann 1986; and see Fig. 3). (d) In the presence of 0.5 mmol/l intracellular HEDTA ((2-hydroxyethyl)-ethylenediamine-N,N,N'-triacetic acid), which chelated all Mg^{2+} ions, but did not prevent the increase in Ca_i^{2+} induced by ACh, there was practically no effect of ACh on gap junction conductance, despite the Ca^{2+} rise (Randriamampita et al. 1988b).

Protein Kinase C

A number of facts converge to support the hypothesis that PKC mediates the effect of ACh on gap junctions. Stimulation of muscarinic receptors in salivary glands (Machado-De Domenech and Söling 1987) and pancreas (Ishizuka et al. 1987) leads to a translocation of PKC (see, however, Hincke 1988). We have shown that activators of PKC such as phorbol dibutyrate or OAG (1-oleoyl-2-acetylglycerol, a permeant analogue of diacylglycerol) elicited a closure of gap junctions (Randriamampita et al. 1988a). The effect of diacylglycerol (after ACh stimulation) was not mediated by products of its metabolism like phosphatidic acid or arachidonic acid (Randriamampita et al. 1988a). When PKC was downregulated or desensitized (Nishizuka 1986) by a prolonged incubation of the cells in OAG, the ability of ACh to uncouple the cells was markedly reduced, as expected if PKC mediates the uncoupling action of ACh (Randriamampita et al. 1988a). The effect of intracellular divalent cations on ACh-induced uncoupling further supports the hypothesis of a direct role of PKC in uncoupling. By comparing the results obtained with high or low concentrations of intracellular EGTA, it appeared that a rise of Ca_i^{2+} facilitated ACh-induced uncoupling in conditions where this uncoupling was only partial (such as after a prolonged pretreatment of the cells with OAG). More striking was the finding that addition of a chelator of Mg^{2+} ions to the intracellular solution inhibited almost completely the ACh-induced uncoupling (Randriamampita et al. 1988a). The reason may be that no phosphorylation can take in the absence of Mg^{2+} ATP.

Arachidonic Acid

We have examined the role of arachidonic acid (AA) on the closure of gap junction in lacrimal glands because it has been shown that AA is produced during stimulation of exocrine glands by various agonists (Dixon and Hokin 1984; I. Llano, A. Marty and M. Whitaker 1988, unpublished experiments). This increase in AA concentration may have resulted from the hydrolysis of diacylglycerol by a diacylglycerol lipase (Berridge 1984) or by the activation of phospholipase A_2 (PLA_2) elicited by the rise in Ca_i^{2+} and/or by the activated PKC (Ho and Klein 1987).

We have shown (Giaume et al. 1989) that AA causes closure of gap junction in lacrimal cells in a dose-dependent way, the half maximal effect being observed with 25 µmol/l AA. This effect was due to the fatty acid itself and not to one its metabolites (eicosanoids) since the AA effect was not prevented by inhibitors of its oxydation, and other fatty acids (even those that are not metabolized) acted similarly to AA. The AA-induced uncoupling was not mediated by a rise in Ca_i^{2+} since AA did not elicit a Ca^{2+} rise in lacrimal cells, as judged by Fura-2 experiments (Giaume et al. 1989). The AA effect was not due to a modulation of the activity of a nucleotide cyclase because the uncoupling efficiency of AA was not modified when cyclic AMP or cyclic GMP was included in the intracellular solution. The activation of a kinase was not involved in AA-induced uncouplings, which took place in the absence of intracellular Mg^{2+} ions (Giaume et al. 1989). Consequently it is conceivable that AA acts directly on the gap junction protein or on its lipid environment. However, when the enzymes that could contribute to the production of AA after muscarinic stimulation were blocked (PLA_2 and diacylglycerol lipase with mepacrine and RHC80267, respectively), the uncoupling efficiency of ACh seemed unaffected (Giaume et al. 1989). Thus, AA does not seem to *mediate* the ACh effect.

In summary (see Fig. 2), the ACh-induced closure of gap junction appears to be mediated primarily by the activation of PKC, at least in rat lacrimal glands. It is, however, likely that the rises in Ca_i^{2+} and in AA concentration that are elicited by ACh contribute to the PKC activation and/or act *in synergy* with PKC to uncouple lacrimal cells. The liver gap junction protein can be phosphorylated in vitro by PKC (Takeda et al. 1987). This suggests, but does not prove, that the physiological effect of this kinase could be exerted directly on the gap junction protein.

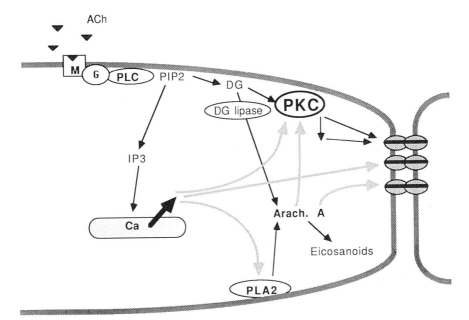

Fig. 2. The main metabolic pathways involved in the modulation of gap junction channels by ACh in lacrimal glands. Some interactions have been omitted for simplicity (e.g., the possible activation of PLA_2 by PKC)

What Is the Function of the Gap Junction Closure Induced by Secretomotor Agonists?

The answer to this question is still controversial. One point of view is that gap junction closure induced by secretomotor agonists is meaningless because it can only be observed at high concentrations of agonists (Maruyama and Petersen 1983) and it does not take place physiologically. The ‚physiological‘ argument is based on the apparent absence of cell uncoupling observed when the nerve endings of pancreatic acinar cells (essentially cholinergic) are stimulated by field stimulation of a piece of the gland (Davison et al. 1980). This argument rests entirely on the changes in gap junction conductance deduced from measurements of the input resistance (R_{in}) of a fragment of gland. R_{in} is, however, a very poor index of the changes in gap junction conductance because it also depends on (and changes with) the resistance of the non-junctional membrane. In an acinar cell, where the non-junctional resistance is almost a hundred times higher than the junctional resistance, a tenfold decrease in gap junction conductance will give a variation of R_{in} of a few percent if the non-junctional conductance is constant. The position will be even worse if channels open in the non-junctional membrane, as normally happens after muscarinic

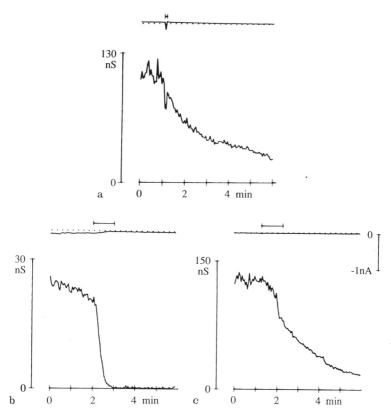

Fig. 3a—c. Uncouplings induced by ACh in pairs of lacrimal cells. The *top traces* give the current measured in one of the cells of each pair at $-50\,\text{mV}$ (*dotted line*, zero current level). **a** Ca_i^{2+} was weakly buffered by 0.5 mmol/l EGTA; a 3-s application of 0.5 µmol/l ACh (*bar*) led to cell uncoupling preceded by a tiny activation of Ca^{2+}-dependent current at $-50\,\text{mV}$. **b** Ca_i^{2+} was strongly buffered (10 mmol/l EGTA) so that no Ca^{2+}-dependent currents (see Marty et al. 1984) were activated by ACh. **c** In the presence of 0.5 mmol/l intracellular EGTA, 50 nmol/l ACh elicited gap junction closure without activating Ca^{2+}-dependent currents. Note the difference in the rate of uncouplings induced by 2 µmol/l and 50 nmol/l ACh

stimulation, and as it appears to do in the recordings of Davison et al. (1980). It is worth mentioning that in these experiments, brief ACh iontophoresis (giving membrane potential changes similar to those elicited by field stimulation) also failed to induce gap junction closure, as judged from R_{in} measurements. On the contrary, in our hands, 0.5 µmol/l ACh applied for a few seconds elicited gap junction closure on almost every occasion (Fig. 3a). Larger ACh concentrations triggered faster uncouplings (Fig. 3b). Longer applications of ACh concentrations as low as 50 nmol/l still caused gap junction closure, even under conditions where no Ca^{2+}-dependent currents were activated (Fig. 3c). These values are very similar to those required for protein and fluid secretion (10–100 nmol/l, see Dartt et al.

1988). Consequently, a closure of gap junctions seems very likely to take place under physiological conditions.

The opposite point of view proposes a causal relation between gap junction closure and protein secretion in exocrine glands (Meda et al. 1986, 1987). First, the observation that dispersed acinar cells do not respond to secretomotor agonists as well as isolated acini (Amsterdam and Jamieson 1974) was used to suggest a role of gap junction in the secretory process (Meda et al. 1986). However, it is quite conceivable that the enzymatic treatment employed to dissociate the acini damaged the cells so that the secretory process was impaired. We suspect that the receptors for the agonist (or some other molecule involved in an early step of cell activation) can be affected by enzymatic treatment since we have observed in dispersed pancreatic cells that trypsin treatment markedly reduces the Ca_i^{2+} rise elicited by ACh or cholecystokinin (Randriamampita et al. 1988 b). Second, it has been argued that long-chain alcohols (like octanol or heptanol), which cause gap junction closure, potentiate amylase secretion induced by low doses of secretomotor agonists in pancreatic acini (Meda et al. 1986), but does this prove that the effects of alcohols on secretion are due to their effect on gap junction coupling? In pancreatic acini, no variation of Ca_i^{2+} was detected in the presence of heptanol (Meda et al. 1986). On the other hand, in lacrimal cells, heptanol provoked a small shift of the current-voltage curve of Ca^{2+}-dependent K^+ channels, presumably due to a small increase in Ca_i^{2+} (C. Randriamampita and A. Trautmann 1988, unpublished results). Consequently, one cannot exclude the possibility that long-chain alcohols affect cellular properties other than gap junction conductance. Obviously, a simultaneous effect of long-chain alcohols on gap junction conductance and protein secretion does not prove that there is a causal relation between the two effects.

In brief, there is no definite proof that gap junctions play a role in secretion. We can only speculate about possible links between gap junction closure and secretion. It is generally thought that in the resting state, gap junctions confer a homogeneity on the different cells of an acinus by allowing the intercellular exchange of small metabolites and by stabilizing membrane potential. It seems logical to conclude that closure of gap junctions could be necessary to confer heterogeneity and metabolic or electrical instability on the different cells of an acinus during secretion. For instance, concentration changes of a substance like Ca^{2+}, which can cross gap junctions in significant amounts (Dunlap et al. 1987), would take place much more rapidly in cells isolated from their neighbours than in the dampened system constituted by an acinus of coupled cells. (This remark does not apply to the initial Ca^{2+} rise, which appears when gap junctions are still open.) It appears in an increasing number of non-excitable cells that the action of hormones or neurotransmitters induces fast changes (often oscillations) in Ca^{2+} concentration (see e.g., Berridge 1987). Oscillations of Ca_i^{2+} in one cell would be transmitted to the neighbours through open gap junctions with a time lag and the resulting phase lag would desynchronize (and eventually suppress) the oscillations in different cells. It can be speculated that if fast rises or regular oscillations of Ca_i^{2+} (or another substance) are necessary for proper secretion in exocrine glands, then gap junction closure is also necessary.

A second rationale for gap junction closure during fluid secretion in exocrine glands can be proposed on slightly different grounds. In endocrine glands, where only protein secretion takes place, no gap junction closure is associated with stimulated secretion, and sometimes an increase in junction coupling is even observed (reviewed in Meda et al. 1984). The gap junction closure in exocrine glands induced by some secretomotor agonists could therefore be relevant for fluid secretion rather than for protein secretion. Intracellular concentrations of Na^+, K^+ and Cl^- are clearly different in resting and in secreting cells (Nakagaki et al. 1984). It is likely that the magnitude of these differences depends on the importance of the ionic fluxes through the acinar cells. If, during secretion, the number of active channels, transporters and pumps is not identical in all the cells, individual cytosolic ionic concentrations will be different. This will create intercellular ionic gradients. If the cells are coupled, part of the fluid entering the cells on the basal side of the most active cells will flow into the neighbouring cells, instead of flowing through the luminal side. Consequently, gap junction closure could play a role during sustained fluid secretion by facilitating transcellular fluid movement. This could explain why gap junction channels close when Ca^{2+}-dependent channels open. On the other hand, tight junctions open when gap junctions close (reviewed in Petersen 1980) because the paracellular fluid movement (allowed by the open tight junctions) takes place at the same time as the transcellular fluid movement (facilitated by the closed gap junctions).

Acknowledgement. We wish to thank A. Marty and J. Neyton for their comments on the manuscript. C.R. was supported by a joined grant from Roussel-Uclaf and the C.N.R.S. (BDI).

References

Amsterdam A, Jamieson JD (1974) Studies on dispersed pancreatic exocrine cells. II. Functional characteristics of separated cells. J Cell Biol 63:1057–1073

Amstrong D, Eckert R (1987) Voltage activated calcium channels that must be phosphorylated to respond to membrane depolarization. Proc Natl Acad Sci USA 84:2518–2522

Berridge MJ (1984) Inositol trisphosphate and diacylglycerol as second messengers. Biochem J 220:345–360

Berridge MJ (1987) Inositol trisphosphate and diacylglycerol: two interacting second messengers. Annu Rev Biochem 56:159–193

Beyer EC, Paul DL, Goodenough DA (1987) Connexin 43: a protein from rat heart homologous to a gap junction protein from liver. J Cell Biol 105:2621–2629

Burt JM, Spray DC (1988) Single channel events and gating behavior of the cardiac gap junction channel Proc Natl Acad Sci USA 85:3431–3434

Chad JE, Eckert R (1986) An enzymatic mechanism for calcium current inactivation in dialyzed *Helix* neurones. J Physiol (Lond) 378:31–51

Chow I, Young SH (1987) Opening of single gap junction channels during formation of electrical coupling between embryonic muscle cells Dev Biol 122:322–337

Cook DI, Day ML, Champion MR, Young JA (1988) Ca^{2+} not cyclic AMP modulates the fluid secretory response to isoproterenol in the rat mandibular salivary gland: whole-cell patch-clamp studies. Pflügers Arch 413:67–76

Dartt D, Shulman M, Gray KL, Rossi SR, Matkin C, Gilbard JP (1988) Stimulation of rabbit lacrimal gland secretion with biologically active peptides. Am J Physiol 254:G300–G306

Davison JS, Pearson GT, Petersen OH (1980) Mouse pancreatic acinar cells: effects of electrical field stimulation on membrane potential and resistance. J Physiol 301:295–305

De Mello W (1984) Effect of intracellular injection of cyclic AMP on the electrical coupling of mammalian cardiac cells. Biochem Biophys Res Commun 119:1001–1007

Dermietzel R, Leibstein A, Frixen U, Jansen-Timmen U, Traub O, Willecke K (1984) Gap junctions in several tissues share determinants with liver gap junctions. EMBO J 3:2261–2270

Dixon JF, Hokin LE (1984) Secretagogue-stimulated phosphatidylinositol breakdown in the exocrine pancreas liberates arachidonic acid, stearic acid, and glycerol by sequential actions of phospholipase C and diglyceride lipase. J Biol Chem 259:14418–14425

Dunlap K, Takeda K, Brehm P (1987) Activation of a calcium dependent phosphoprotein by chemical signalling through gap junctions. Nature 325:60–62

Dupont E, El Aoumari A, Roustiau-Severe S, Briand JP, Gros D (1988) Immunological characterization of rat cardiac gap junctions: presence of common antigenic determinants in hearts of other vertebrate species and various organs. J Membr Biol 104:119–128

Enomoto T, Saski Y, Shiba Y, Kanno Y, Yamasaki H (1981) Tumor promoters cause a rapid and reversible inhibition of the formation and maintenance of electrical cell coupling in culture. Proc Natl Acad Sci USA 78:5628–5632

Findlay I, Petersen OH (1983) The extent of dye coupling between exocrine acinar cells of the mouse pancreas. Cell Tissue Res 232:121–127

Friend DS, Gilula NB (1972) Variation in tight and gap junctions in mammalian tissues. J Cell Biol 53:758–776

Furshpan EJ, Potter DD (1959) Transmission at the giant motor synapses of the crayfish. J Physiol (Lond) 145:289–325

Giaume C, Randriamampita C, Trautmann A (1989) Arachidonic acid closes gap junction channels in rat lacrimal glands. Pflügers Arch 413:273–279

Gorin MB, Yancey SB, Cline J, Revel JP, Horwitz J (1984) The major intrinsic protein (MIP) of the bovine lens fiber membrane characterization and structure based on cDNA cloning. Cell 39:49–59

Green CR, Harfst E, Goudie RG, Severs NJ (1988) Analysis of the rat liver gap junction protein clarification of anomalies in its molecular size. Proc R Soc Lond [Biol] 233:165–174

Hammer MG, Sheridan JD (1978) Electrical coupling and dye transfer between acinar cells in rat salivary glands. J Physiol (Lond) 275:495–505

Hertzberg EL, Skibbens RV (1984) A protein homologous to the 27 kD liver gap junction protein is present in a wide variety of species and tissues. Cell 39:61–69

Hincke MT (1988) Characterization of rat parotid protein kinase C. Int J Biochem 20:303–307

Ho AK, Klein DC (1987) Activation of α_1-adrenoceptors, protein kinase C, or treatment with intracellular free calcium elevating agents increases pineal phospholipase A2 activity. J Biol Chem 262:11764–11770

Ishizuka T, Ito Y, Kajita K, Miura K, Nagao S, Nagata K, Nozawa Y (1987) Redistribution of protein kinase C in pancreatic acinar cells stimulated with caerulein or carbachol. Biochem Biophys Res Commun 144:551–559

Iwatsuki N, Petersen OH (1978a) Electrical coupling and uncoupling of exocrine acinar cells. J Cell Biol 79: 533–545

Iwatsuki N, Petersen OH (1978b) Pancreatic acinar cells: acetylcholine-evoked electrical uncoupling and its ionic dependency. J Physiol (Lond) 274: 81–96

Iwatsuki N, Petersen OH (1979) Pancreatic acinar cells: the effect of carbon dioxide, amonium chloride and acetylcholine on intercellular communication. J Physiol (Lond) 291: 317–326

Jongsma HJ, Rook MB, Van Ginneken ACG (1986) The conductance of single gap junctional channels between cultured rat neonatal heart cells. J Physiol (Lond) 382: 134P

Kater SB, Galvin NJ (1978) Physiological and morphological evidence for coupling in mouse salivary gland cells. J Cell Biol 79: 20–26

Kistler J, Christie D, Bullivant S (1988) Homologies between gap junction proteins in lens heart and liver. Nature 331: 721–723

Kumar NM, Gilula NB (1986) Cloning and characterization of human and rat liver cDNAs coding for a gap junction protein. J Cell Biol 103: 767–776

Loewenstein WR (1975) Permeable junctions. Cold Spring Harbor Symp Quant Biol 40: 49–63

Loewenstein WR (1981) Junctional intercellular communication: the cell-to-cell membrane channel. Physiol Rev 61: 829–913

Loewenstein WR (1985) Regulation of cell-to-cell communication by phosphorylation. Biochem Soc Symp 50: 43–58

Machado-De Domenech E, Söling HD (1987) Effects of stimulation of muscarinic and of β-catecholamine receptors on the intracellular distribution of protein kinase C in guinea pig exocrine glands. Biochem J 242: 749–754

Makowski L (1985) Structural domains in gap junctions: implications for the control of intercellular communication. In: Bennett MVL, Spray DC (eds) Gap junctions. Cold Spring Harbor Lab, New York, pp 5–12

Marty A, Neher E (1983) Tight-seal whole-cell recording. In: Sakmann B, Neher E (eds) Single-channel recording. Plenum. New York, pp 107–122

Marty A, Tan YP, Trautmann A (1984) Three types of calcium-dependent channel in rat lacrimal glands. J Physiol (Lond) 357: 293–325

Maruyama Y, Petersen O (1983) Voltage clamp study of stimulant evoked currents in mouse pancreatic acinar cells. Pflügers Arch 399: 54–62

Meda P, Findlay I, Kolod E, Orci L, Petersen OH (1983) Short and reversible uncoupling evokes little change in the gap junctions of pancreatic acinar cells. J Ultrastruct Res 83: 69–84

Meda P, Perrelet A, Orci L (1984) Gap junctions and cell-to-cell coupling in endocrine glands. In: Satir B (ed) Modern cell biology, vol 3. Liss, New York, pp 131–196

Meda P, Bruzzone R, Knodel S, Orci L (1986) Blockage of cell-to-cell communication within pancreatic acini is associated with increased basal release of amylase. J Cell Biol 103: 475–483

Meda P, Bruzzone R, Chanson M, Bosco D, Orci L (1987) Gap junction coupling modulates secretion of exocrine pancreas. Proc Natl Acad Sci USA 84: 4901–4904

Nakagaki I, Sasaki S, Shiguma M, Imai Y (1984) Distribution of elements in the pancreatic exocrine cells determined by electron probe X-ray microanalysis. Pflügers Arch 401: 340–345

Neyton J, Trautmann A (1985) Single-channel currents of an intercellular junction. Nature 317: 331–335

Neyton J, Trautmann A (1986) Acetylcholine modulation of the conductance of intercellular junctions between rat lacrimal cells. J Physiol (Lond) 377: 283–295

Nicholson B, Dermietzel R, Teplow D, Traub O, Willecke K, Revel JP (1987) Two homologous protein components of hepatic gap junctions. Nature 329: 732–734

Nishizuka Y (1986) Studies and perspectives of protein kinase C. Science 233: 305–312

Paul DL (1986a) Antibody against liver gap junction 27 kD protein is tissue specific and cross-reacts with a 54 kD protein. In: Bennett MVL, Spray DC (eds) Gap junctions. Cold Spring Harbor Lab, New York, pp 107–122

Paul DL (1986b) Molecular cloning of cDNA for rat liver gap junction protein. J Cell Biol 103: 123–134

Peralta EG, Ashkenazi A, Winslow JW, Smith DH, Ramachandran J, Capon DJ (1987) Distinct primary structures, ligand-binding properties and tissue-specific expression of four human muscarinic acetylcholine receptors. EMBO J 6: 3923–3929

Petersen OH (1980) The electrophysiology of gland cells. Academic, London

Piccolino M, Neyton J, Gerschenfeld HM (1984) Decrease of gap junction permeability induced by dopamine and cyclic adenosine $3':5'$-monophosphate in horizontal cells of turtle retina. J Neurosci 4: 2477–2488

Randriamampita C, Giaume C, Neyton J, Trautmann A (1988a) Acetylcholine-induced closure of gap junction channels in rat lacrimal glands is probably mediated by protein kinase C. Pflügers Arch 412: 462–468

Randriamampita C, Chanson M, Trautmann A (1988b) Calcium and secretagogues-induced conductances in rat exocrine pancreas. Pflügers Arch 411: 53–57

Rose B (1971) Intercellular communication and some structural aspect of cell junction in a single cell system. J Membr Biol 5: 1–19

Saez JC, Spray DC, Nairn AC, Hertzberg E, Greengard P, Bennett MVL (1986) Cyclic AMP increases junctional conductance and stimulates phosphorylation of the 27-kDa principal gap junction polypeptide. Proc Natl Acad Sci USA 83: 2473–2477

Saito Y, Ozawa T, Suzuki SR, Nishiyama A (1988) Intracellular pH regulation in the mouse lacrimal gland acinar cells. J Membr Biol 101: 73–81

Schulz I, Schnefel S, Banfic H, Thevenod F, Kemmer T, Eckhardt L (1987) The role of phosphatidylinositides in stimulus-secretion coupling in the exocrine pancreas. In: Mandel LJ, Eaton DC (eds) Cell calcium and the control of membrane transport. Rockefeller University Press, New York, pp 117–131

Simpson I, Rose B, Loewenstein WR (1977) Size limit of permeating the junctional membrane channels. Science 195: 294–296

Somogyi R, Kolb HA (1988) Cell to cell channel conductance during loss of gap junctional coupling in pairs of pancreatic acinar and Chinese hamster ovary cells. Pflügers Arch 412: 54–65

Spray DC, Bennett MVL (1985) Physiology and pharmacology of gap junctions. Annu Rev Physiol 47: 281–303

Spray DC, Harris AL, Bennett MVL (1981) Equilibrium properties of the voltage dependent junctional conductance. J Gen Physiol 77: 75–94

Takeda A, Hashimoto E, Yamamura H, Shimazu T (1987) Phosphorylation of liver gap junction protein by protein kinase C. FEBS Lett 210: 169–172

Teranishi T, Negishi K, Kato S (1983) Dopamine modulates S-potential amplitude and dye-coupling between external horizontal cells in carp retina. Nature 301: 243–246

Trautmann A, Neyton J, Randriamampita C, Giaume C (1988) Role of divalent cations in the control of gap junction conductance in a rat exocrine gland. In: Hertzberg EL, Johnson R (eds) Modern cell biology, vol 7. Gap junctions. Liss, New York, pp 365–374

Veenstra RD, De Haan RL (1986) Measurement of single channel currents from cardiac gap junctions. Science 233: 972–974

Veenstra RD, De Haan RL (1988) Cardiac gap junction channel activity in embryonic chick ventricular cells. Am J Physiol 254: H170–H180

Vigne P, Frelin C, Ladzunski M (1985) The Na/H antiport is activated by serum and phorbol esters in proliferating myoblast but not in differentiated myotubes. J Biol Chem 260: 8008–8013

Williams JA (1987) Regulatory mechanisms in pancreas and salivary acini. Annu Rev Physiol 46: 361–375

Yada T, Rose B, Loewenstein WR (1985) Diacylglycerol down regulates junctional membrane permeability. TMB-8 blocks this effect. J Membr Biol 88: 217–232

Zampighi GA, Simon SA (1985) The structure of gap junctions as revealed by electron microscopy. In: Bennett MVL, Spray DC (eds) Gap junctions. Cold Spring Harbor Lab, pp 13–22

Ion Channels in the Intracellular Organelles of Secretory Cells

H. Gögelein, A. Schmid, T. Kemmer, and I. Schulz

Introduction

It is well-established that the transfer of ions across plasma membranes is mediated by transport proteins embedded in the lipid bilayer. One type of ionic transport mechanism, namely, passage through ion channels, has been studied extensively with the patch-clamp technique (Neher and Sakmann 1976; Hamill et al. 1981). With this method, a variety of channel types has been observed in plasma membranes. Lipid bilayer membranes exist, however, not only to form the plasma membranes of cells, but also to form intracellular organelles, such as mitochondria and sarcoplasmic or endoplasmic reticulum, as well as intracellular vesicles, such as endosomes and zymogen granules. These lipid membranes, separating the intraorganelle compartment from the cytosol, are also capable of mediating transport of various substances and exhibit finite conductances for specific ions. For example, it has been observed in preparations of isolated rough endoplasmic reticulum (RER) from the rat exocrine pancreas that the active reuptake of Ca^{2+} ions is associated with an anion conductance (Bayerdörffer et al. 1984; Kemmer et al. 1987) and it can be assumed that this permeability to anions serves to maintain electrical charge compensation during the uptake of the divalent cations. It is likely that ion channels are responsible for conductances in organelle membranes. Indeed, reconstitution experiments with planar lipid bilayer membranes reveal that K^+ and Cl^- selective ion channels are present in membranes of the sarcoplasmic reticulum (Miller 1978; Tanifuij et al. 1987). Our own attempts to reconstitute ion channels from the RER of the exocrine pancreas into planar lipid bilayer membranes, however, have so far failed to reveal ion channels.

It was a great advance when recently a new method was developed to apply the patch-clamp technique to membranes of intracellular organelles. Criado and Keller (1987) reported that giant liposomes with diameters up to 100 µm formed spontaneously when vesicle preparations were first dehydrated in the presence of artifical lipid vesicles and then subsequently rehydrated. This observation is based on experiments performed by Mueller et al. (1983), demonstrating that giant liposomes are formed when dried phospholipids are rehydrated at low ionic strength. Criado and Keller (1987) applied the method of dehydration/rehydration to vesicles of the sarcoplas-

Young · Wong, Epithelial Secretion of Water and Electrolytes
© Springer-Verlag Berlin · Heidelberg 1990

mic reticulum and of purified postsynaptic membranes from the *Torpedo* electric organ. In addition, the authors demonstrated that the patch-clamp technique can be applied to these large liposomes, and Keller et al. (1988a) showed that K^+ channels are present in giant liposomes derived from reconstituted lipid vesicles of the sarcoplasmic reticulum of rabbit skeletal muscle. The characteristics of this channel were similar to those observed by other methods. This means that the procedure of dehydration and rehydration did not impair channel proteins in this preparation.

Our aim was to apply this novel technique to intracellular organelles of the rat exocrine pancreas. We have demonstrated that giant structures can be obtained from native vesicles of the RER and of zymogen granules and by applying the patch-clamp technique we observed Cl^- channels in the RER preparation, although no channel activity has been observed thus far in zymogen granules.

Preparation of Giant Liposomes

RER vesicles were prepared from isolated rat pancreatic acinar cells by differential centrifugation as described by Imamura and Schulz (1985). Briefly, cells were homogenized in a mannitol buffer and centrifuged twice at $400 \times g$ to separate cell fragments and nuclei. Further centrifugation at 11000 $\times g$ yielded a heavy pellet which was discarded, a loosely attached fluffy layer, and the supernatant. This last was centrifuged at $27000 \times g$. The resulting pellet as well as the fluffy layer from the former centrifugation step were resuspended in mannitol buffer. Both vesicle preparations were stored in liquid nitrogen in small aliquots.

The procedure for formation of large liposomes is outlined in Fig. 1. About 10 µl of native vesicle suspension is dried at 4°C by vacuum

lo µl vesicle suspension

(lo-2o mg protein/ml)

were evaporated in an exsiccator

(4°C; lo-2o min)

to the dried vesicles

~ 2oo µl KCl-solution were added

spontaneous formation of

large liposomes occured

within 1-4 h (4°C)

Fig. 1. Schematic diagram showing formation of giant liposomes from native ER vesicles

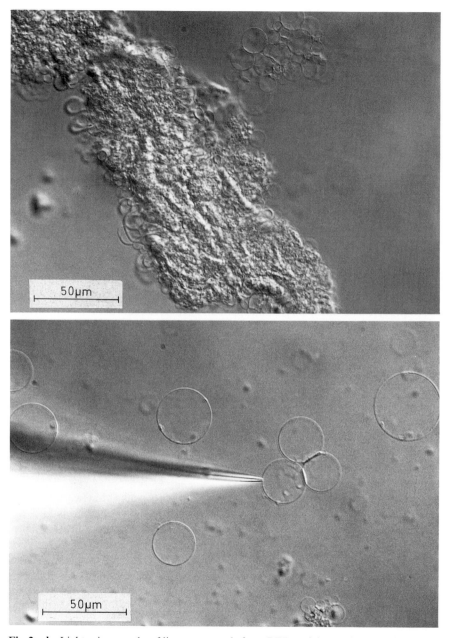

Fig. 2a, b. Light micrographs of liposomes made from RER vesicles. **a** Liposome formation during rehydration of the dried vesicles. **b** A patch pipette in contact with a giant liposome

evaporation. After addition of 200–500 µl KCl buffer (in mmol/l: 140 KCl, 1 $MgCl_2$, 0.01 $CaCl_2$, 10 hydroxyethylpiperazine ethanesulfonic acid (HEPES) adjusted to pH 7.4 with KOH) the formation of liposomes was observed. Figure 2a reveals that groups of small liposomes appear first at the border of the dried lipid. These liposomes enlarge by further fusion and detach from the bulk lipid. As demonstrated in Fig. 2b, the giant liposomes have spherical shape, do not contain any material in their interior, and seem to be unilamellar. They settle down on the coverslip of the measuring chamber and can be approached by a patch pipette (Fig. 2b).

Recording of Cl⁻ Channels

Seals in the range of 1–10 GΩ were obtained after applying very slight suction via the patch pipette. The success rate for formation of stable seals was about 10%. Single ion channels were observed in the attached mode, but were studied in detail only after removing the pipette from the liposome, resulting in an excised inside-out patch configuration. With KCl solution in both pipette and bath, single channel currents were recorded, as demonstrated in Fig. 3. It is characteristic that several channels with similar amplitude and kinetic properties are present in a single membrane patch. As shown in Fig. 3b, the current–voltage curve of one current level can be fitted by linear regression, yielding a single channel conductance of 260 ± 7 pS ($n = 23$). The single channel current recordings in Fig. 3a reveal a voltage dependence of the channels. At low potentials (± 20 mV) the channels are predominantly in their open state but they close more frequently both at higher postitive and negative voltages. Potentials beyond ± 70 mV cause an almost permanent channel closure. This voltage dependence is evident in the current–amplitude histograms (Fig. 4a–d) obtained from the respective channels shown in Fig. 3.

The distribution of the current amplitudes yielded peaks that were fitted by Gaussian curves. The probability that a current level is occupied is given by the relative areas under these peaks. The respective numbers are presented on the plots. Figure 4 shows that the current levels are equally displaced and that lower current levels are favored at higher potentials. With the assumption that the number of channels N in one patch is equal to the highest occuring current level, and that each channel fluctuates with the same mean open probability, the open-state probability of a single channel, P_0, is given by:

$$P_0 = 1/N \sum_{r=1}^{N} r \cdot P(r)$$

where $P(r)$ is the probability that level r is occupied. In Fig. 4e the means of the open-state probabilities from six experiments are plotted as a function of

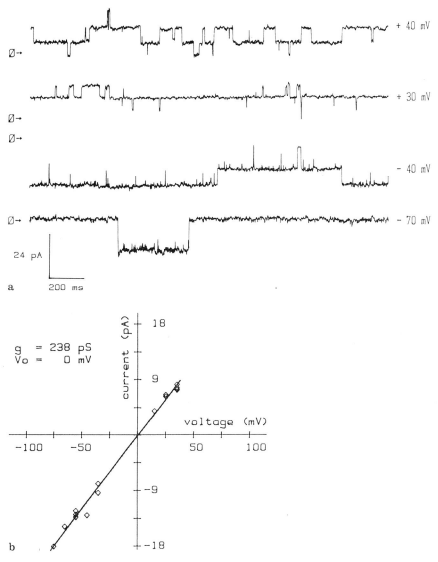

Fig. 3a. Single anion-channel currents of an excised membrane patch of liposomes made from RER vesicles. Pipette and bath contained KCl solution. $0 \rightarrow$ denotes the baseline (all channels closed). The clamp potential is given on the *right* side of each trace. **b** Corresponding current–voltage curve. The data were fitted by linear regression

the clamp potential. The data yield a bell-shaped curve with its maximum shifted slightly to the left. This indicates that the amplitude of the single channel current is dependent on the direction of the current flow. As this was consistently observed, it shows that the channel molecule was oriented in the same manner in the membrane patch.

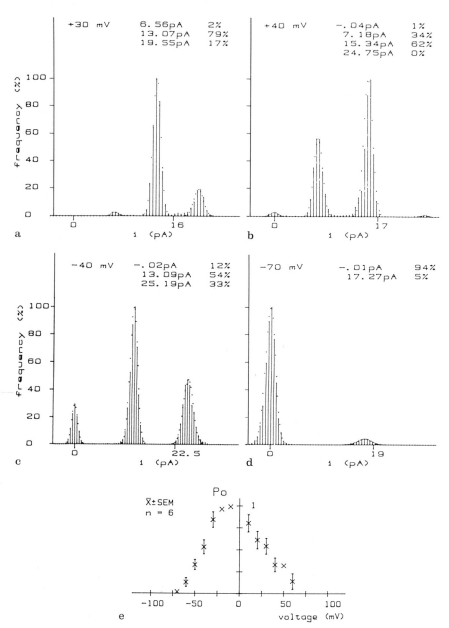

Fig. 4a – e. Current–amplitude histograms (**a – d**) of the single-channel currents shown in Fig. 3, demonstrating the inactivation of channels at higher clamp potentials. The individual *peaks* were fitted with Gaussian curves. The areas under each curve (as a percentage), as well as the absolute value of the corresponding single-channel current, are given on the plots. **e** Means of the open-state probability P_0 from six experiments are plotted as a function of the clamp potential

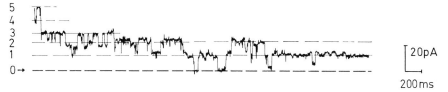

Fig. 5. Inactivation of single-anion channels after a voltage step from $0\,mV$ to $+40\,mV$. The trace demonstrates the successive decrease in the number of occupied current levels. Pipette and bath contained a KCl solution

The voltage dependence of the channels is demonstrated in more detail in Fig. 5, where a voltage jump from 0 to $40\,mV$ has been applied. Immediately after the voltage jump, about five channels are open which inactivate successively. After about 3 s a new steady state is reached, where only one current level is occupied. Another characteristic of this channel is the appearance of sublevels (Fig. 6). These levels occurred only in the presence of the channel main-state activity, and this main state was not composed of multiples of the sublevels. Moreover, direct transitions from the main state to the sublevels were observed. These features demonstrate that the sublevels are not due to different channels, but are substates of one type of channel (Fox 1987). The most frequently observed substate had about 65% of the full amplitude, but sublevels with different amplitudes also occurred irregularly.

The ion selectivity of the channels was evaluated by substitution experiments. Replacing all K^+ with Na^+ on either side of the membrane patch had no influence on the single-channel conductance or on the reversal potential. Substitution of all Cl^- by gluconate, however, caused channel opening in the upward direction at $0\,mV$ clamp potential, indicating that Cl^- ions were moving down their chemical gradient from the pipette into the bath (Fig. 7). The permeability ratio between Cl^- and K^+ ions was assayed by experiments in which a gradient of 140 mmol/l KCl in the pipette versus 30 mmol/lKCl in the bath was established. In four experiments of this kind, a shift of the reversal potential to $-19 \pm 1.6\,mV$ was observed, yielding

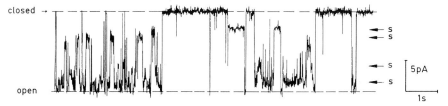

Fig. 6. Single-channel current recording of anion channels, demonstrating the existence of various sublevels (indicated by $s\rightarrow$). Pipette and bath contained a KCl solution. The clamp potential was $-40\,mV$

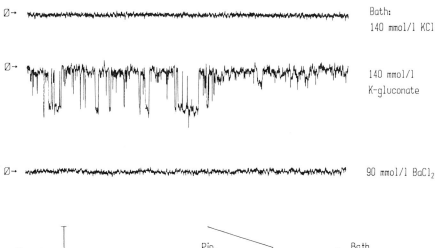

Fig. 7. Single-channel current recordings, demonstrating the selectivity of the channels to anions (*middle*) and the impermeability to Ba^{2+} ions (*bottom*). The pipette contained a KCl solution. The clamp potential was 0 mV *Top:* Control conditions (140 mmol/l KCl both sides, clamp potential 0 mV). The diagram on the lower right side demonstrates the conditions for the middle trace.

a permeability ratio P_{Cl^-}/P_{K^+} of 3.8 ± 0.5. In conclusion, the described channels are mainly permeable to Cl^- ions, but can also conduct K^+ ions.

Experiments with blocker substances showed that the channel could not be blocked by typical Cl^- channel blockers, such as diphenylamine-2-carboxylate (DPC, 1 mmol/l), and 5-nitro-2-(3-phenylpropylamino)-benzoic acid (NPPB, 0.1 mmol/l; Wangemann et al. 1986; Greger et al. 1987), or 4-acetamido-4'-isothiocyanatostilbene-2,2'-disulfonic acid (SITS, 1 mmol/l). In addition, neither the K^+ channel blockers, tetraethylammonium (TEA$^+$, 10 mmol/l) or Ba^{2+} (70 mmol/l), had any effect. The anion channel was not Ca^{2+} sensitive: changing the free Ca^{2+} concentration on either side from 1 mmol/l to less than 10^{-9} mol/l did not affect the channel activity.

The last trace of Fig. 7 demonstrates that replacement of the bath by a 90 mmol/l solution of $BaCl_2$ did not cause current flow. Such experiments where also performed in the presence of inositol-1,4,5-trisphosphate (IP_3). Previously it has been shown that IP_3 induces the release of Ca^{2+} ions from intracellular stores of permeabilized cells of the rat exocrine pancreas (Streb et al. 1983) as well as from isolated vesicles of the RER (Streb et al. 1984). Consequently, Ca^{2+}-selective channels are supposed to exist in the membrane of the RER. So far, however, we have not observed ion channels for Ca^{2+} or Ba^{2+} in our experiments. The lack of Ca^{2+} channels could be due to several reasons: (1) Channels are present in situ, but become inactive during the dehydration/rehydration procedure; (2) the IP_3-induced Ca^{2+} release is due to an electrically silent step, or (3) there exist ion channels for Ca^{2+}, the conductance of which is too small to be detected by the patch-clamp method. At present we favor the last possibility.

As described elsewhere (Schmid et al. 1988), in addition to this large-conductance anion channel, in about 1% of all the experiments in which gigaseals were achieved, we observed a voltage-independent Cl^- channel with a single-channel conductance of about 80 pS. The channels appeared in bursts and had fast closing events (flickering). Thus far, we have not detected K^+-selective channels although a K^+ conductance that is inhibited by tetraethylammonium ions has been observed in an RER preparation from rat liver (Muallem et al. 1985). On the other hand, Keller et al. (1988b) described a cation channel that is selective for K^+ and Na^+ ions in giant liposomes from rat hepatocytes. These authors also observed anion channels with a single-channel conductance of 64 pS in a 50 mmol/l NaCl solution in the RER of liver cells. This corresponds to a conductance of about 190 pS in 150 mmol/l solution, being somewhat less than the single-channel conductance of the large anion channel described in the present paper. On the other hand, the anion channels in the RER of liver cells show a similar voltage dependence to those described here (B. U. Keller, personal communication).

In conclusion, the new method of forming giant liposomes by dehydration and rehydration of vesicle preparations has been applied to vesicles from the RER of hepatocytes (Keller et al. 1988b) and of rat pancreatic cells. In both preparations, voltage-dependent anion channels with a high conductance have been observed. It is assumed that these channels are responsible for the maintenance of charge neutrality during Ca^{2+} release or Ca^{2+} uptake. In order to fulfill this task, there would be no need for regulation of the opening or closing of the anion channels: they could be permanently activated to allow free passage of Cl^- ions through the RER membrane. On the other hand, these anion channels are strongly voltage dependent. Since the electrical potential difference across the membrane of the RER in situ is unknown, the significance of the channel's voltage dependence remains unresolved. More experiments are needed before anything can be said about the presence of cation conductances in RER membranes. In our experiments with RER membranes from the exocrine pancreas no cation-selective channels were observed. On the other hand, the anion channels were not perfectly impermeable to cations. In vesicle preparations of the RER of the rat parotid gland, Thévenod and Schulz (1988) revealed active H^+ uptake that depended on the presence of different cations. In addition, dissipation of the H^+ gradient by the protonophore, CCCP, was slower in the presence of choline$^+$ as compared to K^+. These experiments indicate the existence of a K^+ conductance in the membranes of these organelles. It has yet to be established whether this conductance can be explained by the permeability of the channels to cations described here.

References

Bayerdörffer E, Streb H, Eckhardt L, Haase W, Schulz I (1984) Characterization of calcium uptake into rough endoplasmic reticulum of rat pancreas. J Membr Biol 81: 69–82

Criado M, Keller BU (1987) A membrane fusion strategy for single-channel recordings of membranes usually non-accessible to patch-clamp pipette electrodes. FEBS Lett 224: 172–176

Fox JA (1987) Ion channel subconductance states. J Membr Biol 97:1–8

Greger R, Schlatter E, Gögelein H (1987) Chloride channels in the luminal membrane of the rectal gland of the dogfish (*Squalus acanthias*). Properties of the "larger" conductance channel. Pflügers Arch 409: 114–121

Hamill OP, Marty A, Neher E, Sakmann B, Sigworth FJ (1981) Improved patch-clamp technique for high-resolution current recording from cells and cell-free membrane patches. Pflügers Arch 391: 85–100

Imamura K, Schulz I (1985) Phosphorylated intermediate of $(Ca^{2+}+K^+)$-stimulated Mg^{2+}-dependent transport ATPase in endoplasmic reticulum from rat pancreatic acinar cells. J Biol Chem 260: 11339–11347

Keller BU, Hedrich R, Vaz WLC, Criado M (1988a) Single channel recordings of reconstituted ion channel proteins: an improved technique. Pflügers Arch 411: 94–100

Keller BU, Kleineke J, Criado M, Söling HD (1988b) Single channel recordings from endoplasmic reticulum membranes of rat liver: a patch clamp study on giant vesicles. Pflügers Arch 411: R105

Kemmer TP, Bayerdörffer E, Will H, Schulz I (1987) Anion dependence of Ca^{2+} transport and $(Ca^{2+}+K^+)$-stimulated Mg^{2+}-dependent transport ATPase in rat pancreatic endoplasmic reticulum. J Biol Chem 262: 13758–13764

Miller C (1978) Voltage-gated cation conductance channel from fragmented sarcoplasmic reticulum: steady-state electrical properties. J Membr Biol 40: 1–23

Muallem S, Schoeffield M, Pandol S, Sachs G (1985) Inositol trisphosphate modification of ion transport in rough endoplasmic reticulum. Proc Natl Acad Sci USA 82: 4433–4437

Mueller P, Chien TF, Rudy B (1983) Formation and properties of cell-size lipid bilayer vesicles. Biopyhs J 44: 375–381

Neher E, Sakmann B (1976) Single-channel currents recorded from membrane of denervated frog muscle fibres. Nature 260: 799–802

Schmid A, Gögelein H, Kemmer TP, Schulz I (1988) Anion channels in giant liposomes made of endoplasmic reticulum vesicles from rat exocrine pancreas. J Membr Biol 104: 275–282

Streb H, Irvine RF, Berridge MJ, Schulz I (1983) Release of Ca^{2+} from a nonmitochondrial intracellular store in pancreatic acinar cells by inositol-1,4,5-trisphosphate. Nature 306: 67–69

Streb H, Bayerdörffer E, Haase W, Irvine RF, Schulz I (1984) Effect of inositol-1,4,5-trisphosphate on isolated subcellular fractions of rat pancreas. J Membr Biol 81: 241–253

Tanifuij M, Sokabe M, Kasai M (1987) An anion channel of sarcoplasmic reticulum incorporated into planar bilayers: single-channel behavior and conductance properties. J Membr Biol 99: 103–111

Thevenod F, Schulz I (1988) H^+-dependent calcium uptake into an IP_3 sensitive calcium pool from rat parotid gland. Am J Physiol 255: 6429–6440

Wangemann P, Wittner M, Di Stefano A, Englert HC, Lang HJ, Schlatter E, Greger R (1986) Cl^- channel blockers in the thick ascending limb of the loop of Henle. Structure activity relationship. Pflügers Arch 407: S128–S141

Changes in Membrane Capacitance in Exocrine Secretion*

Y. Maruyama

Introduction

Exocytosis is the process by which vesicular membranes are incorporated into the plasma membrane (Palade 1975). By this means macromolecules forming part of the vesicular contents as well as physiologically functional proteins in the vesicular membranes are transported to the outside of the cell or inserted into the plasma membrane. In pancreatic exocrine cells, the secretory process is triggered and controlled by neurotransmitters and hormones that activate receptors, generating cellular messengers (Gardner and Jensen 1987); of these, the mechanism for an increase in intracellular Ca^{2+} concentration is of particular importance (Hootman and Williams 1987).

Since exocytosis is accompanied by an increase in the area of the cell surface membrane, its occurrence can be monitored by following changes in plasma membrane capacitance, a parameter that, when measured, can be rescaled to give surface area by use of the specific membrane capacitance, 1 $\mu F/cm^2$. The patch-clamp method makes it possible to address some of the underlying mechanisms for exocytosis by providing a means for monitoring changes in membrane capacitance with a high time resolution in a single secretory cell, the cytosolic composition of which can be precisely controlled (Neher and Marty 1982).

This chapter summarizes (a) the method used for monitoring changes in membrane capacitance with its associated problems, (b) the calcium dependence of exocytosis studied with this method, and (c) the receptor control of internal Ca^{2+} concentration in rat exocrine pancreatic acinar cells.

---

* The study was supported by a grant-in-aid for scientific research from the Ministry of Education, Science and Culture of Japan.

The Phase-Sensitive Detection Method in Exocrine Secretion

Monitoring the change in membrane capacitance with a high time resolution can reveal the process of exocytosis in single secretory cells. The whole-cell patch-clamp recording technique combined with a phase-sensitive detection method has been used for this purpose and aplied to chromaffin cells (Neher and Marty 1982; Clapham and Neher 1984), mast cells (Fernandez et al. 1984; Breckenridge and Almers 1987) and pancreatic acinar cells (Maruyama 1986, 1988).

Principle

Based on the equivalent circuit model of the whole-cell assembly (Fig. 1a), small changes in membrane capacitance (dC) and conductance (dG) can be monitored independently by following changes in the complex admittance (dY) using a two-phase lock-in amplifier (Fig. 1b) (Neher and Marty 1982). In the model system, dY can be linearly approximated as:

$$dY = (\partial Y/\partial G)\, dG + (\partial Y/\partial C)\, dC + (\partial Y/\partial Gs)\, dGs$$

where $Y = B(G + j\omega C)$, $\partial Y/\partial G = B^2$, $\partial Y/\partial C = B^2 j$,
$\quad B = 1/(1 + G/Gs + j\omega C/Gs)$, $j = \sqrt{-1}$.

Here, we introduce some assumptions to simplify the problem.

1. Assuming that the access conductance (Gs) of the whole-cell assembly does not change during the experiment, then $\partial Y/\partial Gs$ can be zeroed. Thus,

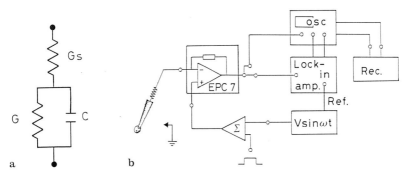

Fig. 1a. The equivalent electrical circuit model of the whole-cell recording assembly and **b** the experimental setup for the measurement of changes in membrane capacitance and conductance. *G*, input conductance; *Gs*, access conductance; *C*, input capacitance; *EPC-7*, a patch-clamp amplifier (EPC-7, List, Darmstadt FRG), *Lock-in amp.*, a two phase lock-in amplifier (Li-574, NF-Electronic Instruments; Yokohama, Japan); *OSC*, oscilloscope; *Rec.*, recticorder; *V* sin ωt, sinusoidal voltage from an oscillator

dY can be modified to:

$$dY = B^2 (dG + j\omega dC).$$

2. Assuming that input capacitance of the cell (C) can be minimized with the C compensation network (C trimmer and Gs trimmer) of patch-clamp amplifiers such as the EPC-5, the EPC-7 (List, Darmstadt, FRG), and the CEZ-2100 (Nihon Koden, Tokyo, Japan), then:

$$B = 1/(1 + G/Gs).$$

3. Assuming that Gs is far larger than input conductance (G, i.e. 100 times larger), then B is approximately equal to 1. Then dY becomes:

$$dY = dY + j\omega dC.$$

In this equation, dG and dC are orthogonal, for they are the real part (0-phase output of the lock-in amplifier) and the imaginary part ($\pi/2$-phase output), respectively, of the complex admittance. In the experiment, the lock-in amplifier locks onto the phase angle of the membrane current at the in phase (0 phase) and at the $\pi/2$-lagged phase of the input to the applied sinusoidal command voltage, so that it produces two mutually independent outputs, representing dG and dC.

Procedure

Experiments begin in the whole-cell recording mode (the patch pipette should be heavily coated with Sylgard, and rippling changes in the solution surface should be minimized to prevent changes in stray capacitance). The capacitance transient should be neutralized by adjusting the C and Gs trimmers of the patch-clamp amplifier by using square command pulses (C neutralization). The command voltage is then switched to the sinusoidal mode, and two outputs (0-phase and $\pi/2$-phase signal) are monitored (Maruyama 1988).

Error Factors Affecting Measurement

The phase-sensitive detection technique has inherent errors since the parameters being set to monitor the system (see assumptions 1–3 above) are fixed, whilst the membrane signal is constantly changing (Joshi and Fernandez 1988).

C neutralization with the patch-clamp amplifier is not perfect in the practical condition, and a small uncompensated C surge remains. Moreover, C as well as G will change steadily during the time course of stimulation.

Strictly speaking, B is no longer assumed as unity in the actual experiments:

$$dY = B^2 (dG + j\omega dC).$$

However, we can minimize the effect of B^2 by searching the optimal phase angle. B^2 is a complex variable. Therefore, it can be rewritten as:

$$B^2 = X (\cos\alpha + j\sin\alpha) \qquad \alpha: \text{phase angle}$$

If α can be nullified ($\alpha-0$), B^2 becomes a real value, a simple real coefficient. The phase angle α is found experimentally with the phase-offset dial of the lock-in amplifier by making small changes in C (C trimmer) and adjusting the phase angle until the 0-phase output produces no deflections, but the $\pi/2$-phase output produces large deflections (Fig. 2, open circles). Thus, the C neutralization and correct phase setting minimize the error due to the C change. In order to maintain the correct phase angle during the experiment, it is necessary to repeat the C neutralization and the correct phase setting frequently (Maruyama 1989).

The 0-phase output artificially produced with the C trimmer (known capacitance) is regarded as a calibrator for dC. A calibrator for dG is obtained simply by multiplying the C calibration by $2\pi f$ (when f is the frequency of the command sinusoidal voltage).

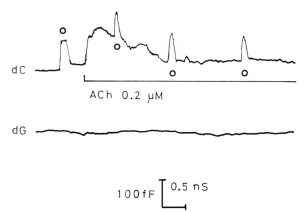

Fig. 2. Ca^{2+}-dependent increase in membrane capacitance (dC) induced by acetylcholine in a single acinar cell of the rat exocrine pancreas. The major electrolytes were replaced by those unable to pass through ion channels. External solution (in mmol/l): N-methyl-D-glucamine methansulfonate, 145; $CaCl_2$, 2.5; $MgCl_2$, 1.13; HEPES, 5.0; pH 7.2. Internal solution (in mmol/l): N-methyl-D-glucamine glutamate, 145; $MgCl_2$, 1.13; EGTA, 0.06; ATP, 1.0; HEPES, 5.0; pH 7.2. *Open circles* show the calibration signals (100 fF) produced by the C trimmer of the patch-clamp amplifier. Individual C changes do not cause detectable change in conductance (dG), indicating that the correct phase setting had been achieved. Cell input capacitance was 8.5 fF, and series resistance 6 $M\Omega$. The time constant of the lock-in amplifier was 300 ms

A change in Gs causes serious errors in the measurement (Joshi and Fernandez 1988). Gs gradually decreases in the usual experiments, leading to drifts in the two output traces of the lock-in amplifier. To minimize the error due to Gs change, it is necessary to use low resistance patch pipettes and to repeat the C neutralization with the C and Gs trimmer frequently throughout the experiment. In practice, it is advisable to select recorded traces not showing marked drifts or trends in order to estimate the system behaviour.

On the whole, the change in C und G can be measured precisely in a limited range and tends to deviate from the real value as it increases. The appropriate error estimation may help us to set the range of estimation, from which we can derive some conclusions in a biological system, both quantitatively and qualitatively.

The Calcium Dependence of Increase in Membrane Capacitance in Exocrine Pancreatic Secretion

Capacitance Flickers

The whole-cell patch-clamp configuration makes it possible to control the composition of the intracellular compartment (Marty and Neher 1983). The influence of $[Ca^{2+}]_i$ on exocytosis has been directly studied by applying the phase-sensitive detection method to the single pancreatic acinar cell subjected to the whole-cell recording (Maruyama 1986). From the study, it was revealed that excess capacitance fluctuations were induced when $[Ca^{2+}]_i$ was adjusted at μM concentrations by an ethylene glycol tetra-acetic acid (EGTA) and Ca^{2+} mixture (an example, Fig. 3). Fluctuations were occasionally seen as steplike alternating increases and decreases and capacitance flickers, and the mean size of both increasing and decreasing steps was 9 and 10 fF, respectively. These values correspond to a vesicle of spherical diameter $0.55\,\mu m$ (rescaled with specific membrane capacitance, $1\,\mu F/cm^2$), which does not deviate from the size of zymogen granules estimated from many electron micrographs in pancreatic acinar cells. The steplike increase in capacitance can be interpreted as due to individual granule fusion with the luminal cell membrane and subsequent fission, and the decrease occurring in similar size as the resealing of the fission (or the closure of the fusion pore; Fig. 3, inset). The capacitance flickers are also observed in chromaffin cells (Neher and Marty 1982) and mast cells (Fernandez et al. 1984; Breckenridge and Almers 1987), suggesting that an alternating fission and resealing process is one of the general features of the exocytotic process. Whether the capacitance flickers are always accompanied by the discharge of macromolecules to some extent remains unanswered, however.

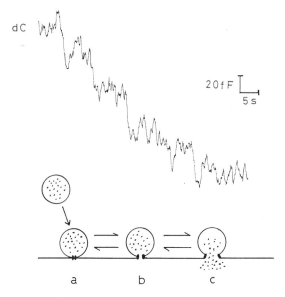

Fig. 3. Excess capacitance fluctuation induced by micromolar concentrations of $[Ca^{2+}]_i$. *Inset* represents a schematic explanation of the steplike changes in membrane capacitance (capacitance flickers). External solution: the normal NaCl solution (N-Methyl-D-glucamine methansulfonate in the solution, described in Fig. 2 legend, was replaced by 145 mmol/l NaCl). Internal solution (in mmol/l): K glutamate, 145; $MgCl_2$, 1.13; ATP, 1.0; $CaCl_2$, 1.0; EGTA, 1.2; HEPES, 5.0; pH 7.2. In the *inset*, *a* represents granular fusion with the plasma membrane, *b* fusion pore formation and *c* the fission (physical dilatation of the fusion pore). These three states probably alternate in the process of exocytosis, leading to the capacitance flickers

The increase of the internal Ca^{2+} facilitates granular fusion and fission since a huge increase in C was induced by externally applied A23187 (Ca^{2+} ionophore) and this can be abolished when the cytosol is dialysed with a high concentration of EGTA (Maruyama 1988, 1989). Furthermore, muscarinic ACh (acetylcholine)- or CCK (cholecystokinin)-receptor stimulation can induce increases in C (of up to 100 fF; an example, Fig. 2), which are synchronous with the activation of Ca^{2+}-dependent ion channels, and a high concentration of EGTA in the cells makes the agonist ineffective. Thus, the membrane capacitance of the acinar cell increases and decreases synchronously with increases and decreases of $[Ca^{2+}]_i$. The peak amplitude of the changes in membrane capacitance in single pancreatic acinar cells induced by physiological doses of ACh or CCK has been estimated as 200 fF, suggesting that about 20 zymogen granules can be transiently incorporated into the luminal cell membrane in response to these agonists.

Ca^{2+}-Mobilizing Receptor Signalling and Guanine-Nucleotide Binding Protein

The change in membrane capacitance (exocytosis) is controlled by $[Ca^{2+}]_i$ in single pancreatic acinar cells. The concept of Ca^{2+}-mobilizing receptor signalling (production of inositol 1,4,5-trisphosphate and diacylglycerol) has been well reviewed elsewhere (Berridge and Irvine 1984; Streb et al. 1984; Downes and Michell 1985). This section summarizes only the electrophysiological evidence for the involvement of guanine-nucleotide binding proteins (G proteins) in the signalling pathway of receptor stimulation with ACh and CCK (Merrit et al. 1986; Maruyama 1988). The increase or decrease of $[Ca^{2+}]_i$ in the acinar cells directly reflects the ionic current through Ca^{2+}-activated ion channels (non-selective cation and Cl^--selective channels) (Maruyama and Petersen 1982; Randriamampita et al. 1988). These channels are regarded as good Ca^{2+} sensors. For example, the non-selective cation channels can be activated when $[Ca^{2+}]^i$ is greater than 0.5 µmol/l (Maruyama and Petersen 1984).

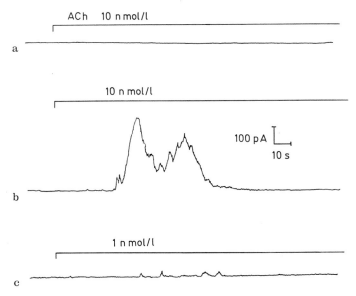

Fig. 4a – c. GTP-γ-S-induced potentiation of the effect of acetylcholine (*ACh*) stimulation. The composition of the internal and external solution is that described in the legend to Fig. 3 except that the concentration of internal $CaCl_2$ and EGTA (the internal solution contained no added Ca^{2+} and EGTA in a concentration of 70 µmol/l). The holding potential was 40 mV, and through the Na^+-K^+ non-selective and Cl^--selective channels there was outward current. **a** The effect of ACh (10 nmol/l) on the membrane current; 10 mmol/l ACh never induced the response (the threshold ACh concentration was about 30–50 nmol/l). **b** The current response induced by ACh 10 nmol/l in a cell dialysed with an internal solution containing 100 µmol/l GTP-γ-S. **c** The current response induced by 1 nmol/l ACh in a cell dialysed with the same solution as in **b**

Single pancreatic acinar cells from rats show transient current responses upon stimulation with physiological concentrations of ACh or CCK (Maruyama 1988). The threshold concentration of these agonists needed to evoke the response is about 30 nmol/l for ACh and 7 pmol/l for CCK. The threshold concentrations, however, are shifted in the lower direction (1 nmol/l in ACh- and 0.2 pmol/l in CCK-stimulation) when the cells are dialysed with a solution containing GTP-γ-S (guanosine-5'-(γ-thio) trisphosphate, a non-hydrolysable GTP analogue; 50–100 µmol/l; Fig. 4). Thus, GTP-γ-S potentiates the effects of ACh and CCK, respectively, by factors of 30 and 140 (Maruyama 1988); similar potentiation has also been reported in lacrimal gland acinar cells (Evans and Marty 1986). Moreover, the cytosolic GTP-γ-S can prolong the response when the cells are stimulated with about 100 nmol/l ACh or 10 pmol/l CCK. The prolonged response occasionally accompanies the oscillatory waves, which can be interpreted as an oscillation of $[Ca^{2+}]_i$. The mechanism of $[Ca^{2+}]_i$ oscillation is at present unknown although it might reflect the interaction of negative and positive feedback loops of the signal network. On the other hand, ACh- or CCK-induced responses are all diminished when the cells are dialysed with GDP-β-S (guanosine 5-(β-thio) diphosphate, a non-hydrolysable analogue of GDP). On the whole it is clear that G proteins mediate between receptor stimulation and Ca^{2+} mobilization (Maruyama 1988). One likely interpretation is that G proteins couple the receptor with phospholipase C, which hydrolyses phosphoinositide, generating inositol-trisphosphate (IP_3) and diacylglycerol. IP_3 has been shown to mobilize Ca^{2+} from the intracellukar storage site (Streb et al. 1984).

Acknowledgement. The author would like to thank Professor J.A. Young (University of Sydney, Australia) for his critical reading of the manuscript.

References

Berridge MJ, Irvine RF (1984) Inositol trisphosphate, a novel second messenger in cellular signal transduction. Nature 312: 315—321

Breckenridge LJ, Almers W (1987) Current through the fusion pore that forms during exocytosis of a secretory vesicle. Nature 328: 814–817

Clapham DE, Neher E (1984) Trifluoperazine reduces inward ionic currents and secretion by separate mechanisms in bovine chromaffin cells. J Physiol (Lond) 353: 541–564

Downes CP, Michell RH (1985) Inositol phospholipid breakdown as a receptor-controlled generator of second messengers. In: Cohen P, Hauslay MD (eds) Molecular mechanisms of transmembrane signalling. Elsevier Biomedical, Amsterdam, pp 3–56

Evans MG, Marty A (1986) Potentiation of muscarinic and alpha-adrenergic responses by an analogue of guanosine triphosphate. Proc Natl Acad Sci USA 83: 4099–4103

Fernandez JM, Neher E, Gomperts BD (1984) Capacitance measurements reveal stepwise fusion events in degranulating mast cells. Nature 312: 453–455

Gardner JD, Jensen RT (1987) Secretagogue receptors on pancreatic acinar cells. In: Johnson LR (ed) Physiology of the gastrointestinal tract, 2nd ed. Raven, New York, pp 1109–1127

Hootman SR, Williams JA (1987) Stimulus-secretion coupling in the pancreatic acinus. In: Johnson LR (ed) Physiology of the gastrointestinal tract, 2nd ed. Raven, New York, pp 1129–1146

Joshi A, Fernandez JM (1988) Capacitance measurements: an analysis of the phase detector technique used to study exocytosis and endocytosis. Biophys J 53: 885–892

Maruyama Y (1986) Ca^{2+}-induced excess capacitance fluctuation studied by phase-sensitive detection method in exocrine pancreatic acinar cells. Pflügers Arch 407: 561–563

Maruyama Y (1988) Agonist-induced changes in cell membrane capacitance and conductance in dialysed pancreatic acinar cells of rats. J Physiol (Lond) 406: 299–313

Maruyama Y (1989) Control of exocytosis in single cells. NIPS (in press)

Maruyama Y, Petersen OH (1982) Cholecystokinin activation of single-channel currents is mediated by internal second messenger in pancreatic acinar cells. Nature 300: 61–63

Maruyama Y, Petersen OH (1984) Single calcium dependent cation channels in mouse pancreatic acinar cells. J Membr Biol 81: 83–87

Marty A, Neher E (1983) Tight-seal whole-cell recording. In: Sakmann B, Neher E (eds) Single-channel recording, Plenum, New York, pp 107–122

Merritt JE, Taylor CW, Rubin RP, Putney JW (1986) Evidence suggesting that a novel guanine nucleotide regulatory protein couples receptors to phospholipase C in exocrine pancreas. Biochem J 236: 337–343

Neher E, Marty A (1982) Discrete changes of cell membrane capacitance observed under conditions of enhanced secretion in bovine adrenal chromaffin cells. Proc Natl Acad Sci USA 79: 6712–6716

Palade, G (1975) Intracellular aspects of the process of protein synthesis. Science 189: 347–352

Randriamampita C, Chanson M, Trautmann A (1988) Calcium and secretagogues-induced conductances in rat exocrine pancreas. Pflügers Arch 411: 53–57

Streb H, Irvine RF, Berridge MJ, Schulz I (1984) Release of Ca^{2+} from a non-mitochondrial intracellular store in pancreatic acinar cells by inositol-1,4,5-trisphosphate. Nature 306: 67–69

The Coupling of Stimuli to the Secretion of Protein in Exocrine Glands

M. L. Roberts

Many different cell types secrete protein by regulated exocytosis. It is not known to what extent stimulus-secretion coupling mechanisms are common to the various situations and to what extent the findings in one tissue can be applied to others. It is known that there are significant differences; for example, the exocrine glands lack the voltage-gated channels responsible for initiating secretion by nerve terminals and some endocrine glands, and secretion in exocrine glands results from activation of intracellular enzymatic pathways by cell surface receptors. In this review, current understanding of the mechanisms leading to exocytosis in exocrine cells will be described, concentrating on the salivary glands and pancreas because these have been investigated most extensively.

The major advance in this area in recent years has the been the description of the initial events that follow receptor activation. Both of the major pathways of cellular control, cyclic AMP-dependent mechanisms and Ca^{2+}/protein kinase C-dependent mechanisms, can produce secretion, and the relative importance of each of these varies among glands and among species.

Intracellular Activators of Protein Secretion

Cyclic AMP

There is considerable evidence from both salivary glands and pancreas that indicates that cyclic AMP is an activator of exocytosis. This subject has been reviewed recently (Young et al. 1987) and will only be summarized here. Secretomotor agonists that evoke a Ca^{2+}-independent secretion stimulate an increase in the concentration of cyclic AMP within the secretory cells. Derivatives of cyclic AMP that can cross membranes induce exocytosis when added to the extracellular medium of glands incubated in vitro. Cholera toxin, which produces persistent activation of adenylate cyclase, and forskolin, which directly activates adenylate cyclase, stimulate secretion in both pancreas and salivary gland.

Despite this evidence which supports a role for cyclic AMP in activating protein secretion, there are some experimental results which indicate that the

Young · Wong, Epithelial Secretion of Water and Electrolytes
© Springer-Verlag Berlin · Heidelberg 1990

nucleotide may not act alone. In the salivary glands, where it has been accepted for many years that β-adrenoceptors produce exocytosis through a cyclic AMP-dependent pathway, it is possible to show a lack of correlation between the abilities of β_1- and β_2-selective agonists to elevate cyclic AMP and to stimulate protein secretion (Carlsöö et al. 1982; Henriksson 1982; Yoshimura et al. 1984). One possible explanation for these results would be that β-adrenoceptors produce another intracellular mediator in addition to cyclic AMP and that the subclasses of β-receptors differ in their ability to mobilize this additional agent. Calcium fluxes in salivary glands are changed by β-adrenoceptor agonists (Butcher 1980), and it will be necessary to re-examine the involvement of this ion in the β-receptor response in the light of recent studies that show that Ca^{2+}, and not cyclic AMP, controls the ion channels responsible for β-adrenoceptor-stimulated fluid secretion (Cook et al. 1988) and that β-adrenoceptor stimulation causes inositol trisphosphate production and Ca^{2+} mobilization from an intracellular pool in rat parotid acinar cells (Horn et al. 1988).

Ca^{2+} and Protein Kinase C

Douglas and Poisner (1963) noted that secretion of fluid and protein by salivary glands was reduced by incubation in a Ca^{2+}-free medium and suggested that Ca^{2+} was involved in stimulus-secretion coupling. Many papers have been published since then demonstrating that agonists can alter Ca^{2+} fluxes in exocrine gland cells, that the ionophores A23187 and ionomycin can mimic the effects of agonists in many situations, as can the addition of Ca^{2+} to permeabilized exocrine cells, and that in many situations, stimulation of glands in Ca^{2+}-free solutions leads to an initial secretory response which rapidly declines, all of which support the concept of a Ca^{2+}-dependent pathway in secretion. Putney (1977) showed that the initial responses observed in Ca^{2+}-free solutions were due to the release of Ca^{2+} from intracellular stores and that continued responses were dependent on the entry of Ca^{2+} from the extracellular fluid.

Over the last few years, studies with intracellular fluorescent indicators of calcium concentration ($[Ca^{2+}]$), such as Quin-2 and Fura-2, have provided direct evidence of an elevation of $[Ca^{2+}]$ by agonists and of the kinetics of this rise. In their studies on rat parotid gland acinar cells stimulated with carbachol, Merritt and Rink (1987) found that the $[Ca^{2+}]$ of the cytosol rose from a resting level of just under 200 nmol/l to 780 nmol/l within 800 to 900 ms before falling over the next 2 min to a plateau of about 500 nmol/l. In the absence of extracellular Ca^{2+}, the cytoplasmic $[Ca^{2+}]$ rose more slowly, reached a somewhat lesser peak value (about 630 nmol/l), and decayed to resting levels despite continuous stimulation. Clearly, the early peak arose from the release of Ca^{2+} stored within the cell, while for prolonged responses, the entry of Ca^{2+} from the extracellular fluid was required. Similar results have been obtained in pancreatic acini (Ochs et al. 1983).

Measurements with $^{45}Ca^{2+}$ show that the influx and efflux of Ca^{2+} across the plasma membrane are increased during the sustained phase of exocrine secretion (Dormer et al. 1981). Alkon and Rasmussen (1988) consider that the $[Ca^{2+}]$ in the bulk cytosol measured by Quin-2 may not indicate the $[Ca^{2+}]$ in the important region adjacent to the plasma membrane. If this is so, it would explain apparently anomalous results such as those of Bruzzone et al. (1986), which indicate caerulein- and carbachol-stimulated amylase secretion by rat pancreatic acini apparently at resting levels of cytosolic free $[Ca^{2+}]$.

A significant advance in understanding stimulus-secretion coupling has occurred with the unravelling of the events that couple receptor activation to the release of intracellular Ca^{2+}, and with this has come the knowledge that another intracellular activator, diacylglycerol (DAG), is formed during the reaction which leads to Ca^{2+} release. This area has been reviewed extensively in the last two years and only a summary of it will be given here. More detailed coverage, particularly in relation to exocrine physiology, can be found in reviews by Young et al. (1987) and Putney (1987). In 1953, Hokin and Hokin described changes in the metabolism of an inositol-containing phospholipid in the exocrine pancreas. Subsequent work showed that such changes in the turnover of inositol phospholipids occur in many tissues, and Michell (1975) proposed that they were related to the control of the concentration of Ca^{2+} in the cytosol. In recent years it has been determined that the initial agonist-stimulated event is the hydrolysis of the membrane lipid phosphatidylinositol-4,5-bisphosphate, PIP_2, with the formation of inositol-1,4,5-trisphosphate, IP_3, and diacylglycerol DAG. This response is seen with all agonists that cause Ca^{2+}-dependent exocytosis in exocrine glands.

In a seminal experiment, Streb et al. (1983) showed that IP_3 causes the release of Ca^{2+} from a non-mitochondrial compartment in permeabilized pancreatic acinar cells. In subsequent studies with subcellular fractions of the exocrine pancreas, they found that the IP_3-sensitive compartment appeared to correspond to the endoplasmic reticulum (Streb et al. 1984).

IP_3 is metabolized through the action of kinases and phosphatases. One product of the kinases is inositol-1,3,4,5-tetrakisphosphate (IP_4) and some evidence indicates that this may have a function as an intracellular mediator. Morris et al. (1987) have demonstrated that IP_4 may produce the agonist-stimulated entry of Ca^{2+} into lacrimal gland acinar cells. Another prominent product of the metabolic pathway is IP_3, which appears to result from the action of a phosphatase on IP_4. So far, there is no evidence that this trisphosphate acts as an intracellular mediator.

DAG liberated by the hydrolysis of PIP_2 can act as an intracellular messenger by activating protein kinase C. An understanding of the role of DAG in cell function is still developing and some recent ideas about its involvement in sustained stimulation of cellular responses are discussed by Alkon and Rasmussen (1988). Phorbol esters, which can substitute for DAG in activating protein kinase C, stimulate exocytosis in the exocrine pancreas

(Gunther 1981; Merritt and Rubin 1985), but the role of protein kinase C in stimulus-secretion coupling in exocrine glands has not been clearly defined. The results of Merritt and Rubin (1985) indicate considerable potentiation of the effect of the ionophore ionomycin by phorbol esters or DAG, while Burnham et al. (1986) believe that synergism between Ca^{2+} and protein kinase C is of limited importance in stimulating amylase secretion. On the other hand, the results of Pandol and Schoeffield (1986) indicate that protein kinase C may inhibit amylase secretion, accounting for the reduced secretion seen in the presence of high concentrations of secretomotor agonists.

Interaction of Ca^{2+} and Cyclic AMP

In both salivary gland and pancreas, simultaneous activation of the cyclic AMP-dependent pathway and the Ca^{2+}-dependent pathway produces a potentiated response, the secretion of protein being greater than the sum of that produced by either pathway alone (Gardner and Jackson 1977; Dreux et al. 1987). The potentiation occurs subsequent to the generation of second messengers in these pathways (Dreux et al. 1987). The discovery of the mechanisms involved in this interaction would help to unravel the events in stimulus-secretion coupling that occur subsequent to second messenger generation.

Derivatives of Unsaturated Fatty Acids

Arachidonic acid is released when the exocrine pancreas is stimulated with caerulein (Dixon and Hokin 1984), and the saliva of a number of species contains metabolic products of arachidonic acid (Rigas et al. 1983). It has been proposed that such metabolites may be involved in stimulus-secretion coupling. However, studies using inhibitors of prostaglandin synthesis indicate that these products are not involved in activation of exocytosis (Putney et al. 1981). More recently it has been shown that AA861, an inhibitor of 5-lipoxygenase, reduces amylase secretion by rat pancreatic acini stimulated with carbachol or CCK, suggesting that products of this pathway may be involved in secretion (Sato et al. 1988). Putney et al. (1981) found that exogenous arachidonic acid did not initiate pancreatic amylase secretion, but they did not test whether it modified the agonist-induced response.

G Proteins in Stimulus-Secretion Coupling

It is now recognized that guanine nucleotide-binding proteins, the G proteins, are involved in many aspects of stimulus-response coupling in cells. The first G protein described was that which links the receptors, including the β-adrenoceptor, which can activate adenylate cyclase, to the enzyme; this protein is now known as G_s. Cholera toxin causes ADP ribosylation of G_s, producing persistent activation of the adenylate cyclase independent of receptor occupation. Receptors exist that can inhibit the activation of adenylate cyclase. An example of this in exocrine glands is the inhibition by somatostatin of vasoactive intestinal peptide (VIP)-induced amylase secretion from the pancreas (Esteve et al. 1983). The receptors for the inhibitory hormone are linked to adenylate cyclase by another G protein, G_i. Pertussis toxin causes ADP ribosylation of G_i, which prevents this G protein from linking the receptor to adenylate cyclase, removing the inhibitory action of the hormone.

Indirect evidence from recent work has demonstrated that a G protein (G_p) is probably involved in linking receptors to the phospholipase C responsible for the formation of IP_3 and DAG. Analogues of guanine nucleotides activate PIP_2 hydrolysis in membranes of secretory cells (Cockcroft and Gomperts 1985; Merritt et al. 1986). Fluoride, which indirectly causes dissociation of G_s into the α (active) and $\beta\gamma$ subunits, activates phospholipase C in rat parotid glands (Taylor et al. 1986). In some secretory cells, for example the neutrophil, the G protein involved in PIP_2 hydrolysis appears to be similar to G_i in that pertussis toxin inhibits the effects of receptor occupation by agonists (Molski et al. 1984). Antibodies raised against G_i do not, however, cross-react with the G protein from neutrophils (Gierschik et al. 1986). In addition, in many cell types, the activity of the G protein that leads to hydrolysis of PIP_2 is not affected by pertussis toxin or cholera toxin (Merritt et al. 1986). It appears from this that the G proteins responsible for coupling receptors to phospholipase C differ from G_s and G_i and that they might be of two types, distinguished by their sensitivity to pertussis toxin.

Cockcroft et al. (1987) have shown that a further G protein may be involved in exocytosis. In permeabilized mast cells in which phospholipase C was inhibited to prevent the formation of DAG, analogues of GTP stimulated exocytosis, suggesting a role for a G protein in stimulus-secretion coupling at a stage subsequent to the generation of second messengers.

Events in Stimulus-Secretion Coupling Subsequent to Generation of the Intracellular Activators

Now that the details of the initial events that follow receptor activation have been defined in reasonable detail, attention can be focussed on subsequent events in the coupling mechanisms. Remarkably little is known about these, but it is likely that this situation will change quickly now that access to the cytoplasm is available by use of permeabilized cells and patch-clamp techniques.

Vesicular Swelling and Exocytosis

In exocrine glands, the granules fuse with the plasma membrane at the luminal surface of the cells, but not with that at the basal or lateral surfaces. This restriction of fusion to the luminal membrane probably reflects specializations in the composition of the plasma membrane in this region. Freeze-fracture studies of guinea-pig pancreatic acinar cells have shown that the luminal membrane and the zymogen granule have few intramembraneous particles compared to the basal and lateral surfaces (De Camilli et al. 1977). In addition, the luminal membrane contains less cholesterol than the basal and lateral membranes (Orci et al. 1983).

Studies with phosopholipid bilayers and vesicles show that fusion takes place in two stages (Wilschut and Hoekstra 1984). In the first step the structures aggregate, providing close contact between the membranes. In the next step, tightly bound water must be removed from the surface of the phospholipid structures to allow hydrophobic contact and fusion. Removal of water from the polar head groups of phospholipids is energetically costly. It has been suggested that the energy for removal of the water may be provided by osmotic swelling of the vesicles and, in the case of secretory cells, of the granules. Granule swelling would require the existence of stimulus-regulated ionic permeabilities in the membrane of the zymogen granules, and some evidence for such pathways has been presented recently (Fuller et al. 1988).

The granules of mast cells in beige mice have been observed to undergo swelling during exocytosis, and secretion can be inhibited by incubation in a hypertonic medium which prevents granule swelling (Curran et al. 1984). However, hypertonic media can have diverse effects on intact cells, including a reduction of the Ca^{2+} signal, making the interpretation of these experiments difficult (Kazilek et al. 1988). Holz (1986) has argued that the results obtained using permeabilized cells do not support the idea that osmotic stress plays a role in exocytosis.

Recently, fusion in mast cells has been studied with patch-clamp techniques, using the whole-cell configuration and measuring membrane capacitance, which is proportional to membrane area. When this technique was used on the mast cells of beige mice and combined with studies with Nomarski optics, it was demonstrated that fusion preceded swelling, indicating that in this situation at least, swelling does not provide the energy for fusion (Zimmerberg et al. 1987).

The Cytoskeleton and Exocytosis

The possibility that elements of the cytoskeleton may be involved in regulating exocytosis has been considered for many years (Orci et al. 1972). In the exocrine pancreas and parotid gland, immunocytochemical studies reveal a narrow band beneath the luminal membrane which stains strongly for many cytoskeletal proteins (Drenckhahn and Mannherz 1983). It is possible that the cytoskeleton prevents access of the granules to the luminal membrane. As Linstedt and Kelly (1987) have pointed out, if access of the granules to the plasma membrane is regulated by Ca^{2+}, the fusion of the two membranes need not be a regulated event. Much of the recent work on the cytoskeleton and secretion has been on adrenal chromaffin cells. In these cells, disassembly of the actin filaments takes place in the first 15 s of stimulation with nicotinic agonists (which stimulate secretion of catecholamines by the cells; Cheek and Burgoyne 1986). A particularly interesting finding concerns fodrin, a non-erythroid form of spectrin. Fodrin occurs close to the secretory granules and plasma membrane of chromaffin cells, and when these cells are permeabilized, the application of antibodies to fodrin reduces exocytosis by 50% (Perrin et al. 1987). The use of permeabilized cells together with antibodies to specific cytoskeletal proteins is likely to demonstrate the role that these proteins play in exocytosis in the near future.

Enzymatic Activation of Exocytosis

The involvement of protein hydrolysis at some stage in the events leading to exocytosis has been proposed by a number of workers. The formation of fusogenic peptides (Lucy 1984) and the involvement of Ca^{2+}-activated neutral proteinase either in the disassembly of the cytoskeleton (Burgoyne and Cheek 1987) or in the conversion of protein kinase C to its soluble Ca^{2+}-independent form (Pontremoli et al. 1986) have been suggested as possible events in stimulus-secretion coupling.

Metallo-endopeptidases have been implicated in the Ca^{2+}-dependent fusion of membranes in secretion from adrenal chromaffin and mast cells (Mundy and Strittmatter 1985). In adrenal chromaffin cells, inhibitors of metallo-endopeptidases do reduce secretion, but this is apparently a result of interference with the mechanisms responsible for elevation of the cytosolic $[Ca^{2+}]$ rather than by inhibition of membrane fusion (Harris et al. 1986). In the exocrine pancreas, 1,10-phenanthroline, an inhibitor of metallo-endopeptidases, inhibits CCK- and bombesin-stimulated amylase secretion, but does not affect A23187 or cyclic AMP-stimulated amylase secretion (Collins and Roberts 1988). These results show that the metallo-endopeptidase inhibitor does not prevent membrane fusion in these exocrine cells, and the reduction in CCK- and bombesin-induced secretion appears to result from a reduced hydrolysis of inositol phospholipids in the presence of 1,10-phenanthroline (Collins and Roberts 1988).

Cyclic AMP, DAG and Ca^{2+} each activate protein kinases that phosphorylate proteins in exocrine cells (Roberts and Butcher 1983; Wrenn ans Wooten 1984). Phosphorylation of proteins regulates metabolic activity in many situations, and its possible involvement in stimulus-secretion coupling is discussed in this volume by Quissell.

References

Alkon DL, Rasmussen H (1988) A spatial-temporal model of cell activation. Science 239: 998–1005

Bruzzone R, Pozzan T, Wollheim CB (1986) Caerulein and carbamylcholine stimulate pancreatic amylase release at resting cytosolic free Ca^{2+}. Biochem J 235: 139–143

Burgoyne RD, Cheek TR (1987) Role of fodrin in secretion. Nature 326: 448

Burnham DB, Munowitz P, Hootman SR, Williams JA (1986) Regulation of protein phosphorylation in pancreatic acini. Distinct effects of Ca^{2+} ionophore A23187 and 12-O-tetradecanoylphorbol 13-acetate. Biochem J 235: 125–131

Butcher FR (1980) Regulation of calcium efflux from isolated rat parotid cells. Biochim Biophys Acta 630: 254–260

Carlsöö B, Danielsson A, Henriksson R, Idahl L-A (1982) Dissociation of β-adrenoceptor-induced effects on amylase secretion and cyclic adenosine 3'-5'-monophosphate accumulation. Br J Pharmacol 75: 633–638

Cheek TR, Burgoyne RD (1986) Nicotine-evoked disassembly of cortical actin filaments in adrenal chromaffin cells. FEBS Lett 207: 110–114

Cockcroft S, Gomperts BD (1985) Role of guanine nucleotide binding protein in the activation of polyphosphoinositide phosphodiesterase. Nature 314: 534–536

Cockcroft S, Howell TW, Gomperts BD (1987) Two G-proteins act in series to control stimulus-secretion coupling in mast cells: use of neomycin to distinguish between G-proteins controlling polyphosphoinositide phosphodiesterase and exocytosis. J Cell Biol 105: 2745–2750

Collins SP, Roberts ML (1988) Metallo-endoprotease inhibitors and stimulus-secretion coupling in mouse exocrine pancreas. In: Wong PYD, Young JA (eds) Exocrine secretion. Hong Kong University Press, Hong Kong, pp 49–50

Cook DI, Day ML, Champion MP, Young JA (1988) Ca^{2+} not cyclic AMP mediates the fluid secretory response to isoproterenol in the rat mandibular salivary gland. Pflügers Arch 413: 67–76

Curran MJ, Brodwick MS, Edwards C (1984) Direct visualization of exocytosis in mast cells. Biophys J 45: 170A

De Camilli P, Peluchetti D, Meldolesi J (1977) Structural difference between luminal and lateral plasmalemma in pancreatic acinar cells. Nature 248: 245–247

Dixon JF, Hokin LE (1984) Secretogogue-stimulated phosphatidylinositol breakdown in the exocrine pancreas liberates arachidonic acid, stearic acid, and glycerol by sequential actions of phospholipase C and diglyceride lipase. J Biol Chem 259: 14418–14425

Dormer RL, Poulsen JH, Licko V, Williams JA (1981) Calcium fluxes in isolated pancreatic acini: effects of secretagogues. Am J Physiol 240: G38–G49

Douglas WW, Piosner AM (1963) The influence of calcium on the secretory response of the submaxillary gland to acetylcholine or to noradrenaline. J Physiol (Lond) 165: 528–541

Drenckhahn D, Mannherz HG (1983) Distribution of actin and the actin-associated proteins myosin, tropomyosin, alpha-actinin, vinculin, and villin in rat and bovine exocrine glands. Eur J Cell Biol 30: 167–176

Dreux C, Imhoff V, Rossignol B (1987) [^{3}H]protein secretion in rat parotid gland: substance P-β-adrenergic synergism. Am J Physiol 253: C774–C782

Esteve JP, Vaysse N, Susini C, Kunsch JM, Fourmy D, Pradayrol L, Wunsch E, Moroder L, Ribet A (1983) Bimodal regulation of pancreatic exocrine function in vitro by somatostatin-28. Am J Physiol 245: G208–G216

Fuller CM, Eckhardt L, Schulz I (1988) Ionic dependence of exocytosis from permeabilized acini of the rat pancreas. In: Wong PTD, Young JA (eds) Exocrine secretion. Hong Kong University Press, Hong Kong, pp 65–67

Gardner JD, Jackson MJ (1977) Regulation of amylase release from dispersed pancreatic acinar cells. J Physiol (Lond) 270: 439–454

Gierschik P, Falloon J, Milligan G, Pines M, Gallin JI, Spiegel A (1986) Immunochemical evidence for a novel pertussis toxin substrate in human neutrophils. J Biol Chem 261: 8058–8062

Gunther GR (1981) Effect of 12-O-tetradecanoyl-phorbol-13-acetate on Ca^{2+} efflux and protein discharge in pancreatic acini. J Biol Chem 256: 12040–12045

Harris B, Cheek, TR, Burgoyne RD (1986) Effects of metallo-endoproteinase inhibitors on secretion and intracellular free calcium in bovine adrenal chromaffin cells. Biochim Biophys Acta 889: 1–5

Henriksson R (1982) β^1- and β^2-adrenoceptor agonists have different effects on rat parotid acinar cells. Am J Physiol 242: G481–G485

Hokin MR, Hokin LE (1953) Enzyme secretion and the incorporation of P^{32} into phospholipides of pancreas slices. J Biol Chem 203: 967–977

Holz RW (1986) The role of osmotic forces in exocytosis from adrenal chromaffin cells. Annu Rev Physiol 48: 175–189

Horn VJ, Baum BJ, Ambudkar IS (1988) β-Adrenergic receptor stimulation induces inositol trisphosphate production and Ca^{2+} mobilization in rat parotid acinar cells. J Biol Chem 263: 12454–12460

Kazilek CJ, Merkle CJ, Chandler DE (1988) Hyperosmotic inhibition of calcium signals and exocytosis in rabbit neutrophils. Am J Physiol 254: C709–C718

Linstedt AD, Kelly RB (1987) Overcoming barriers to exocytosis. Trends Neurosci 10: 446–448

Lucy JA (1984) Do hydrophobic sequences cleaved from cellular polypeptides induce membrane fusion reactions in vivo? FEBS Lett 166: 223–231

Merritt JE, Rink TJ (1987) Rapid increases in cytosolic free calcium in response to muscarinic stimulation of rat parotid acinar cells. J Biol Chem 262: 4958–4960

Merritt JE, Rubin RP (1985) Pancreatic amylase secretion and cytoplasmic free calcium. Effects of ionomycin, phorbol dibutyrate and diacylglycerols alone and in combination. Biochem J 230: 151–159

Merritt JE, Taylor CW, Rubin RP, Putney JW (1986) Evidence suggesting that a novel guanine nucleotide regulatory protein couples receptors to phospholipase C in exocrine pancreas. Biochem J 236: 337–343

Michell RH (1975) Inositol phospholipids and cell surface receptor function. Biochim Biophys Acta 415: 81–147

Molski TFP, Naccache PH, Marsh ML, Kermode J, Becker EL, Sha'afi RI (1984) Pertussis toxin inhibits the rise in the intracellular concentration of free calcium that is induced by chemotactic factors in rabbit neutrophils: possible role of the "G proteins" in calcium mobilization. Biochem Biophys Res Commun 124: 644–650

Morris AP, Gallacher DV, Irvine RF, Petersen OH (1987) Synergism of inositol trisphosphate and tetrakisphosphate in activating Ca^{2+}-dependent K^+ channels. Nature 330: 653–655

Mundy DI, Strittmatter WJ (1985) Requirement for metallo-endoprotease in exocytosis: evidence in mast cells and adrenal chromaffin cells. Cell 40: 645–656

Ochs DL, Korenbrot JI, Williams JA (1983) Intracellular free calcium concentrations in pancreatic acini: effects of secretagogues. Biochem Biophys Res Commun 117: 122–128

Orci L, Gabbay KH, Malaisse W (1972) Pancreatic beta-cell web: its possible role in insulin secretion. Science 175: 1128–1130

Orci L, Perrelet A, Montesano R (1983) Differential filipin labeling of the luminal membranes lining the pancreatic acinus. J Histochem Cytochem 31: 952–955

Pandol SJ, Schoeffield MS (1986) 1,2-diacylglycerol, protein kinase C, and pancreatic enzyme secretion. J Biol Chem 261: 4438–4444

Perrin D, Langley OK, Aunis D (1987) Anti-α-fodrin inhibits secretion from permeabilized chromaffin cells. Nature 326: 498–501

Pontremoli S, Melloni E, Michetti M, Sacco O, Salamino F, Sparatore B, Horecker BL (1986) Biochemical responses in activated human neutrophils mediated by protein kinase C and a Ca^{2+}-requiring proteinase. J Biol Chem 261: 8309–8913

Putney JW (1977) Muscarinic, alpha-adrenergic and peptide receptors regulate the same calcium influx sites in the parotid gland. J Physiol (Lond) 268: 139–149

Putney JW (1987) Formation and actions of calcium-mobilizing messenger, inositol 1,4,5-trisphosphate. Am J Physiol 252: G149–G157

Putney JW, De Witt LM, Hoyle PC, McKinney JS (1981) Calcium, prostaglandins and the phosphatidylinositol effect in exocrine gland cells. Cell Calcium 2: 561–571

Rigas B, Lewis RA, Austen KF, Corey EJ, Levine L (1983) Identification and quantitation of arachidonic-acid metabolic products in rabbit, rat and human saliva. Arch Oral Biol 28: 1031–1035

Roberts ML, Butcher FR (1983) The involvement of protein phosphorylation in stimulus-secretion coupling in the mouse exocrine pancreas. Biochem J 210: 353–359

Sato S, Adachi H, Noguchi M, Honda T, Onishi S, Aoki E, Torizuka K (1988) Effect of AA861, a 5-lipoxygenase inhibitor, on amylase secretion from rat pancreatic acini. Biochim Biophys Acta 968: 1–8

Streb H, Irvine RF, Berridge MJ, Schulz I (1983) Release of Ca^{2+} from a non-mitochondrial intracellular store in pancreatic acinar cells by inositol-1,4,5-trisphosphate. Nature 306: 67–69

Streb H, Bayerdörffer E, Haase W, Irvine RF, Schulz I (1984) Effect of inositol-1,4,5-trisphosphate on isolated subcellular fractions of rat pancreas. J Membr Biol 81: 241–253

Taylor CW, Merritt JE, Putney JW, Rubin RP (1986) A guanine-nucleotide dependent regulatory protein couples substance P receptors to phospholipase C in rat parotid gland. Biochem Biophys Res Commun 136: 362–368

Wilschut J, Hoekstra D (1984) Membrane fusion: from liposomes to biological membranes. Trends Biochem Sci 9: 479–483

Wrenn RW, Wooten MW (1984) Dual calcium-dependent protein phosphorylation systems in pancreas and their differential regulation by polymyxin B. Life Sci 35: 267–276

Yoshimura K, Nezu E, Yoneyama T (1984) Mechanism of regulation of amylase release by α- and β-adrenergic agonists in rat parotid tissue. Jpn J Physiol 34: 655–667

Young JA, Cook DI, van Lennep EW, Roberts ML (1987) Secretion by the major salivary glands. In: Johnson LR (ed) Physiology of the gastrointestinal tract, 2nd edn. Raven, New York, pp 2501–2543

Zimmerberg J, Curran M, Cohen FS, Brodwick M (1987) Simultaneous electrical and optical measurements show that membrane fusion precedes secretory granule swelling during exocytosis of beige mouse mast cells. Proc Natl Acad Sci USA 84: 1585–1589

Ion Transport in Mutant Cell Lines: Possibilities for Analysis*

A. W. Cuthbert

Two reasons can be identified which make a study of ion transport in mutant cell lines of importance. First, mutants provide the first stage for molecular genetic studies from which the molecular identification of the transporting proteins can eventually be derived. Incidentally, if the phenotypic characteristics of the mutant are sufficiently different from the wild type, then important aspects of cell function overall may be revealed. The second reason, which is not unconnected with the first, is that a number of identifiable disease states appear to be associated with a mutation affecting cellular transport mechanisms. The obvious examples are cystic fibrosis and chloridorrhoea.

These introductory remarks are based on the premise that transport proteins and their variants are uniquely encoded by structural genes. Having isolated a cell line showing an aberrant transport function of interest, subsequent analysis will be easier if all of the phenotypic changes can be attributed to a single mutation event.

As Gargus (1987a) points out in his excellent review, the principles involved in mutant selection and molecular genetics are commonplace in prokaryotic systems, while only now are similar approaches being used with eukaryotes, although the principles remain the same. There are, of course, significant advantages using prokaryotic systems with rapid growth, but perhaps the most crucial aspect with either eukaryotes or prokaryotes is obtaining a rapid and simple screening assay for mutant selection. This, as will be shown later, is not always an easy matter.

What follows are some examples of how the approaches outlined above are being used to uncover the properties of membrane macromolecules involved in the transport of inorganic ions across eukaryotic cell membranes. Some examples concern the transport of ions into or out of the cell, while others concern transepithelial ion transport when ions are moved across two membrane barriers in series, movements characteristic of transepithelial absorptive or secretory processes. In the latter group I shall include an example from my own laboratory.

---

* Work from the authors laboratory referred to in this review was supported by NIH HL17705.

Abnormal Potassium Transport

Using the thymidine kinase-deficient murine fibroblast line, (LM(TK$^-$), and mutagenising first with ethyl methane sulphonate, two mutants, LTK-1 and LTK-5, were isolated that showed abnormal potassium handling (Gargus et al. 1978). The phenotype of both mutants allowed survival in low K (0.2 mmol/l), maintaining high internal K$^+$ and low Na$^+$ concentrations. Further analysis showed that neither mutant had an altered Na$^+$-, K$^+$-ATPase, yet LTK-5 cells showed enhanced K$^+$-influx via the furosemide-sensitive Na$^+ - K^+ - $2Cl$^-$ cotransporter, while LTK-1 had a reduced K$^+$ efflux. The K$^+$ channels in LTK-1 had a conductance of only 20 pS, compared with 50 pS in the wild type, and showed enhanced K$^+$ selectivity (Gargus and Coronado 1985).

Using another mouse L-cell line (501C) carrying the hypoxanthine guanine phosphoribosyl transferase (HGPRT$^-$) marker, somatic cell hybrids were formed which grew in hypoxanthine, aminopterin and thymidine (HAT) medium (Table 1). However, only hybrids of 501C with either LTK-1 or LTK-5 could survive in both HAT medium and low K$^+$ medium. This indicates that both mutations were dominant (Gargus 1987b).

By extracting high-molecular-weight DNA from the mutants and mixing with excess plasmid DNA carrying the TK$^+$ gene it has proved possible to transfect LMTK$^-$ cells using the calcium phosphate method. Primary transformants can then be isolated by selection in low K$^+$ HAT medium (Mitas and Gargus 1985). Secondary transformants are then selected using DNA from the primary transformant, but without a plasmid. These secondary transformants will then have both the TK$^+$ and Low K$^+$ resistant genes reasonably close together in the genome. Using DNA from the secondary transformant, formation of a genomic library and cloning with a viral vector leads eventually to the isolation of the genes responsible for low K$^+$ resistance. Further progress with this fascinating approach is awaited.

Table 1. Growth rate in parent and hybrid cell lines (generations/day, from Gargus 1987b)

	Medium	
	0.2 mmol/l K$^+$	6 mmol/1 K$^+$ + HAT
Parents		
LMTK$^-$	0	0
LTK-1	0.7	0
LTK-5	0.6	0
501-C	0	0
Hybrids		
LMTK$^-$ × 501 C	0	1.0
LTK-1 × 501 C	0.7	1.0
LTK-5 × 501 C	0.75	1.0

Selection of mutants using low K^+ resistance has been used in a number of cell lines, for instance BALB/c3T3 preadipose cells (Sussman and O'Brien 1985) and in Madin-Darby canine kidney cells (McRoberts et al. 1983). In both instances there was reduced activity of the $Na^+ - K^+ - 2Cl^-$ cotransporter system. In the case of the BALB/c3T3 cell mutant this was due, apparently, to a reduced affinity to K^+ and Na^+, but not to Cl^-. Both types of mutant cells have been used to ask questions about the role of the furosemide-sensitive transporter system in cell volume regulation. Binding studies with another loop diuretic, ^3H-piretanide, showed two different sites with different affinities, correlating with the presence or absence of $Na^+ - K^+ - 2Cl^-$ cotransporter activity in normal and mutant MDCK cell lines. However, it is difficult to ascribe transporter activity exclusively to a particular binding site (Giesen-Crouse and McRoberts 1987).

A fascinating example of a point mutation affecting both K^+ transport and behaviour is found in a *Paramecium* mutant (Schaefer et al. 1987). In the mutant there is failure to activate a calcium-sensitive potassium channel plus exaggerated backward swimming in response to environmental stimuli. The defect can be corrected by injection of wild type calmodulin. Calmodulin from the mutant strain differs from that of the wild type by replacement of serine by phenylalamine at residue 101. The mutant calmodulin, however, is able to activate phosphodiesterase from bovine brain.

Sodium–Hydrogen Exchanger

The ubiquitous sodium-proton exchanger in its normal mode exchanges extracellular Na^+ for intracellular protons, a process driven by the sodium gradient, with a coupling ratio of $1:1$, that is, an electroneutral process. The system is reversible, it can take up protons in exchange for sodium efflux if the correct gradients are imposed. At the external site H^+, Na^+, Li^+, NH_4^+ and amiloride compete for binding, while internally H^+, Na^+ and Li^+ can be transported outwards, but H^+ also can activate the system. The system shuts off as pH_i reaches 7.3, but is activated in an allosteric manner as pH_i falls, reaching a maximum rate at a pH_i of around 6.0.

The lethal effects of reduced pH_i have been used to select mutants with altered exchanger activity. The Na^+-H^+ exchanger can function as a cell killer if H^+ uptake is promoted or as a survival mechanism when H^+ efflux is enhanced (Pouysségur 1985).

Mutants lacking the Na^+-H^+ exchanger have been developed using Chinese hamster lung fibroblasts (CCL39) (Pouysségur et al. 1984). Cells were first mutagenised with ethyl methane sulphonate and the resulting cultures loaded with Li^+. Afterwards the cells were exposed for up to 60 min in a saline without Li^+, Na^+ or bicarbonate and at pH 5.5 and subsequently cultured in normal medium. Only cells without the exchanger could survive the fall in pH_i occasioned by exchange of the internal Li^+ for protons.

Repeated treatments of this type gave mutant cells without the exchanger that were stable over many passages in the absence of the selective pressure. Cell viability in the wild type cells CCL39 was reduced to zero when using the same protocol as for the mutagenised cells, although protection was afforded by dimethylamiloride.

Clones of fibroblast cells which were fully resistant to repeated proton-suicide testing (PS10, PS12, PS20 and PS21) had no amiloride-sensitive sodium influx, whereas in the wild type cells 95% of sodium influx was amiloride sensitive. A further mutant, PS6, which survived a less rigorous acid-suicide protocol, expressed diminished exchanger activity and had an amiloride-sensitive sodium influx of some 10% of the wild type.

Hybrids cells formed from crosses of PS12 and PS20 with 023 − 61, a CCL39 derivative, expressing ouabain resistance and HGPRT deficiency were selected, after fusion with polyethylene glycol (PEG), in HAT medium containing 3 mmol/l ouabain. Hybrids showed 44% of the exchanger activity of the parent cell line and with an intermediate type phenotype. One conclusion is that the mutation is codominant.

The proton-suicide technique can be used in another mode in which cells are first loaded with protons using an NH_4^+ prepulse (Baron 1983). When cells are then suspended in normal medium, the chances of survival depend upon an ability to raise pH_i rapidly. Obviously cells without the exchanger cannot do this, and furthermore, wild type cells will also be killed if either low external sodium or a submaximal concentration of amiloride is present. Cells which over express exchanger activity or have a reduced affinity for amiloride will therefore be selectable. A mutant AR300 was found which 'over expresses' exchanger activity recovering from an acid load in 5 s compared with 15 min in wild type hamster lung cells. In this variant the exchanger had a 20-fold reduction in affinity for methylpropyl amiloride, a 2.5-fold increased affinity for Na^+ and a V_{max} that was 4−5-fold that of the wild type (Franchi et al. 1986a).

In order to gain some insight into the molecular structure of the transporter, mutants lacking the gene can be used to express a foreign exchanger gene using DNA-mediated gene transfer protocols. To do this use is made both of the proton-suicide and survival regimens described earlier (Franchi et al. 1986b).

Starting with a mouse fibroblast line, L 929, which is TK^+ deficient, the proton-suicide method was used to establish a mutant, LAP1, which was deficient in the Na^+–H^+ exchanger. Human genomic DNA plus plasmid TK^+DNA was used to transform LAP1, using the calcium phosphate precipitation method. To select mutant clones which contained the human Na^+–H^+ exchanger gene, selection was made on the basis of ability to grow in HAT medium (i.e. contained TK^+) and to survive an acid load imposed following NH_4^+ prepulse (contained the human exchanger gene). As it was not necessarily true that the human Na^+–H^+ exchanger would be expressed so well in LAP1, compared with the wild type cells, the selection procedure following the NH_4^+ prepulse was modified by varying the sodium

Table 2. $Na^+ - H^+$ exchanger activity in mutants and transformants (modified from Franchi et al. 1986b)

Cell line	Na^+-H^+ exchanger activity	Donor DNA
L929 (LTK$^-$)	+	
LAP1	−	
AR300	+ +	
PT2, PT11	+	Human genomic DNA
ST31	+	PT11 mouse DNA
ST34	+	PT2 mouse DNA
TT1	+	ST31 mouse DNA
TAR8	+ +	AR300 hamster DNA

concentration of the external bathing medium. This allowed transformants with 0%, 15%, 50% and 100% of the activity of the parent L929 line to be selected. Secondary and tertiary transformants were also produced using genomic DNA from the primary transformants. The results of this study are given in Table 2.

The kinetic characteristics of the exchanger found in AR300 and TAR cell lines were similar, and different from that of the parent cell, providing good evidence that the transformants express the donor DNA. This was supported by demonstration of repeated sequences of human DNA on polycrylamide gel electrophoresis (PAGE) gels prepared from the transformants. It would appear that the human Na^+-H^+ transporter gene is stably expressed in mouse L cells, providing a basis for further cloning approaches. That all this has been achieved when the "only information available about this membrane transporter was its biological function" (Franchi et al. 1986b) illustrates the power of the approach.

Even though little has yet been learned of the molecular nature of the Na^+-H^+ exchanger, the genetic approach has had an important impact upon the understanding of the functional responsibilities of this membrane macromolecule. The Na^+-H^+ exchanger appears to be activated rapidly in cells following application of external stimuli as variable as sperm, a multitude of growth-promoting agents and tumour promoters. Internal alkalisation of sea urchin eggs following fertilisation was shown to be blocked by amiloride, which also blocked subsequent development (Johnson et al. 1976). At first there was some confusion because the amiloride concentrations required were far greater than those blocking conductive, nonelectrically excitable sodium channels (Cuthbert and Cuthbert 1978). It later became apparent that amiloride at high concentrations could inhibit both Na^+-H^+ and Na^+-Ca^{2+} exchange mechanisms and the ubiquitous nature of these transporters was discovered fulfilling an earlier prediction of the need for an exchanger (Kirschner 1979).

It now appears that a rapid sodium influx coupled with an increase in pH_i may be a general response to growth-promoting agents. The latter may activate the exchanger by stimulating phosphatidylinositol hydrolysis, generating inositol phosphates and diacylglycerol, explaining why phorbol esters promote a similar type of response.

In wild type Chinese hamster lung fibroblasts blockade of the Na^+–H^+ exchanger with amiloride analogues prevents DNA synthesis when grown in HCO_3^--free media (L'Allemain et al. 1984). With mutants lacking the exchanger, DNA synthesis is prevented without the need for amiloride. While the wild type grows in a pH range of 6.5 to 8.3, the mutants fail to grow below pH 7.2 and have an optimum rate in the range pH 8–8.3 (Pouysségur et al. 1984). Reinitiation of DNA synthesis by growth factors follows upon early stimulation of the Na^+–H^+ exchanger and protein phosphorylation, including that of the ribosomal S6 proteins. Amiloride or procedures which acidify cells prevent both of these events (Pouysségur et al. 1982). It appears, therefore, that sodium-proton exchange may have a signal role in the genesis of these mitogenic responses.

Other Transporters

With the two major examples so far considered, the transporters of interest, the Na^+–K^+–$2Cl^-$ cotransporter and the Na^+–H^+ exchanger, are widely distributed in cells. This has allowed a genetic approach with cells that are

Table 3. Characteristics of HCA-7, Colony 1 and Colony 3 cells

	HCA-7	Colony 1	Colony 3
Dome forming ability	+	+	−
Transepithlial resistance ($\Omega\,cm^2$)	78 ± 7	42 ± 5	117 ± 14
Lysylbradykinin 100 nmol/l ($\mu A/cm^2$)	43 ± 6	9 ± 3	0
A 23187 1 $\mu mol/l$, nmol	13.0 ± 0.7	1.0 ± 1.0	12.5 ± 1.1
Forskolin 10 $\mu mol/l$, nmol	6.8 ± 1.4	27.5 ± 2.9	1.1 ± 0.3
Forskolin 10 $\mu mol/l$, pmol/mg	142 ± 10	195 ± 12	1428 ± 54
Forskolin 10 $\mu mol/l$ pmol/mg/h	4125	6600	5700
PKA %	134 ± 34	13 ± 6	51 ± 22

Taken from Cuthbert et al. (1987) and unpublished data. Responses to lysylbradykinin are transient and are given as peak SCC (short circuit current) ($\mu A/cm^2$). Responses to A 23187 and forskolin were maintained and are given as nmol in eight minutes, by integrating the SCC time curve. Basal cyclic AMP content of the cells was around 10 pmol/mg protein. Values given are after exposure to forskolin, 10 $\mu mol/l$, for 15 min. Adenylate cyclase activity was measured in membrane preparations and is given as pmol cyclic AMP formed per mg protein per h. Protein kinase A measurements were based on the phosphorylation of histone. The percentage increase in phosphorylation caused by cyclic AMP, 10 $\mu mol/l$ is given. PKA, cAMP activated protein kinase A.

easy to manipulate in tissue culture. However, some of the rarer macromolecules which are involved in more specialist ion transport functions occur only in particular tissues. Furthermore, specialist transporters, such as epithelial chloride and sodium channels, occur with relatively low abundance so that isolation and partial characterisation as an approach to cloning has not, so far, been successful. An alternative approach is to obtain mutants which can be selected and then, by developing hybrids or using DNA transfection, to move to molecular cloning by techniques illustrated in earlier sections.

A number of epithelial mutants has been described with altered transport phenotypes. For example, the LLC-PK$_1$ cell line is heterogenous, but has been cloned into three phenotypically stable mutants. Whether these arose from independent mutations in a phenotypically stable monoclonal population or whether the original line was polyclonal is unknown. Evidence of transporting activity in epithelial monolayers comes from dome formation. It was found for the mutants that dome formation correlated with transepithelial resistance (Table 4; Wohlwend et al. 1986).

Epithelial Chloride Channels

Cystic fibrosis (CF) is a human disease due to a single gene defect on chromosome 7. A defect in the ability of CF epithelia to secrete chloride ions electrogenically has been demonstrated and in recent times interest has focussed, almost exclusively, upon chloride channels. These are found in the apical membranes of secretory and absorptive epithelia such as airway epithelia, pancreatic duct, coil and duct of sweat glands and the intestinal lining.

It is beyond the scope of this article to review the findings in detail here, particularly as other articles in this volume deal with them explicitly. In brief, CF epithelia fail to secrete chloride in response to cyclic AMP-dependent agonists (Welsh and Liedtke 1986; Frizzell et al. 1986; Boucher et al. 1986), but do respond to A23187. In isolated patches from CF tissues chloride channels are found with electrical properties characteristic of normal channels, which either open and close spontaneously or do so in response to calcium. They do not respond to cyclic AMP or the catalytic subunit of protein kinase A (Welsh and Liedtke 1986; Frizzell et al. 1986; Li et al. 1988; Barthelson and Widdicombe 1987). While the defect in CF may reside in the chloride channel itself, there is further confusion following the recent demonstration that the intestinal epithelium responds neither to calcium nor to cyclic AMP-dependent signals (Berschneider et al. 1988). This suggests that the regulation of chloride channels in CF epithelia is indeed subtle and will require a subtle approach to unravel. While there have been brief reports of immortalised CF cell lines, these mutants have not become generally available for investigation. Stable mutant cell lines would provide a considerable boost to CF research which, thus far, is highly dependent on a supply of tissue from CF donors.

A variety of human cell lines which effect chloride secretion in response to various agonists have been described, such as T_{84} and Caco-2. In addition, a number of mutant cell lines derived from a single human adencarcinoma have become available, one of which has a phenotype with some of the characteristics of CF epithelia.

The cell line HCA-7 was described first by Kirkland (1985) from which a number of distinct lines (Colony 1, Colony 3, Colony 29) have been obtained either by mutagenisation with sodium butyrate or by isolating epithelial cells with different morphologies. These cell lines have been maintained in continuous culture for over 1 year without losing their phenotypes. Characterisation of these phenotypes has been based upon functional responses, i.e. the ability to transport anions (Cuthbert et al. 1987).

All the mutant cell lines referred to above can be grown on pervious supports to form epithelial sheets capable of transepithelial transport. Furthermore, they respond to a variety of agonists, all of which stimulate electrogenic chloride secretion, the epithelial monolayers having the characteristics of crypt cells. Secretory responses are partially blocked by loop diuretics such as furosemide and piretanide, the remaining current being sensitive to acetazolamide. The result indicates that bicarbonate ions can be secreted as well as chloride ions.

To investigate the intracellular mechanisms controlling anion secretion, receptors were bypassed by using forskolin and A23187, respectively, to increase cyclic AMP content and raise Ca_i^{2+} within the cells (recently thapsigargin has been used as an alternative way to increase Ca_i^{2+}) (Brayden et al. 1989). There are highly significant differences in the responses to the two mutant lines compared to the parent line, set out in Table 3. It is seen that while HCA-7 and Colony 3 monolayers respond to A23187, the response in Colony 1 cells is minimal. By contrast, the parent line and Colony 1 monolayers respond to forskolin, while Colony 3 monolayers have small responses. At a superficial level failure to respond to forskolin while responding to A23187 is characteristic of airway epithelia in CF.

Further understanding of the failure to respond to forskolin was followed by measuring the accumulation of cyclic AMP in the cells. As is shown in Table 4 the nucleotide accumulated to concentrations 9–10 times greater than in the other two cell lines. As cyclic AMP was measured in cell extracts and not the supernatant, it might be that leakage from cells was reduced in Colony 3 cells compared to Colony 1, while the activity of the cyclase might be abnormally low in Colony 3. Measurement of adenylate cyclase activity showed the activity to be rather similar in all three cell lines. Finally deficiency in protein kinase A was sought, but not found in Colony 3 monolayers.

It is notable that Colony 1 layers not only accumulate the least cyclic AMP and have barely detectable levels of protein kinase A, but show the most vigorous responses to forskolin. There remains, however, a number of

Table 4. Dome formation in LLC-PK cell clones (from Wohlwend et al. 1986)

Cell line	Dome formation	Transepithelial resistance ($\Omega\,cm^2$)
LLC-PK$_1$ (parent)	+	98 ± 18
D-	−	37 ± 9
D + Sc	+	230 ± 16

unexplained differences between the mutants. Lysylbradykinin (LBK) in many systems operates by stimulating phosphatidylinositol metabolism, a consequence of which is to increase Ca_i^{2+} (Shayman and Morrison 1985; Shayman et al. 1986). Recently we have shown that LBK causes a transient rise in Ca_i^{2+} in HCA-7 cells (Pickles and Cuthbert, unpublished). Colony 1 cells resond significantly better to LBK than do either HCA-7 or Colony 3 cells, yet this line is unresponsive to A23187. This may mean that other aspects of LBK effects are responsible for the increase in short-circuit current, although involvement of prostaglandins has been eliminated.

One way in which chloride secretion can be induced following upon an increase in Ca_i^{2+} is by the activation of Ca^{2+}-sensitive potassium channels. The consequent hyperpolarisation of the apical membrane increases the electrochemical gradient for chloride efflux through the apical membrane. Thus, Colony 3 monolayers might respond to A23187 by this mechanism without the activity of the apical chloride channels per se being modified by cyclic AMP, Ca_i^{2+} or transmembrane voltage. However, Ca^{2+}-sensitive chloride channels have been demonstrated in Colony 3 cells by patch clamping (Henderson and Cuthbert, unpublished).

In summary, the mutant cell lines, Colony 1 and Colony 3, offer some unique opportunities for a molecular genetic approach, for example, for kinin receptors or for control mechanisms for the epithelial chloride channel. However, the problems are significantly greater than with the examples given earlier where cells were selected by survival in low K^+ medium or following proton attack. Clearly, measuring SCC in cultured monolayers or patch clamping apical membranes are not suitable screening techniques for massive numbers of clones. However, DNA-mediated transfection along with a selectable marker gene, such as an engineered neomycin gene (Southern and Berg 1982) provides some selection. Since the location of the CF gene is known, further selection would be achieved by transfection with choromosone 7 fragments. Complementation analysis of the Colony 3 transformants in relation to chloride secretion might then be possible, but would rely on a bioassay in which functional chloride transport is measured. The urgent need, therefore, in eukaryotic systems is to discover simple life or death screening procedures such as are described earlier here. Use of toxic anions that pass through the chloride channel is a possible way forward.

References

Baron WF (1983) Transport of H^+ and of ionic weak acids and bases. J Membr Biol 72: 1–16

Barthelson R, Widdicombe J (1987) Cyclic adenosine monophosphate-dependent kinase in cystic fibrosis tracheal epithelium. J Clin Invest 80: 1799–1802

Berschneider HM, Knowles MR, Azizkhan RG, Boucher RC, Tobey NA, Orlando RC, Powell DW (1988) Altered intestinal chloride transport in cystic fibrosis. FASEB J 2: 2625–2629

Boucher RC, Stutts MJ, Knowles MR, Cautley L, Gatzy JT (1986) Sodium transport in cystic fibrosis epithelia: abnormal basal rate and response to adenylate cyclase activation. J Clin Invest 78: 1245–1252

Brayden DJ, Hanley MR, Thastrup O, Cuthbert AW (1989) Thapsigargin, a new calcium dependent epithelial anion secretagogue. Br J Pharmacol 98: 809–816

Cuthbert A, Cuthbert AW (1978) Fertilization acid production in psammechinus eggs under pH-clamp conditions, and the effects of some pyrazine derivatives. Exp Cell Res 114: 409–415

Cuthbert AW, Egleme C, Greenwood H, Hickman ME, Kirkland SC, McVinish LJ (1987) Calcium- and cyclic AMP-dependent chloride secretion in human colonic epithelia. Br J Pharmacol 91: 503–515

Franchi A, Cragoe E, Pouysségur J (1986a) Isolation and properties of fibroblast mutants over expressing an altered Na^+/H^+ antiporter. J Biol Chem 261: 14614–14620

Franchi A, Perucca-Lostaneen D, Pouysségur J (1986b) Functional expression of a human Na^+/H^+ antiporter gene transfected into antiporter-deficient mouse L cells. Proc Natl Acad Sci USA 83: 9388–9392

Frizzell RA, Rechkemmer G, Shoemaker RL (1986) Altered regulation of airway epithelial cell chloride channels in cystic fibrosis. Science 233: 558–560

Gargus JJ (1987a) Mutant isolation and genes transfer as tools in study of transport proteins. Am J Physiol 252: C457–C467

Gargus JJ (1987b) Selectable mutations altering two mechanisms of mammalian K^+ transport are dominant. Am J Physiol 252: C515–C522

Gargus JJ, Coronado A (1985) A selectable mutation alters the conductance of a mammalian K^+ channel. Fed Proc 44: 1901

Gargus JJ, Miller JL, Slageman CW, Adelberg EA (1978) Genetic alterations in potassium transport in L-cells. Proc Natl Acad Sci USA 75: 5589–5593

Giesen-Crouse EM, McRoberts JA (1987) Coordinate expression of piretanide receptors and Na^+, K^+, Cl cotransport activity in Madin-Darby canine kidney cell mutants. J Biol Chem 262: 17393–17397

Johnson J, Epel D, Paul M (1976) Intracellular pH and activation of sea urchin eggs after fertilisation. Nature 262: 661–664

Kirkland SC (1985) Dome formation by a human adenocarcinoma cell line (HCA-7). Cancer Res 45: 3790–3795

Kirschner LB (1979) Extrarenal action of amiloride in aquatic animals. In: Cuthbert AW, Fanelli GM, Scriabine A (eds) Amiloride and epithelial sodium transport. Urban and Schwarzenberg, Baltimore, pp 41–49

L'Allemain G, Franchi A, Cragoe E, Pouysségur J (1984) Blockade of the Na^+/H^+ antiport abolishes growth factor-induced DNA synthesis in fibroblasts. J Biol Chem 259: 4313–4319

Li M, McCann JD, Leidtke CM, Nairn AC, Greengard P, Welsh MJ (1988) Cyclic-AMP-dependent protein kinase opens chloride channels in normal but not cystic fibrosis airway epithelium. Nature 331: 358–360

McRoberts JA, Tran CT, Saier MH (1983) Characterisation of low potassium-resistant mutants of the Madin-Darby kidney cell line with defects in NaCl/KCl symport. J Biol Chem 258: 12320–12326

Mitas M, Gargus JJ (1985) Successful DNA-mediated transfer of a mammalian gene encoding a potassium transport system. J Gen Physiol 86: 34A

Pouysségur J (1985) The growth factor-activatable Na^+/H^+ exchange system: a genetic approach. Trends in Biochem Sci 10: 453–455

Pouysségur J, Chambard JC, Franchi A, Paris S, van Obberghen-Schilling E (1982) Growth factor activation of an amiloride-sensitive Na^+/H^+ exchange system in quiescent fibroblasts: coupling to ribosomal protein S6 phosphorylation. Proc Natl Acad Sci USA 79: 3935–3939

Pouysségur J, Sardet C, Franchi A, L'Allemain G, Paris S (1984) A specific mutation abolishing Na^+/H^+ antiport activity in hamster fibroblasts precludes growth at neutral and acidic pH. Proc Natl Acad Sci USA 81: 4833–4837

Schaefer WH, Hinrichsen RD, Burgess-Cassler A, Ching Kung Blair IA, Watterson DM (1987) A mutant paramecium with a defective calcium-dependent potassium conductance has an altered calmodulin: A non-lethal selective alteration in calmodulin regulation. Proc Natl Acad Sci USA 84: 3931–3935

Shayman JA, Morrison AR (1985) Bradykinin-induced changes in phosphatidyl inositol turnover in cultured rabbit papillary collecting tubule cells. J Clin Invest 76: 978–984

Shayman JA, Hruska KA, Morrison AR (1986) Bradykinin stimulates increased intracellular calcium in papillary collecting tubules of the rabbit. Biochem Biophys Res Commun 134: 299–304

Southern PJ, Berg P (1982) Transformation of mammalian cells to antibiotic resistance with a bacterial gene under control of the SV40 early region promoter. J Mol Appl Genet 1: 327–341

Sussman I, O'Brien TG (1985) Characterisation of a BALB/c3T3 preadipose cell mutant with altered $Na^+K^+Cl^-$ cotransport activity. J Cell Physiol 124: 153–159

Welsh MJ, Liedtke CM (1986) Chloride and potassium channels in cystic fibrosis airway epithelia. Nature 322: 467–470

Wohlwend A, Vassalli JD, Belin D, Orci L (1986) LLC-PK_1 cells: cloning of phenotypically stable subpopulations. Am J Physiol 250: C682–C687

Use of Nuclear Magnetic Resonance Spectroscopy in the Study of Exocrine Secretion

M. Murakami, Y. Seo, M. C. Steward and H. Watari

Introduction

The ultimate goal in the study of exocrine secretion is to explain the phenomenon in vivo at a molecular level. Such an approach requires non-invasive methods to measure ion and water movements and energy metabolism. Nuclear magnetic resonance (NMR) spectroscopy provides one such method (see e.g. Gadian 1982; Farrar and Becker 1971).

NMR is a physical phenomenon, first observed in 1946, exhibited by certain atomic nuclei when they are placed in a strong magnetic field. The phenomenon is confined to those nuclei that are said to possess 'spin'. Some of the nuclei of biological importance showing this property are listed in Table 1.

When an aqueous solution or a sample of biological tissue is placed in a strong, uniform magnetic field and exposed to a pulse of radio frequency (RF) radiation of the appropriate frequency, particular nuclei in the sample will absorb some of the radiation. The frequency at which this occurs, the resonance frequency, depends on the strength of the magnetic field (Table 1).

For various reasons, identical nuclei present at different locations within a particular molecule absorb at slightly different frequencies. Thus, for

Table 1. NMR characteristics of biologically important nuclei

Nucleus	Spin quantum number	Resonance frequency at 4.7 amd 8.45 T (MHz)		Natural abundance (%)	Relative sensitivity
		4.7 T	8.45 T		
^{1}H	1/2	200.07	360.06	99.985	1
^{7}Li	3/2	77.75	139.93	92.58	0.295
^{13}C	1/2	50.31	90.54	1.108	0.0159
^{17}O	$-5/2$	27.29	49.07	0.037	0.0291
^{19}F	1/2	188.23	338.42	100	0.833
^{23}Na	3/2	52.92	95.24	100	0.0925
^{31}P	1/2	80.99	145.75	100	0.0664
^{35}Cl	3/2	19.6	35.25	75.53	0.0047
^{39}K	3/2	9.34	16.80	93.10	0.00051
^{43}Ca	$-7/2$	13.44	24.18	0.145	0.064

Young · Wong, Epithelial Secretion of Water and Electrolytes
© Springer-Verlag Berlin · Heidelberg 1990

example, the ^{31}P nuclei in a molecule of ATP display a characteristic absorption spectrum in which the three phosphate groups appear as three separate resonance peaks. The differences in frequency, referred to as 'chemical shifts', are very small and are usually measured in parts per million (ppm) of the observation frequency.

Absorption is detected by a receiver coil placed around the sample, in which an electric current is induced as the nuclei recover to their equilibrium state after the RF pulse has been applied. This recovery process, referred to as 'relaxation', is characterized by two time constants, T_1 and T_2.

The great power of NMR for the biologist lies in its ability to detect and identify molecules non-invasively and with great precision in isolated tissues or even whole animals or human subjects. Intracellular events can thus be followed in a single preparation without the need for freeze clamping, tissue digestion and chemical assay. The only drawback of NMR is its relatively low sensitivity. At best it is only possible to detect a compound with good time resolution or in a small sample of tissue if it is present at a fairly high concentration – usually in the millimolar range.

Exocrine glands are particularly well suited to investigation by NMR, especially those, such as the major salivary glands, that are compact, approximately spherical and fairly homogeneous. It is relatively easy to maintain an isolated gland within the magnet of an NMR spectrometer by conventional vascular perfusion methods. The gland can then be stimulated to secrete, transport inhibitors can be applied and extracellular ions substituted during the course of the NMR measurements.

Energy Metabolism

Following the demonstration that ^{31}P NMR could be used to measure ATP, creatine phosphate and inorganic phosphate in skeletal muscle (Hoult et al. 1974), applications in the biological sciences have spread rapidly. ^{31}P NMR has been used to study the kinetics of phosphorus energy metabolites in various epithelia, including the kidney (Balaban et al. 1981), toad urinary bladder (Bond et al. 1981) and frog skin (Lin et al. 1982; Nunnally et al. 1983). The first successful ^{31}P NMR studies of exocrine glands were performed on the isolated perfused dog mandibular gland (Murakami et al. 1982, 1983).

The ^{31}P Spectrum

Seven main resonance peaks are observed in the ^{31}P NMR spectra of mammalian salivary glands (Fig. 1). By comparing the chemical shifts of the resonance peaks with those of pure samples in solution, six peaks have been identified as follows:

1) sugar phosphates (SP) and nucleotide monophosphates (NMP),
2) inorganic phosphate (Pi),
3) creatine phosphate (PCr),
4) γ-phosphate of nucleotide triphosphates (γ-NTP) and β-phosphate of nucleotide diphosphates (β-NDP),
5) α-NTP and α-NDP, nicotinamide adenine dinucleotide (NAD^+) and reduced NAD (NADH),
7) β-NTP.

The areas and the heights of the phosphorus peaks have been found to remain stable during perfusion for at least 48 h, indicating that the viability of the isolated gland can be maintained for long periods.

Although ^{31}P NMR spectroscopy can measure the total amount of nucleotide phosphate, it cannot discriminate between the different bases since ATP, GTP and UTP have similar spectra. Although the ATP system is known as the major energy carrier, GTP is also recognized as the energy donor to several biosynthetic pathways such as those for cellulose, porphyrin, protein, etc. (Lehninger 1975). By use of high performance liquid chromatography (HPLC) of perchloric acid extracts of the rat mandibular gland (Murakami et al. 1987), 80%–90% of the NTP resonance has been found to be due to ATP (1.86 ± 0.03 mmol/kg wet weight) and the rest to GTP (0.37 ± 0.01 mmol/kg). Although UTP is known to act as a phosphate donor for polysaccharide synthesis and may possibly participate in mucin synthesis in salivary glands, it was present at less than the noise level of the HPLC measurement, viz. 0.05 mmol/kg.

Comparing the ^{31}P NMR spectrum of the rat mandibular gland (Fig. 1) with that of the dog gland (Murakami et al. 1983, 1984; Nakahari et al. 1985), many similarities are observed. However, the phosphodiester resonances present in the dog gland are not observed in the rat gland, and while the sugar phosphate of the dog gland is observed as a composite resonance of several components, that of the rat gland appears to be just a single

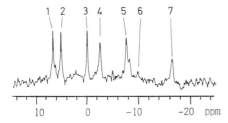

Fig. 1. ^{31}P NMR spectrum of the perfused rat mandibular gland. Seven resonance peaks, of which six were identified, were observed: (*1*) sugar phosphates and nucleotide monophosphate, (*2*) inorganic phosphate, (*3*) creatine phosphate, (*4*) γ-phosphate of nucleotide triphosphate (γ-NTP) and β-phosphate of nucleotide diphosphate (β-NDP), (*5*) α-NTP and α-NDP, NAD^+ and NADH, (*6*) an unidentified peak, and (*7*) β-NTP. In this spectrum the area of each resonance is proportional to the content of the respective component in the gland

component. The rabbit mandibular gland (Seo et al. 1988b) shows a similar ^{31}P spectrum (Fig. 10a) to the rat gland.

In the isolated perfused rat pancreas (Matsumoto et al. 1988), the levels of phosphodiesters and sugar phosphates are higher than those of the mandibular gland. PCr is present in the pancreas, but not in the isolated perfused liver (Tsukamoto et al. 1988), while the isolated perfused kidney contains only a small amount (Takano et al. 1988).

Measurement of Absolute Concentrations

The signal areas of the ^{31}P NMR spectrum are proportional to the concentrations of the ^{31}P nuclei in the sample. Consequently, a simple estimation of the concentration of a metabolite is possible by comparison with a reference solution. However, biological material does not usually fill the sample volume completely, and the intracellular volume of the sample may be unknown. Consequently, the estimation of intracellular concentration in biological tissues and organs is not simple.

One possible approach is by comparison with another method such as tissue analysis by HPLC (Table 2). This is satisfactory for organs in which energy metabolism is slow, such as skeletal muscle, but in organs with rapid metabolism, more refined techniques are required for chemical analysis. Another method is to use a compound indicating the size of the extracellular space. Dawson et al. (1977) used a 10 mmol/l phosphate buffer to determine the volume fraction of the extracellular space in skeletal muscle, and a similar method can be used for perfused glands.

Table 2. Tissue concentrations of phosphorus compounds in perfused rat mandibular salivary gland

Concentrations of nucleotides measured by HPLC (mmol/kg wet weight)[a]

ATP	GTP	ADP	GDP	AMP	GMP
1.86 ±0.03	0.37 ±0.01	0.47 ±0.02	0.10 ±0.004	0.37 ±0.01	0.40 ±0.02

Concentrations of phosphorus compounds measured by ^{31}P NMR (mmol/kg wet weight)[b]

Pi	PCr	NDP	ADP	NTP	ATP
3.6	3.3	0.5	0.4	2.2[b]	1.86[b]

Pi, inorganic phosphate; PCr, creatine phosphate; NDP, ADP+GDP; NTP, ATP+GTP
[a] Values are means ±SEM for five glands.
[b] Values of NTP and ATP were measured by HPLC and values of other phosphorus compounds are estimated from relative concentrations determined from ^{31}P NMR spectra of 26 glands.

Relaxation Times

The relaxation time constants, T_1 and T_2, are important for the following reasons:

(a) the values of T_1 and T_2 contain information about the structure and mobility of the molecule in the living tissue;
(b) the T_1 value determines the amount of saturation occurring at a given pulse repetition rate and may be used to correct for this effect;
(c) the line shape and line width are partly determined by T_2;
(d) saturation transfer NMR techniques, which can be used to measure the rate of chemical exchange, depend upon a knowledge of the T_1 values of the intermediates.

Unfortunately, the low sensitivity of the ^{31}P nucleus is a hindrance for the measurement of the spin-lattice relaxation times (T_1) in biological systems. The standard inversion recovery method, used widely in ^1H NMR, requires a prohibitively long time. To overcome this difficulty, the variable nutation method (Homer and Beevers 1985; Seo et al. 1988a) has been used. This reduces the time required for the measurement to 10% of that required for the inversion-recovery method. The method has been applied to several tissues, including the rat mandibular gland (Suzuki et al. 1989).

Compartmentation

In general, if the motion of the nuclei is restricted, the T_2 relaxation time will be shorter and the resonance peak broader. For example, the less-mobile phosphate groups, such as those of the phospholipids of the cell membrane and ADP bound to actin filaments, are detected as extremely broad resonances with a line width at half height of 1–5 kHz. The ^{31}P NMR signals of ATP in mitochondria may be broadened by the restricted mobility of ATP and also by the presence of paramagnetic ions (Ogawa et al. 1978). These observations suggest that both bound and mitochondrial ATP in living cells may be invisible to ^{31}P NMR.

Compartmentation of ATP has recently been suggested in the rat mandibular gland (Murakami et al. 1987). The ATP content of the hypoxic gland (after perfusion had been stopped for 20 min) was measured by HPLC as 60% of that of the aerobic resting gland, whereas a 50% decrease in the ATP content of the gland was observed by ^{31}P NMR after 15 min of hypoxia. This observation suggests the presence of a small fraction of NMR-invisible ATP in the mandibular gland, but, as a fraction of the total ATP, it may be somewhat less than in myocardium (Takami et al. 1988).

Effects of Perfusion Rate

Changes in the tissue content of creatine phosphate and ATP reflect an imbalance in the supply and consumption of the common energy source, ATP. Cessation of perfusion, for example, causes hypoxia and reduces the supply of ATP from oxidative metabolism. Figure 2 shows the changes in the ^{31}P spectrum that occurred in the canine mandibular gland when perfusion was stopped (Murakami et al. 1983). The level of PCr decreased more quickly than that of ATP, suggesting that PCr donates high energy phosphate to ATP via the Lohmann reaction. This pathway seems to contribute substantially to energy metabolism in the salivary gland. The

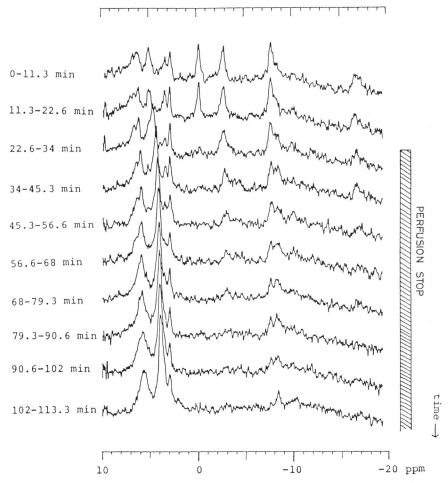

Fig. 2. Metabolic changes in the ^{31}P NMR spectrum of the perfused canine mandibular salivary gland induced by cessation of perfusion. Sequential 11-min spectra were collected before and after the arterial perfusion line was clamped (*hatched bar*)

same phenomenon was observed in the rat pancreas (Matsumoto et al. 1986, 1988). When perfusion was stopped, the levels of ATP and PCr decreased, while the levels of PME and Pi increased. In addition, the Pi resonance shifted to a lower frequency, indicating that the tissue pH decreased (see below). On reperfusion, the levels of phosphorus compounds and the tissue pH were restored to their resting values.

Changes during Secretion

Stimulation of secretion increases the oxygen consumption in the salivary gland (Terroux et al. 1959; Murakami 1981), indicating that the supply of ATP from oxidative metabolism is increased during salivary secretion. In the canine mandibular gland, 1 μmol/l acetylcholine caused no change in the ATP content, but decreased the content of PCr, suggesting that the increase in the supply of ATP was mainly via the Lohmann reaction and that it compensated quite well for the increase in the consumption of ATP. It is widely believed that an increase in Na^+ entry due to acetylcholine stimulation (Imai 1965; Burgen 1956; Poulsen 1974; Goto 1981) increases the activity of the Na^+-, K^+-ATPase, thus increasing the consumption of ATP.

In the rat pancreas, continuous infusion of 0.1 μmol/l acetylcholine caused marked and sustained increases in the flow of pancreatic juice (4.8 ± 0.5 μl/g-min, mean $\pm$ SEM) and protein output (190 ± 43 μg/g-min) although the tissue levels of phosphorus compounds remained unchanged (Matsumoto et al. 1988). This suggests that the consumption of ATP during secretion in the pancreas may be compensated immediately by ATP production from oxidative metabolism.

In salivary glands, continuous stimulation with 1 μmol/l acetylcholine causes 'tachyphylaxis', a time-dependent decrease in secretory rate. This is more pronounced at higher concentrations of acetylcholine (Case et al. 1980; Murakami et al. 1986b) and has been attributed to the accumulation of excess cytosolic Ca^{2+} (Putney 1978). Since higher doses of acetylcholine may also have effects on energy metabolism, these have also been investigated (Murakami et al. 1986b, 1988). Stimulation of the rat mandibular gland with 1 μmol/l acetylcholine induced a tachyphylactic secretory response, a persistently elevated oxygen consumption, and decreased PCr and ATP (Fig. 3a). In contrast, 1 mmol/l acetylcholine caused an initial burst of secretion that was followed by suppression of secretion. Oxygen consumption increased to the same level as that with 1 μmol/l acetylcholine, indicating a dissociation between secretion and oxygen consumption. During stimulation with 1 mmol/l acetylcholine, the level of PCr first decreased and then partially recovered (Fig. 3b), but the level of ATP continued to decrease and the levels of Pi and SP increased markedly. These observations suggest compartmentation of creatine phosphokinase (CPK) isoenzymes (Furuyama et al. 1980) and the possibility that a high concentration of acetylcholine

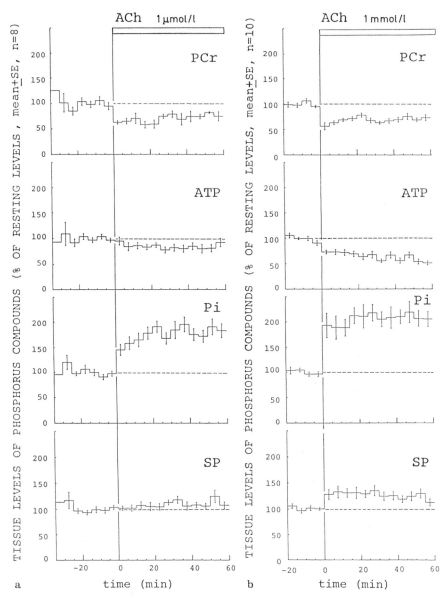

Fig. 3a, b. Time courses of the changes in content of creatine phosphate (PCr), ATP, inorganic phosphate (Pi) and sugar phosphates (SP) of the perfused rat mandibular gland induced by acetylcholine (ACh). Means $\pm$SEM are presented as percentages of the resting level. Eight and ten glands were used for **a** 1.0 μmol/l and **b** 1.0 mmol/l of ACh stimulation, respectively

interferes with the intracellular transport of PCr, possibly between one CPK system near the Na^+-, K^+-ATPase and another system near the mitochondria in the acinar cells.

^{31}P NMR has also been used to study energy metabolism in the rabbit mandibular gland (Seo et al. 1988b). The content of high-energy phosphates and the ratio of MgATP to total ATP (from the chemical shift of β-ATP; Gadian et al. 1979) were measured during stimulation with 10^{-9} to 10^{-4} mol/l acetylcholine. Even during stimulation with the higher doses of acetylcholine, PCr decreased more than ATP, indicating no significant retardation of the Lohmann reaction. In addition, there was no evidence of any inhibition of ATP usage caused by a decrease in MgATP availability.

The Effects of Na^+ Replacement

In most epithelial transport systems, the Na^+-, K^+-ATPase is believed to establish the Na^+ gradient across the cell membrane which provides the driving force for Na^+-coupled transport systems. The dependence of fluid secretion and the levels of phosphorus compounds on extracellular Na^+ have thus been studied in the perfused canine mandibular gland (Murakami et al. 1984). If the Na^+ gradient across the basolateral membrane is reduced by depletion of the extracellular Na^+, the entry of Na^+ into the cell during secretion should be decreased. Reduced Na^+ entry will reduce the activity of the Na^+-, K^+-ATPase and may thus change the levels of ATP and PCr.

When the Na^+ in the perfusate was completely replaced with Li^+, acetylcholine induced only a minimal rate of salivary secretion and no change in the ATP and PCr levels. Restoration of Na^+ to the perfusate, even without added acetylcholine, caused a decrease in ATP and PCr and a small increase in salivary secretion. These results suggest that the activity of the Na^+-,K^+-ATPase is increased via a rise in the intracellular Na^+ concentration and that salivary secretion may be stimulated not only by added secretomotor agonists, but also by an increase in Na^+ entry alone.

In Vivo Studies

The technique of topical magnetic resonance (TMR) was developed for in situ NMR spectroscopy. It uses a method of magnetic focussing (Tanaka et al. 1974) to obtain ^{31}P NMR signals selectively from a small volume within the intact animal, including organs deep within the body (Gordon et al. 1980). ^{31}P TMR has been applied to two preparations of the canine mandibular gland (Nakahari et al. 1985): one with a normal blood supply (in situ) and the other an isolated gland perfused with artificial perfusate (in vitro). Salivary secretion was found to be greater in situ than in vitro. In situ, only the PCr content decreased during secretion, whereas in vitro both PCr and ATP decreased, possibly as the result of inadequate perfusion.

Electrolyte Transport

In exocrine glands, electrolytes such as Na^+, K^+, and Cl^- play important roles in the transport mechanisms mediating water and electrolyte secretion. The nuclear spins of these electrolytes are all 3/2 and their resulting 'quadrupole moments' show different NMR characteristics from nuclei of spin 1/2, such as ^{31}P, ^{13}C and ^1H. Their more complex relaxation behaviour has been discussed by Hubbard (1970) and Berendsen and Edzes (1973).

Tissue Na^+ content has been measured by ^{23}Na NMR in various biological tissues: skeletal muscle, frog skin, kidney, brain, liver and nerve bundle (e.g. Civan and Shporer 1978). The values obtained by ^{23}Na NMR from these tissues were about 60% of the values obtained from the ashed material dissolved in water. This result was explained as follows: Na^+ ions interact with macromolecules in the tissue and their motion is restricted, resulting in the broadening of the resonance and underestimation of the resonance area. Initially, this problem was further complicated by the difficulty of discriminating between Na^+ in the intracellular and extracellular compartments. As mentioned below, more recent NMR studies using chemical shift reagents have been able to discriminate between the two compartments and have demonstrated that more than 80% of the intracellular Na^+ in erythrocytes is visible to NMR (Boulanger et al. 1985).

Total Gland Content

Using a tunable, broad-band probe, multinuclear magnetic resonance can be applied to a single gland. In this way, the total content of Na^+, Li^+ and Cl^- has been measured non-invasively in the perfused rat mandibular gland, continuously and with good time resolution (20 s or better; Murakami et al. 1986a).

Figure 4 shows ^{23}Na, ^7Li, ^{35}Cl NMR spectra obtained from the gland during an experiment in which one half or all of the extracellular Na^+ was replaced with Li^+. When the peristaltic pump was stopped briefly at the beginning of the experiment, the ^{23}Na signal decreased after 10 s to about

---

Fig. 4a – c. Total content of Na, Li and Cl of the perfused rat mandibular gland measured by ^{23}Na, ^7Li and ^{35}Cl NMR during an experiment in which one half or all of the extracellular Na was replaced with Li. **a** ^{23}Na NMR spectra were obtained at 95.24 MHz every 15 or 20 s. Accumulations of 12 or 17 transients (free induction decay, FID) were collected with a recycling time of 1 s using a 45° RF pulse; the additional 3 s were necessary for computer processing and data storage. **b** $^7Li^+$ NMR spectra were simultaneously obtained at 139.9 MHz every 15 s. The recycling time was 1 s, using a 5° pulse, and 12 scans were accumulated. **c** ^{35}Cl NMR spectra were obtained at 35.28 MHz every 15 s, using a recycling time of 0.5 s and a 60° pulse, and accumulations of 24 FID. Na and Li concentrations are mmol/l. Asterisks indicate spectra obtained during cessation of perfusion (see text)

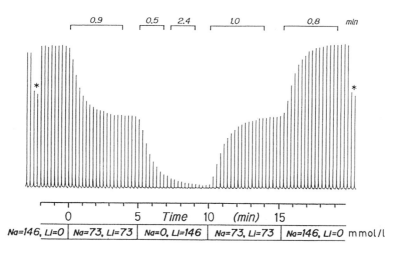

a

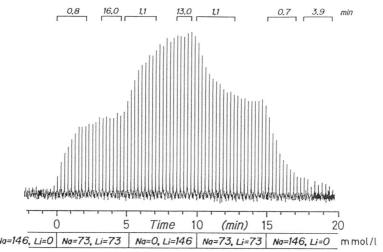

b

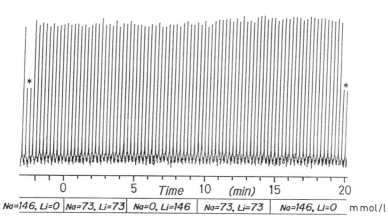

c

65% of the initial value. This decrement was also observed in the ^{35}Cl signal and could be due to shrinkage of the oedema that developed during perfusion. The ^{23}Na signal changed predictably when the Na^+ concentration of the perfusate was reduced. The time course had a single time constant of 0.9 min when the Na^+ concentration of the perfusate remained above 73 mmol/l. However, when Na^+ was completely replaced with Li^+, a slow component (2.4–2.7 min) appeared in addition to the faster component (0.5–0.7 min). The absence of the slow component during partial Na^+ replacement suggests that 73 mmol/l perfusate Na^+ is enough to maintain the normal intracellular Na^+ concentration in the unstimulated mandibular gland.

When all of the extracellular Na^+ was replaced with Li^+, the ^7Li signal increased exponentially with two time constants of about 1 and 8 min. When the extracellular Li^+ was restored to Na^+, Li^+ decreased quickly with a time constant of about 1.3 min. This value is in the same range as that for Na^+ restoration. However, some Li^+ remained in the gland, presumably in an intracellular compartment, and was slow to leave because of the absence of a Li^+ extrusion system.

The Cl^- level in the gland remained almost constant throughout the Na^+ replacement experiment. When the peristaltic pump was stopped, the ^{35}Cl signal decreased quickly due to shrinkage of the oedema.

^{23}Na Studies

Separation of Intracellular and Extracellular Signals

To understand secretory mechanisms, it is important to be able to determine the concentrations of intracellular ions and to trace their changes during secretion. In order to discriminate the intracellular Na^+ signal from that due to the extracellular Na^+ in the rat mandibular gland, an aqueous chemical shift reagent, dysprosium triethylenetetramine-N,N,N',N'',N''',N'''-hexaacetic acid, $Dy(TTHA)^{3-}$, has been used (Seo et al. 1987a). $Dy(TTHA)^{3-}$ shifts the Na^+ resonance frequency to a higher frequency in proportion to the concentration of $Dy(TTHA)^{3-}$. Since its physical properties are similar to those of Cr ethylenediaminetetra acetate, Cr(EDTA), the complex cannot enter the intracellular space and only the signal from Na^+ in the extracellular fluid is shifted to a higher frequency. Thus, it is possible to discriminate intracellular and extracellular Na^+ from the difference in their chemical shifts.

Another chemical shift reagent, dysprosium tripolyphosphate $(Dy(PPP)_2^{7-})$, has also been used to determine intracellular and extracellular Na^+ concentrations, both in frog skin (Civan et al. 1983) and in human erythrocytes (Gupta and Gupta 1982). $Dy(PPP)_2^{7-}$ can produce shifts large enough to allow the intracellular and extracellular Na^+ to be discriminated, but in its biological applications, several problems arise as a result of its low stability: (a) free tripolyphosphate chelates Ca^{2+} and decreases the extracellular free Ca^{2+} (Gullans et al. 1985), and (b) free Dy^{3+} accumulates in the cells (Boulanger et al. 1985). By using $Dy(TTHA)^{3-}$, one of the most stable lanthanide complexes, these problems can largely be overcome (Bryden and Reilley 1981; Masuda et al. 1978; Chu et al. 1984).

The viability of the rat salivary gland and pancreas, when perfused with a modified Krebs solution containing 10 mmol/l $Dy(TTHA)^{3-}$, has been assessed by determining the secretory responses of the glands and the tissue levels of high-energy phosphates (Seo et al. 1987a). When the $Dy(TTHA)^{3-}$-perfused mandibular gland was stimulated with acetylcholine, the initial secretion was found to be similar to that of the gland perfused with normal Krebs solution, but the plateau phase of secretion was depressed to a rate as low as one half of that of the gland perfused without $Dy(TTHA)^{3-}$. The amounts of pancreatic juice secreted and the output of protein from the $Dy(TTHA)^{3-}$-perfused pancreas were also smaller than the values obtained in the control gland. This inhibition is explained by the fact that free $TTHA^{6-}$ chelated Ca^{2+} ions and reduced the extracellular free Ca^{2+} concentration to 0.4 mmol/l.

During perfusion with $Dy(TTHA)^{3-}$, ATP and creatine phosphate were measured by ^{31}P NMR spectroscopy. Although the ^{31}P spectrum showed a slight broadening of the resonances, the content of high energy phosphates was maintained. $Dy(TTHA)^{3-}$ is thus thought to have only a small effect on the physiological functions of the perfused salivary gland and pancreas, mainly as a result of the reduced Ca^{2+} activity of the perfusate.

Changes in Intracellular Na^+ During Secretion

A typical ^{23}Na NMR spectrum from the rat mandibular gland perfused with 10 mmol/l $Dy(TTHA)^{3-}$ is shown in Fig. 5. The spectrum appears to consist of three components. The resonance at 0.0 ppm was assigned as the signal from intracellular Na^+ (Na^+_{in}) although it could include some contamination from Na^+ in a compartment inaccessible to $Dy(TTHA)^{3-}$. Although $Dy(TTHA)^{3-}$ did not appear in the saliva, the Na^+ content of the luminal fluid of the gland can be estimated as only amounting to 5%–8% of Na^+_{in} from stereological (Tamarin and Sreebny 1965) and micropuncture data (Young and Schögel 1966). Such a small component would lie within the error of determination of Na^+_{in} from the resonance.

Measured in this way, the Na^+_{in} of resting glands ranged from around 5 mmol/l intracellular fluid (ICF) to over 40 mmol/l ICF, with a median value of around 15 mmol/l ICF. In spite of the broad distribution, the mean value of Na^+_{in} was similar to that measured by flame photometry (Schneyer and Schneyer 1962; Imai 1965), but was lower than that obtained by electron probe X-ray microanalysis (Sasaki et al. 1983).

Following the onset of stimulation with acetylcholine (1 µmol/l), Na^+_{in} increased by 9.1 ± 1.5 mmol/l ICF and remained at this level during sustained stimulation (Seo et al. 1987b, Fig. 6a). In the initial phase of

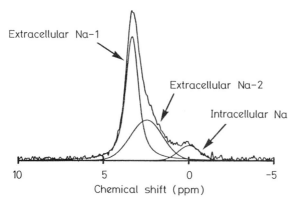

Extracellular Na-1

Extracellular Na-2

Intracellular Na

10   5   0   -5

Chemical shift (ppm)

Fig. 5. ^{23}Na NMR spectrum of the rat mandibular salivary gland perfused with the aqueous chemical-shift reagent, Dy(TTHA)$^{3-}$: original spectrum and the result of line shape analysis. The spectrum consists of three components: one intracellular and two extracellular. The difference in chemical shift between the two resonances (3.23 and 2.20 ppm) suggests two compartments in the extracellular space containing different concentrations of Dy(TTHA)$^{3-}$

secretion (0–5 min), about 50 mmol min^{-1}l^{-1} ICF of Na$^+$ was secreted into the luminal space (estimated from the secretory rate by assuming an isotonic primary secretion), but, in spite of the higher secretory rate, Na$_{in}^+$ increased at an initial rate of only 4.1 mmol min^{-1}l^{-1} ICF.

During the plateau phase of secretion (15–30 min), ouabain (1 mmol/l) caused an increment in Na$_{in}^+$ of 44±8 mmol min^{-1}l^{-1} ICF (Fig. 6b). From the rate of increase of Na$_{in}^+$, the influx of Na$^+$ during the plateau phase was estimated to be 4.5 mmol min^{-1}l^{-1} ICF. This corresponds with about 50% of the secretory rate for Na$^+$ during the plateau phase of secretion as estimated from the fluid secretory rate. This is consistent with the operation of the Na$^+$–K$^+$–2Cl$^-$ cotransport system from which one would expect a Na$^+$ influx rate equal to one half of the overall rate of Na$^+$ and Cl$^-$ secretion.

^{39}K Studies

Separation of Intracellular and Extracellular Signals

^{39}K is one of the least sensitive nuclei for NMR. Its relative sensitivity compared with ^{23}Na is $5 \cdot 10^{-3}$. In addition, strong acoustic ringing in the RF coil and the broad resonance of the intracellular K$^+$ reduce the Signal-to-noise (S/N) ratio of the spectrum. It is therefore quite difficult to measure K$^+$ quickly and accurately. Nonetheless, the use of ^{39}K NMR to measure intracellular K$^+$ by means of chemical shift reagents has recently received attention as a way of studying epithelial K$^+$ transport in vivo (Pike et al. 1983; Ogino et al. 1985; Gullans et al. 1985).

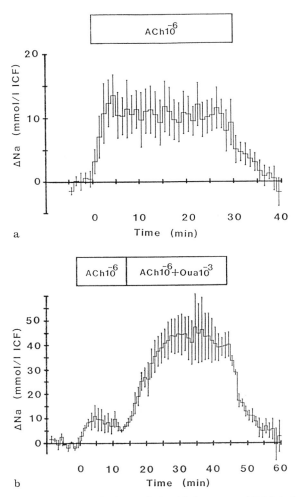

Fig. 6a. Changes in intracellular Na^+ content (ΔNa) induced by 1 µmol/l acetylcholine (ACh 10^{-6}) in the perfused rat mandibular salivary gland at 24 °C. Means and SEM of 5 to 13 glands are presented. **b** Changes in ΔNa induced by 1 µmol/l acetylcholine with 1 mmol/l ouabain (ACh 10^{-6} + Oua 10^{-3}) at 24 °C. Means and SEM of four glands are presented

The ^{39}K NMR spectrum of the perfused rat mandibular gland consists of two components (Fig. 7; Seo et al. 1987c): one is a broad resonance with a line width of 120 Hz and the other is a sharp resonance with line width of 10 Hz. By using $Dy(TTHA)^{3-}$, Seo et al. (1987c) were able to assign the broad resonance as the intracellular K^+ and the sharp resonance as the extracellular K^+.

These two components also show a significant difference in their T_1 relaxation times. The sharp resonance has a long T_1 (ca. 55 ms), whereas the broad resonance has a short T_1 (ca. 3 ms). This suggests that there is some

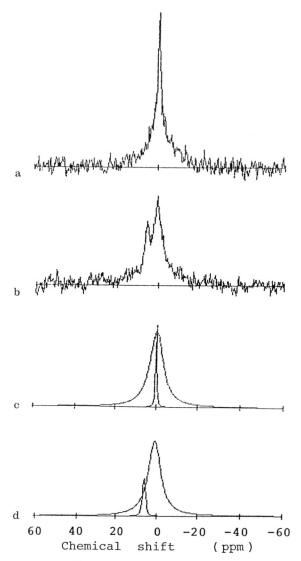

a

b

c

d

60   40   20   0   -20   -40   -60
Chemical   shift   (ppm)

Fig. 7a – d. ^{39}K NMR spectrum of the perfused rat mandibular gland. **a** The spectrum of the gland perfused without shift reagent consists of two components: one is a broad resonance with a line width of 120 Hz and the other is a sharp resonance with line width of 10 Hz. The result of using a line-shaped fitting routine is shown in **c. b** Spectrum of the gland perfused with the aqueous chemical-shift reagent, $Dy(TTHA)^{3-}$. The sharp resonance from K^+ in the perfusate is shifted 5 ppm down field, whereas the broad resonance from the intracellular K^+ retains its original chemical shift and its area is unchanged (**d**)

interaction between the K^+ and large molecules in the cytosol. On the other hand, the significant difference in the T_1 values offers an alternative to the use of shift reagents for discriminating between intra- and extracellular K^+.

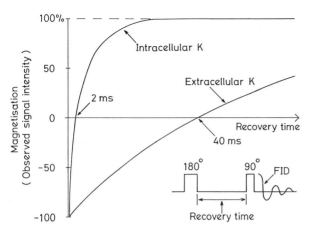

Fig. 8. Discrimination between intracellular and extracellular K^+ using a ^{39}K NMR inversion recovery pulse sequence. Initially, a $180°$ pulse is applied to invert the magnetisation. Thereafter, the magnetisation starts to relax to its original value according to its relaxation time constants. The magnetisation of the intracellular K^+ relaxes quickly with a relaxation time of 3 ms and returns to its original value after 15 ms. The extracellular K^+ relaxes with a relaxation time of 55 ms and passes through zero at around 40 ms. Thus a $90°$ pulse applied 40 ms after the $180°$ pulse will excite only the intracellular K^+. *FID*, free induction decay

This is achieved by using an inversion recovery pulse sequence, as shown in Fig. 8 (Seo et al. 1987c). With this method it is possible to obtain a spectrum consisting only of the intracellular K^+ without having to use a chemical shift reagent.

Simultaneous Measurement of Net Fluxes

NMR spectroscopy can thus provide useful information about the intracellular content of ^{23}Na and ^{39}K in perfused glands. Stimulation of secretion alters the ion fluxes across the cell membranes, and the resulting imbalance of influx and efflux may cause changes in the intracellular content. By the law of mass balance, the change in intracellular content should match the cumulative value of the net flux and vice versa.

It is well established that the mechanism of fluid secretion in the salivary gland involves substantial net movements of K^+. Since Burgen (1956) first noticed that the secreting salivary gland lost K^+ both to the saliva and to the blood perfusing the gland, the handling of K^+ by the salivary acinar cells has been studied by various methods including flame photometry (Schneyer and Schneyer 1962; Goto 1981), ion-selective microelectrodes (Poulsen and Oakley 1978; Mori et al. 1984) and electron probe X-ray microanalysis (Sasaki et al. 1983). The great advantage of the NMR method is that it can be carried out simultaneously with net flux measurements by flame photometry or with ion-selective electrodes (Murakami et al. 1989).

In the rat mandibular gland, the net fluxes of K^+ to the venous blood and to the saliva have been calculated from the flow rates and K^+ concentrations of the saliva and venous effluent during stimulation with 1 µmol/l acetylcholine (Murakami et al. 1989). K^+ was initially released to the vascular side and subsequently taken up from vascular side during sustained stimulation. The amount of K^+ taken up from the vascular side was the same as that secreted in the saliva. The Na^+ fluxes were obtained by the same procedure. Although the sensitivity of the method used to measure changes in Na^+ concentration was relatively low compared with that for K^+, the behaviour of Na^+ was the mirror image of that of K^+ (Murakami et al. 1989).

Changes in Intracellular K^+ During Secretion

Changes in the intracellular K^+ content (K_{in}^+) of the rat mandibular gland during stimulation with 1 µmol/l acetylcholine have been observed by ^{39}K NMR using the method based on the difference of the intracellular and extracellular T_1 values (Fig. 9a, Murakami et al. 1989). K_{in}^+ decreased to about 70% of the control level within 5 min and remained at a steady level (66%) during sustained stimulation. Ion analysis of the venous effluent and saliva, as described above, had indicated that the K_{in}^+ was maintained at a steady level during sustained stimulation. This was thus confirmed by ^{39}K NMR.

Withdrawal of acetylcholine caused a transient increase in K^+ uptake. The amount of K^+ taken up during the recovery phase compensated for the initial loss of K^+ from the gland. ^{39}K NMR showed directly that after removal of acetylcholine, K_{in}^+ returned to its original level. Furthermore, the changes in K_{in}^+ caused by stimulation with acetylcholine were the mirror image of the changes in Na_{in}^+.

The change in K_{in}^+ visible to ^{39}K NMR was also compared with the amount of K^+ released, as determined by flame photometry. ^{39}K NMR gave a value of 34% for the decrement in K_{in}^+ upon stimulation with acetylcholine, whilst flame photometry gave 27 mmol/kg as the amount of K^+ released from the gland. Using measured values for the intracellular volume fraction and the solid mass fraction of the gland, K_{in}^+ was calculated to be 167 mmol/l ICF, which agrees well with a previously reported value of 157 mmol/l ICF (Schneyer and Schneyer 1960).

Blocking the Na^+-, K^+-ATPase during the plateau phase of secretion with 1 mmol/l ouabain reduced oxygen consumption to 20 µl/g per min and stopped secretion quickly. This was accompanied by a transient release of K^+ to the vascular side, measured by flame photometry, which decreased exponentially to zero over a period of 15 min. ^{39}K NMR revealed a 40% decrease in K_{in}^+ to a steady level equivalent to 29% of the resting level (Fig. 9b, Murakami et al. 1989). The cumulative K^+ loss to the effluent and saliva was measured as about 84.8 ± 4.7 mmol/kg by flame photometry.

Removal of ouabain and acetylcholine transiently increased the oxygen consumption of the gland to 40 ml/kg per min. It then recovered to the

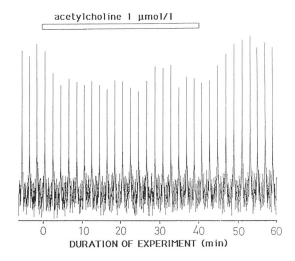

a

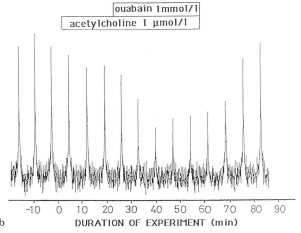

b

Fig. 9a. Changes in intracellular K^+ content (K_{in}^+) of the perfused rat mandibular gland induced by 1 µmol/l acetylcholine at 25 °C. ^{39}K NMR spectra of the intracellular K^+ were collected every 2 min using the inversion recovery pulse sequence shown in Fig. 8, and data from 11 series of experiments with the same protocol were summed. **b** Changes in K_{in}^+ induced by 1 µmol/l acetylcholine with the further addition of 1 mmol/l ouabain. Data from six series of experiments with the same protocol were summed

resting level after a further 15 min. During this recovery period, K^+ was taken up from the vascular side at a rate that declined to zero after 15 min. The cumulative K^+ uptake during the recovery period was 81.9 ± 11.2 mmol/kg, which indicates a complete compensation of K^+ loss. ^{39}K NMR showed that K_{in}^+ recovered to the resting level within 20 min. The recovery process is apparently dominated by active transport since the rate of recovery of K_{in}^+ was increased by a factor of approximately two when the temperature was raised from 24 °C to 37 °C.

Intracellular pH

Another parameter that may be measured by NMR spectroscopy is intracellular pH (pH_i). Much may be learnt about the mechanisms of electrolyte transport in exocrine tissues by studying the changes in pH_i that accompany secretion (e.g. Lau et al., this volume). Absolute values of pH_i provide information about transmembrane H^+ and HCO_3^- gradients, whilst changes in pH_i reflect the net fluxes of H^+ and HCO_3^- in and out of the cells.

NMR Methods

The most commonly used NMR method is based on information that is already present in the ^{31}P NMR spectrum. Other methods depend on the introduction of pH-sensitive, NMR-detectable indicator molecules into the cytosol.

Using ^{31}P NMR, pH_i may be determined from the chemical shift of the endogenous Pi (Fig. 10). The reliability of this method and the problems of calibration have been discussed extensively elsewhere (e.g. Gillies et al. 1982; Seo et al. 1983; Adler et al. 1984). Briefly, HPO_4^{2-} and $H_2PO_4^-$ ions have different chemical shifts in the ^{31}P NMR spectrum, but because exchange between the two is rapid, a single resonance with an intermediate chemical shift appears in the spectrum. The chemical shift of Pi (δ), usually measured with reference to the PCr resonance, is related to pH according to:

$$pH = pK_a + \log \frac{\delta - \delta_1}{\delta_2 - \delta}$$

as illustrated in Fig. 10b. The values of δ_1 and δ_2, the chemical shifts of $H_2PO_4^-$ and HPO_4^{2-}, respectively, and the value of pK_a in the intracellular environment may be measured using tissue homogenates or solutions made up to resemble the composition of the cytosol. The greatest degree of uncertainty concerns the value of pK_a because this parameter is sensitive to ionic strength, Mg^{2+} concentration and temperature (Seo et al. 1983). As a result, absolute values of pH_i measured by this method are subject to an uncertainty of about 0.1 pH units. Changes in pH_i, however, are quite accurately determined in the physiological range.

Unless extracellular pH is so different from pH_i that the two Pi resonances can be separately resolved, it is necessary to work with phosphate-free perfusion media. In addition, the low concentration of intracellular Pi often observed in well-perfused tissues sets a limit to the time resolution that may be achieved by this method. Reliable measurements of pH_i in an unstimulated rabbit mandibular gland in a 4.7 T spectrometer, for example, may require 5 to 10 min of signal accumulation.

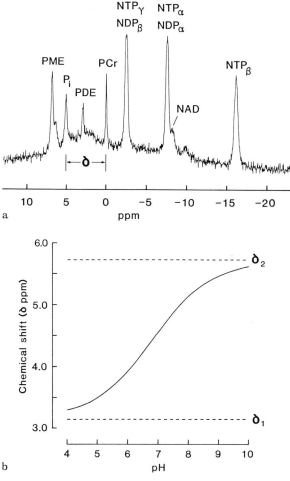

a

b

Fig. 10a. ^{31}P NMR spectrum of the isolated, perfused rabbit mandibular salivary gland at 37°C. The chemical shift (δ) of Pi with respect to PCr is indicated by the *arrows*. *PME*, phosphomonoesters; *Pi*, inorganic phosphate; *PDE*, phosphodiesters; *PCr*, creatine phosphate; *NAD*, nicotinamide adenine dinucleotide; *NTP/NDP*, nucleoside tri/diphosphates (mainly ATP and ADP). Data from Steward et al. (1989). **b** Relation between chemical shift of Pi (referred to PCr) and pH as described by the formula given in the text. δ_1 and δ_2 (*broken lines*) are the chemical shifts of $H_2PO_4^-$ and HPO_4^{2-}, respectively. The pKa was taken to be 6.8 in this example

Another problem arises in tissues that contain heterogeneous cell populations. Because the NMR method pools Pi signals from all of the cells in the sample, the measured value of pH_i may be a weighted average of a range of different values. In salivary glands this is not a serious problem because the acinar cell population greatly outnumbers other cell types. The ductal cells in the rabbit parotid gland, for example, occupy only about 5% of the total gland volume (Cope 1978).

The first measurements of pH_i by ^{31}P NMR in intact mammalian salivary glands were obtained from the dog mandibular gland, both in vitro (Murakami et al. 1983) and in vivo (Nakahari et al. 1985), the latter study using the technique of TMR. More recent studies, described below, have used ^{31}P NMR to investigate in detail the changes in pH_i that accompany secretion in the isolated, perfused rabbit mandibular gland (Seo et al. 1988b; Steward et al. 1989).

If the tissue content of Pi is too low for the required time resolution, SP resonances, which are also pH sensitive, provide an alternative approach (e.g. Civan et al. 1986). Alternatively, fluorine-containing indicator molecules are available that show pH-dependent chemical shifts in the ^{19}F spectrum. These include α-difluoromethyl-alanine (Taylor and Deutsch 1988) and fluoroquene (Metcalfe et al. 1985). The good sensitivity of NMR to the ^{19}F nucleus and the very low 'background' of endogenous fluorine compounds in animal tissues allow relatively low concentrations of these compounds to be detected. In order to load the indicator molecules into the cytosol, tissues are exposed to the relatively permeable acetoxymethyl or parachlorophenyl esters which, after crossing the cell membrane, are then cleaved by endogenous esterases.

It is also possible to measure pH_i using proton NMR. Early experiments by Chapman et al. (1982) used the pH-dependent chemical shift of imidazole which had been loaded into isolated acini prepared from the rat mandibular gland. Their estimate of 7.2 for pH_i in the unstimulated gland is in good agreement with most subsequent measurements.

Alternative Methods

NMR faces strong competition from other techniques in the measurement of pH_i. In tissues where it is technically possible to impale the cells with microelectrodes and at the same time maintain good oxygenation and substrate supply, the use of ion-selective microelectrodes may be preferred (e.g. Saito et al. 1988). pH microelectrodes may be calibrated accurately and offer good time resolution. The only disadvantage, as with other single-cell methods, is that the responses of many different cells have to be recorded in order to obtain an average response.

Recent years have seen the introduction of pH-sensitive fluorescent dyes, such as the fluorescein derivative, 2′,7′-bis(carboxyethyl)-5(6)-carboxyfluorescein (BCECF), which may be loaded into the cytosol as the acetoxymethyl ester and used to measure pH_i in cell suspensions and single cells by spectrofluorimetry (e.g. Lau et al., this volume). This method, too, offers excellent time resolution, although leakage of dye from the cells, quenching artefacts and difficulties of calibration may cause problems. While it may prove possible to perform fluorescence measurements in perfused exocrine glands, most work so far has used isolated cells or acini.

Apart from the NMR methods described above, the only other established technique for measuring pH_i in perfused glands involves the measurement of the partitioning of a weak acid (or weak base) between the cytosol and perfusate (Pirani et al. 1987). To do this, an isotopically labelled weak acid such as DMO (5,5-dimethyl-2,4-oxazolidinedione) is added to the perfusate together with an extracellular marker. The distribution of the weak acid is then determined after a period of time by radioassay following chemical digestion of the whole gland. For time course studies, many series of glands have to be set up since each gland yields only a single value. The method is thus laborious and costly, but, like NMR, has the advantage that it is relatively non-invasive and does not require prior fragmentation of the tissue.

Changes in pH_i During Salivary Secretion

As discussed elsewhere (Lau et al., this volume), the rabbit mandibular salivary gland generates a primary secretion in response to cholinergic stimulation which, under certain conditions, may be very rich in HCO_3^-. Using the fluorescent dye BCECF loaded into isolated acini, Lau et al. (1989) found that the onset of secretion was accompanied by a HCO_3^--dependent, transient intracellular acidification most probably due to HCO_3^- efflux through anion channels in the luminal membrane.

Measurements of pH_i by ^{31}P NMR in the intact, perfused gland (Steward et al. 1989) have confirmed several of the findings of the fluorescence studies. Because the onset of secretion is accompanied by an increase in the Pi content of the gland (Seo et al. 1988b), the time required to accumulate ^{31}P spectra for pH_i estimation is substantially shorter than in the unstimulated gland. Consequently, the time resolution required to detect the changes in pH_i occurring at the onset of secretion lies within the reach of a 4.7 T spectrometer.

As was observed in the fluorescence studies, stimulation of the rabbit mandibular gland with 1 µmol/l acetylcholine elicited a transient intracellular acidification (Fig. 11a) which was absent when the gland was perfused with a HCO_3^--free solution (Fig. 11b). The results of the NMR and fluorescence studies differ, however, in the subsequent changes in pH_i observed during continuous stimulation with acetylcholine. In isolated acini, fluorescence measurements showed a recovery of pH_i to its resting value. In the intact gland, the transient acidification was followed by a change in pH_i to a more alkaline value (Fig. 11a) which was sustained for the duration of the stimulation period. Furthermore, in the absence of HCO_3^-, the response to acetylcholine was a rapid and sustained alkalinisation (Fig. 11b). No such change in pH_i was observed in the fluorescence studies.

Using ^{31}P NMR it was also found that the alkalinisation phase of the response to acetylcholine was abolished by amiloride (Fig. 11c). We have therefore proposed that this component of the response results from

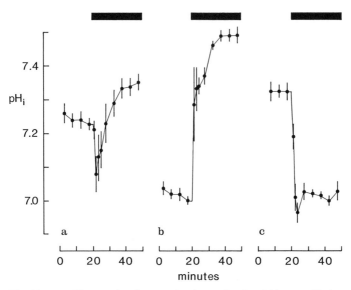

Fig. 11 a – c. Changes in the pH_i in the perfused rabbit mandibular gland on sustained stimula-tion with 1 µmol/l acetylcholine (*solid bar*) during perfusion **a** with HCO_3^-/CO_2-buffered Krebs solution, **b** with a HCO_3^--free, HEPES-buffered solution and **c** with HCO_3^-/CO_2-buffered Krebs solution containing 1 mmol/l amiloride. Data (*solid circles*; taken from Steward et al. 1989a) are means and SEM from three to five experiments

activation of $Na^+ - H^+$ exchange. The lack of effect of amiloride on the resting pH_i, in contrast, suggests that the exchanger is less active in the unstimulated gland.

It remains to be seen whether the differences in response that are observed using the two techniques are due to technical artefacts or to differences in the behaviour of the cells in the isolated acini and in the intact gland. Despite its relatively poor time resolution, the NMR method may have an important role to play in assessing the validity of more invasive techniques.

Water Transport

Biological fluids contain water at a concentration that approaches 56 mol/l – several orders of magnitude greater than the concentrations of most solutes. Since, in addition, the proton (^1H) is the nucleus to which NMR is most sensitive, water can be studied by NMR in ways that are impossible with most solutes. For example, measurements of the relaxation time constants, T_1 and T_2, of water protons in biological tissues provide useful information about the physical state of intracellular water (Mathur-De Vre 1979). It is also possible to use proton NMR both to distinguish between intracellular and extracellular water and to measure the rate of diffusive exchange between them (see below, *Measurement of Membrane Water Permeability*).

Transepithelial Water Flow During Secretion

Although it is widely accepted that exocrine glands secrete water by osmosis, uncertainty remains with regard to the route of water flow across the secretory epithelium. Water is clearly drawn into the lumen by actively secreted electrolytes, but it is not clear whether the water flows mainly through the basolateral and luminal membranes (the transcellular pathway) or through the intercellular junctional complexes (the paracellular pathway). Although exocrine epithelia are often presumed to fall into the low resistance, 'leaky' category, the electrical leakiness of the paracellular pathway does not necessarily imply that it provides a major pathway for water transport. There are several absorptive epithelia, for example, where the evidence lies in favour of transcellular water flow despite the well-established leakiness of the paracellular pathway (e.g. gall bladder epithelium; Spring 1983).

Studies of the rabbit mandibular gland, in which solvent drag of non-electrolytes has been demonstrated during secretion, have helped to define the effective pore size of the channels through which water is secreted (Case et al. 1985). But the location of those channels remains to be determined. One approach that may help to resolve this question is to measure the osmotic water permeability of the epithelial cell membranes and calculate whether the measured permeability is sufficient to explain the generation of a near-isosmotic primary secretion.

Measurement of Membrane Water Permeability

Proton NMR offers a convenient method for measuring the rate of diffusive water exchange across the cell membrane. This is achieved by including a relaxation reagent, such as the paramagnetic Mn^{2+} ion, in the extracellular fluid and by following the time course of the relaxation of the water protons. The technique has been applied successfully to several tissues (e.g. Fabry and Eisenstadt 1975; Steward and Garson 1985) and has recently been used to determine the water permeability of salivary gland cell membranes (Steward et al. 1990).

The time constant of longitudinal relaxation (T_1) is most conveniently measured by using an inversion-recovery pulse sequence similar to that described above in the context of ^{39}K NMR. A radio frequency pulse is applied in order to invert the net magnetisation of the water protons along the axis of the magnet. Then, after a delay (D), a second pulse is applied to rotate the remaining magnetisation into the plane of the receiver coil so that it can be detected and measured. Using a range of values for D, it is possible to reconstruct the time course of the recovery (relaxation) to equilibrium. In a sample of pure water, the relaxation of the protons is a slow exponential process with a time constant of a few seconds. In the presence of Mn^{2+}, however, relaxation is accelerated by two or three orders of magnitude.

By including a relaxation reagent in the perfusate supplying the isolated rabbit mandibular gland, Steward et al. (1990) were able to measure the rate constant of diffusive water efflux from the cytosol into the extracellular fluid of the gland. The paramagnetic complex gadolinium diethylenetriamine-N,N,N',N'',N''-penta acetic acid, $Gd(DTPA)^{2-}$, was used as the relaxation reagent for this study, because, unlike Mn^{2+} (Young et al. 1987), it does not interfere with the secretory response of the gland and it remains confined to the extracellular space for long periods of time.

In the absence of $Gd(DTPA)^{2-}$, the water protons in the perfused gland relaxed very slowly with a time constant (T_1) of about 2.9 s (Fig. 12a). The T_1 of water in a 10 mmol/l solution of $Gd(DTPA)^{2-}$ was around 32 ms (Fig. 12b), nearly 100 times faster. When the glands were perfused with a solution containing 10 mmol/l $Gd(DTPA)^{2-}$, the relaxation time course showed two exponential components with T_1 values of 32 ms and 217 ms (Fig. 12c). The fast component was clearly due to the rapid relaxation of the extracellular water protons. The slower component, however, probably arose as a result of water diffusing from the slowly relaxing cytosolic compartment into the more rapidly relaxing extracellular population. In support of this interpretation, the initial magnitude of the slow component was found to correspond closely with the fractional volume occupied by the intracellular water, and its magnitude changed in the expected fashion when the cells were exposed to anisotonic perfusates (see below, *Cell Volume Changes*).

From the time constants of the two components of relaxation and an estimate of the surface area: volume ratio of the acinar cells, the diffusive

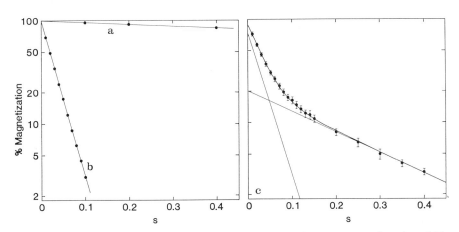

Fig. 12. Longitudinal (spin-lattice) relaxation time courses of water protons in *a* the rabbit mandibular salivary gland perfused with a HEPES-buffered Ringer, *b* a sample of perfusate to which 10 mmol/l $Gd(DTPA)^{2-}$ has been added and *c* glands perfused with the $Gd(DTPA)^{2-}$-containing solution (means and SEM from four glands) at 37°C. An inversion-recovery pulse sequence was used in each case, and the rate constants $(1/T_1)$ shown in the figure were determined by least-squares regression. In **c**, the fast and slow components of the biexponential relaxation time course are also shown (data from Steward et al. 1990)

water permeability (P_d) of the acinar cell membranes was calculated to be $3 \cdot 10^{-3}$ cm/s. This is comparable with values obtained for other biological membranes known to be moderately permeable to water (House 1974).

Previous work has shown that the secretory response of the perfused gland to continuous acetylcholine stimulation is an initially brisk flow (approximately 250 µl/min) that declines over the following 20 min to a plateau rate (approximately 40 µl/min) that may be sustained for several hours (Case et al. 1980). Making a number of reasonable assumptions, it seems that an osmotic gradient of less than 10 mosmol/l could be sufficient to account for the plateau rate. The more rapid initial flow, however, would require a much larger gradient, which would be inconsistent with the production of a near-isosmotic primary secretion.

Cell Volume Changes

In addition to the measurement of the water permeability of cell membranes, proton NMR may also be used to follow changes in cell volume with time. This is because the initial magnitude of the slow component of relaxation in glands perfused with $Gd(DTPA)^{2-}$ is closely related to the size of the intracellular water population. Although a full set of relaxation data such as that shown in Fig. 12c may take several minutes to collect, the slow component intercept can be determined much more quickly by using just a

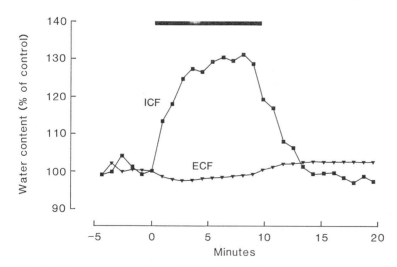

Fig. 13. Changes in intracellular (*ICF*) and extracellular (*ECF*) water content of a perfused rabbit mandibular salivary gland during exposure to a hypotonic perfusate (*solid bar*) made by omitting 50 mmol/l sucrose which was included in the control perfusate. Changes in water content were determined by the proton relaxation method described in the text, in which the T_1 of the extracellular water was shortened by the inclusion of 10 mM $Gd(DTPA)^{2-}$ in the perfusate

few time points and by making the justifiable assumption that the time constant remains unchanged during the experiment. Preliminary experiments suggest that by using just two pulse delays (0.2 and 2 s), it is possible to determine changes in the intracellular and extracellular water content of the gland with a time resolution of around 20 s.

The response of cell volume to changes in perfusate osmolality has been studied using the method, in the intact rabbit mandibular gland. For example, exposure to a hypotonic perfusate (by removal of 50 mmol/l sucrose initially present in the perfusate) caused cell swelling as shown in Fig. 13. Although the rate at which changes in the extracellular osmolality in the gland can be made is limited by the time required for the new perfusate to equilibrate with the extracellular space, this method does provide an opportunity for studying cell volume regulation, if it occurs, in the intact tissue. The only alternative method currently available for doing this in intact glands is by electrical impedance measurements (Nakahari et al. 1986).

Future Developments

NMR methodologies and instrumentation have evolved rapidly over the last 15 years, and it is difficult to predict the state of the art even five years from now. However, with the advent of high field, superconducting magnets large enough to accommodate human subjects, much interest now centres on the clinical possibilities afforded by in vivo magnetic resonance spectroscopy (MRS) used in conjunction with the more established techniques of magnetic resonance imaging (MRI). Methods for obtaining localised ^{31}P and proton spectra from particular human organs such as the brain, liver and heart are now well developed. At the opposite extreme, high-resolution, narrow-bore instruments, previously used only for spectroscopy, are being equipped with gradient coils and used as NMR 'microscopes'. These can produce proton images of small samples of biological tissue with a spatial resolution of the order of 10 µm.

The greatest drawback of NMR lies in its intrinsically low sensitivity. This has serious repercussions both for temporal and spatial resolution. With the single exception of water, the use of NMR to follow changes in tissue content with a time resolution of a few minutes is restricted to solutes present at millimolar concentrations in tissue volumes of not much less than 1 cm^3. Solutes present at lower concentrations may be detected, but only at the expense of temporal or spatial resolution. Technical advances are unlikely to have much impact on this problem because it is due to the theoretical limit set by the physical laws governing the resonance phenomenon. Increases in magnetic field strength will only help a little.

For the investigation of exocrine secretory mechanisms, in vivo studies are of relatively limited value. The experimentalist's need to alter ionic gradients and apply transport inhibitors in order to probe transport mechanisms and their regulation often rules out the whole-animal approach. Perhaps the greatest promise of NMR currently lies in multinuclear spectroscopic studies of isolated gland preparations carried out in conjunction with other methods: on-line analysis of secretion and venous effluent, and possibly the simultaneous use of fluorescent probes for the measurement of intracellular ions which are less accessible to NMR, such as Ca^{2+}.

References

Adler S, Shoubridge E, Radda GK (1984) Estimation of cellular pH gradients with ^{31}P-NMR in intact rabbit renal tubular cells. Am J Physiol 247: C188–C196

Balaban RS, Gadian DG, Radda GK (1981) Phosphorus nuclear magnetic resonance study of the kidney in vivo. Kidney Int 20: 575–579

Berendsen HJC, Edzes HT (1973) The observation and general interpretation of sodium magnetic resonance in biological material. Ann N Y Acad Sci 204: 459–485

Bond M, Shporer M, Petersen K, Civan MM (1981) ^{31}P nuclear magnetic resonance analysis of toad urinary bladder. Mol Physiol 1: 243–263

Boulanger Y, Vinay P, Desroches M (1985) Measurement of a wide range of intracellular sodium concentrations in erythrocytes by ^{23}Na nuclear magnetic resonance. Biophys J 47: 553–561

Bryden CC, Reilley CN, Desreux JF (1981) Multinuclear nuclear magnetic resonance study of three aqueous lanthanide shift reagents: Complexes with EDTA and axially symmetric macrocyclic polyamino polyacetate ligands. Anal Chem 53: 1418–1425

Burgen ASV (1956) The secretion of potassium in saliva. J Physiol (Lond) 132: 20–39

Case RM, Conigrave AD, Novak I, Young JA (1980) Electrolyte and protein secretion by the perfused rabbit mandibular gland stimulated with acetylcholine or catecholamines. J Physiol (Lond) 300: 467–487

Case RM, Cook DI, Hunter M, Steward MC, Young JA (1985) Transepithelial transport of nonelectrolytes in the rabbit mandibular salivary gland. J Membr Biol 84: 239–248

Chapman BE, Cook DI, Gerrard J, Healey AP, Kuchel PW, Young JA (1982) Proton nuclear magnetic resonance spectroscopy (NMR) of rat salivary gland endpieces. J Physiol (Lond) 330: 36P

Chu SC, Pike MM, Fossel ET, Smith TW, Balschi JA, Springer CS (1984) Aqueous shift reagents for high resolution cationic nuclear magnetic resonance III. Dy(TTHA)$^{3-}$, Tm(TTHA)$^{3-}$, and Tm(PPP)$_2^{7-}$. J Magn Reson 56: 33–47

Civan MM, Shporer M (1978) NMR of sodium-23 and potassium-39 in biological systems. In: Berliner LJ, Reuben J (eds) Biological magnetic resonance, vol. 1. Plenum, New York

Civan MM, Degani H, Malgalit Y, Shporer M (1983) Observations of ^{23}Na in frog skin by NMR. Am J Physiol 245: C213–C219

Civan MM, Williams SR, Gadian DG, Rozengurt E (1986) ^{31}P NMR analysis of intracellular pH of mouse 3T3 cells: effects of extracellular Na$^+$ and K$^+$ and mitogenic stimulation. J Membr Biol 94: 55–64

Cope GH (1978) Stereological analysis of the duct system of the rabbit parotid gland. J Anat 126: 591–604

Dawson MJ, Gadian DG, Wilkie DR (1977) Contraction and recovery of living muscles studied by ^{31}P nuclear magnetic resonance. J Physiol (Lond) 267: 703–735

Fabry ME, Eisenstadt M (1975) Water exchange between red cells and plasma: measurement by nuclear magnetic relaxation. Biophys J 15: 1101–1110

Farrar TC, Becker ED (1971) Pulse and Fourier transform NMR. Academic, New York

Furuyama S, Abe M, Yokoyama N, Sugiya H, Fujita Y (1980) Mitochondrial creatine kinase in rat submandibular gland. Int J Biochem 11: 259–264

Gadian DG (1982) Nuclear magnetic resonance and its applications to living systems. Oxford University Press, New York

Gadian DG, Radda GK, Richards RE, Seeley PJ (1979) ^{31}P NMR in living tissue: the road from a promising to an important tool in biology. In: Shulman RG (ed) Biological applications of magnetic resonance. Academic, London, pp 463–535

Gillies RJ, Alger JR, den Hollander JA, Shulman RG (1982) Intracellular pH measured by NMR: methods and results. In: Nuccitelli R, Deamer DW (eds) Intracellular pH: its measurement, regulation, and utilization in cellular functions. Liss, New York, pp 79–104

Gordon RE, Hanley PE, Shaw D, Gadian DG, Radda GK, Styles P, Bore PJ, Chan L (1980) Localization of metabolites in animals using ^{31}P topical magnetic resonance. Nature 287: 736–738

Goto T (1981) Studies of sodium transport during secretion in the perfused dog submandibular gland. J Physiol Soc Jpn 43: 31–43

Gullans SR, Avison MJ, Ogino T, Giebisch G, Shulman RG (1985) NMR measurements of intracellular sodium in the rabbit proximal tubule. Am J Physiol 249: F160–F168

Gupta RK, Gupta P (1982) Direct observation of resolved resonances from intra- and extracellular sodium-23 ions in NMR studies of intact cells and tissues using dysprosium (III)tripolyphosphate as paramagnetic shift reagent. J Magn Reson 47: 344–350

Homer J, Beevers MS (1985) Driven-equilibrium single-pulse observation of T1 relaxation. A reevaluation of a rapid "new" method for determining NMR spin-lattice relaxation times. J Magn Reson 63: 287–297

Hoult DI, Busby RJW, Gadian DG, Radda GK, Richards RE, Seeley BJ (1974) Observation of tissue metabolites using ^{31}P nuclear magnetic resonance. Nature 252: 285–287

House CR (1974) Water transport in cells and tissues. Arnold, London

Hubbard PS (1970) Nonexponential nuclear magnetic relaxation by quadrupole interactions. J Chem Phys 53: 985–987

Imai Y (1965) Study of the secretion mechanism of the submaxillary gland of dog; part 2. Effects of exchanging ions in the perfusate on salivary secretion and secretory potential, with special reference to the ionic distribution in the gland tissue. J Physiol Soc Jpn 27: 313–324

Lau KR, Elliott AC, Brown PD (1989) Acetylcholine-induced intracellular acidosis in rabbit salivary gland acinar cells. Am J Physiol 256: C288–C295

Lehninger AL (1975) Biochemistry, 2nd edn. Worth, New York

Lin L-E, Shporer M, Civan MM (1982) ^{31}P nuclear magnetic resonance analysis of frog skin. Am J Physiol 243: C74–C80

Masuda Y, Nakamori T, Sekido E (1978) Polarographic studies of the exchange reaction between a cadmium(II)-triethylene-tetramine-1-hexaacetic acid complex and lanthanoid(III). J Chem Soc Jpn 204–207

Mathur-De Vre R (1979) The NMR studies of water in biological systems. Prog Biophys Mol Biol 35: 103–134

Matsumoto T, Kanno T, Seo Y, Murakami M, Watari H (1986) ^{31}P NMR studies of the isolated perfused pancreas of the rat. Biomed Res 7 (Suppl 2): 29–31

Matsumoto T, Kanno T, Seo Y, Murakami M, Watari H (1988) Phosphorus nuclear magnetic resonance in isolated perfused rat pancreas. Am J Physiol 254: G575–G579

Metcalfe JC, Hesketh TR, Smith GA (1985) Free cytosolic Ca^{2+} measurements with fluorine labelled indicators using ^{19}F NMR. Cell Calcium 6: 183–195

Mori H, Nakahari T, Imai Y (1984) Intracellular K activity in canine submandibular gland cells in resting and its change during stimulation. Jpn J Physiol 34: 1077–1088

Murakami M (1981) Heat production, blood flow, O_2 uptake and CO_2 output in the secretory process of the dog submandibular gland. J Physiol Soc Jpn 43: 135–147

Murakami M, Imai Y, Seo Y, Watari H (1982) Assays of phosphorus compounds in perfused salivary gland by ^{31}P-NMR. J Physiol Soc Jpn 44: 334

Murakami M, Imai Y, Seo Y, Morimoto T, Shiga K, Watari H (1983) Phosphorus nuclear magnetic resonance of perfused salivary gland. Biochim Biophys Acta 762: 19–24

Murakami M, Seo Y, Nakahari T, Mori H, Imai Y, Watari (1984) Effects of Na^+ depletion on fluid secretion and levels of phosphorus compounds as measured by ^{31}P-NMR in perfused canine mandibular gland. Jpn J Physiol 34: 587–597

Murakami M, Seo Y, Matsumoto T, Ichikawa O, Ikeda A, Watari H (1986a) Continuous measurement of Na, Li, and Cl in the perfused salivary gland by use of NMR. Jpn J Physiol 36: 1267–1274

Murakami M, Novak I, Young JA (1986b) Choline evokes fluid secretion by the perfused rat mandibular gland without desensitization. Am J Physiol 251: G84–G89

Murakami M, Seo Y, Watari H, Ueda H, Hashimoto T, Tagawa K (1987) ^{31}P NMR studies on the isolated perfused mandibular gland of the rat. Jpn J Physiol 37: 411–423

Murakami M, Seo Y, Watari H (1988) Dissociation of fluid secretion and energy supply in rat mandibular gland by high dose of ACh. Am J Physiol 254: G781–G787

Murakami M, Suzuki E, Miyamoto S, Seo Y, Watari H (1989) Direct measurement of K movement by ^{39}K NMR during secretion with acetylcholine in perfused rat mandibular salivary gland. Pflügers Arch 414: 385–392

Nakahari T, Seo Y, Murakami M, Mori H, Miyamoto S, Imai Y, Watari H (1985) ^{31}P-NMR study of dog submandibular gland in vivo and in vitro using the topical magnetic resonance. Jpn J Physiol 35: 729–740

Nakahari T, Yoshida H, Miyamoto M, Imai Y (1986) Measurement of extracellular fluid change in salivary gland using an impedance method. Jpn J Physiol 36: 565–583

Nunnally RL, Stoddard JS, Helman SI, Kokko JP (1983) Response of ^{31}P-nuclear magnetic resonance spectra of frog skin to variations in pCO_2 and hypoxia. Am J Physiol 245: F792–F800

Ogawa S, Rottenberg H, Brown TR, Shulman RG, Castillo CL, Glynn P (1978) High-resolution ^{31}P nuclear magnetic resonance study of rat liver mitochondria. Proc Natl Acad Sci USA 75: 1796–1800

Ogino T, Shulman GI, Avison MJ, Gullans SR, den Hollander JA, Shulman RG (1985) ^{23}Na and ^{39}K NMR studies of ion transport in human erythrocytes. Proc Natl Acad Sci USA 82: 1099–1103

Pike MM, Yarmush DM, Balschi JA, Lenkinski RE, Springer CS (1983) Aqueous shift reagents for high-resolution cationic nuclear magnetic resonance. 2. ^{25}Mg, ^{39}K, and ^{23}Na resonances shifted by chelidamate complexes of dysprosium(III) and thulium(III). Inorg Chem 22: 2388–2392

Pirani D, Evans LAR, Cook DI, Young JA (1987) Intracellular pH in the rat mandibular salivary gland: the role of $Na-H$ and $Cl-HCO_3$ antiports in secretion. Pflügers Arch 408: 178–184

Poulsen JH (1974) Acetylcholine-induced transport of Na^+ and K^+ in the perfused cat submandibular gland. Pflügers Arch 349: 215–220

Poulsen JH, Oakley II B (1978) Intracellular potassium ion activity in resting and stimulated mouse pancreas and submandibular gland. Proc R Soc Lond [Biol] 204: 99–104

Putney JW (1978) Role of calcium in the fade of the potassium release response in the rat parotid gland. J Physiol (Lond) 281: 383–394

Saito Y, Ozawa T, Suzuki S, Nishiyama A (1988) Intracellular pH regulation in the mouse lacrimal gland acinar cells. J Membr Biol 101: 73–81

Sasaki S, Nakagaki I, Mori H, Imai Y (1983) Intracellular calcium store and transport of elements in acinar cells of the salivary gland determined by electron probe X-ray microanalysis. Jpn J Physiol 33: 69–83

Schneyer LH, Schneyer CA (1960) Electrolyte and inulin spaces of rat salivary glands and pancreas. Am J Physiol 199: 649–652

Schneyer LH, Schneyer CA (1962) Electrolyte and water transport by salivary gland slices. Am J Physiol 203: 567–571

Seo Y, Murakami M, Watari H, Imai Y, Yoshizaki K, Nishikawa H, Morimoto T (1983) Intracellular pH determination by a ^{31}P-NMR technique. The second dissociation constant of phosphoric acid in a biological system. J Biochem (Tokyo) 94: 729–734

Seo Y, Murakami M, Matsumoto T, Nishikawa H, Watari H (1987a) Application of aqueous shift reagent, Dy(TTHA), for ^{23}Na NMR studies of exocrine glands. Viabilities of organs perfused with shift reagent. J Magn Reson 72: 341–346

Seo Y, Murakami M, Matsumoto T, Nishikawa H, Watari H (1987b) Direct measurement of Na influx by ^{23}Na NMR during secretion with acetylcholine in perfused rat mandibular gland. Pflügers Arch 409: 343–348

Seo Y, Murakami M, Suzuki E, Watari H (1987c) A new method to discriminate intracellular and extracellular K by ^{39}K NMR without chemical-shift reagents. J Magn Reson 75: 529–533

Seo Y, Murakami M, Suzuki E, Maeda M, Watari H (1988a) An experimental approach to ^{31}P spin-lattice relaxation time measurement in biological systems. Magn Reson Med 6: 430–434

Seo Y, Steward MC, Mackenzie IS, Case RM (1988b) Acetylcholine-induced metabolic changes in the perfused rabbit mandibular salivary gland studied by ^{31}P-NMR spectroscopy. Biochim Biophys Acta 971: 289–297

Spring KR (1983) Fluid transport by gallbladder epithelium. J Exp Biol 106: 181–194

Steward MC, Garson MJ (1985) Water permeability of *Necturus* gallbladder epithelial cell membranes measured by nuclear magnetic resonance. J Membr Biol 86: 203–210

Steward MC, Seo Y, Case RM (1989) Intracellular pH during secretion in the perfused rabbit mandibular salivary gland measured by ^{31}P NMR spectroscopy. Pflügers Arch 414: 200–207

Steward MC, Seo Y, Rawlings JM, Mackenzie IS, Case RM (1990) Water permeability of cell membranes in the perfused rabbit mandibular salivary gland measured by ^{1}H NMR spectroscopy (to be published)

Suzuki E, Maeda M, Kuki S, Tsukamoto K, Kawakami T, Seo Y, Murakami M, Watari H (1989) ^{31}P spin-lattice relaxation time measurements in biological systems: heart, liver, kidney and erythrocytes of rat. Jpn J Magn Reson Mea 9: 115–120

Takami H, Furuya E, Tagawa K, Seo Y, Murakami M, Watari H, Matsuda H, Hirose H, Kawashima Y (1988) NMR-invisible ATP in rat heart and its change in ischemia. J Biochem (Tokyo) 104: 35–39

Takano K, Miyazaki Y, Nakata K, Seo Y, Murakami M, Watari H, Suzuki E, Mandel LJ (1988) ^{31}P-NMR measurement of perfused rat kidney. Jpn J Magn Reson Med 8 S-1: 108

Tamarin A, Sreebny LM (1965) The rat submaxillary salivary gland. A correlative study by light and electron microscopy. J Morphol 117: 295–352

Tanaka K, Yamada Y, Shimizu T, Sano F, Abe Z (1974) Fundamental investigations for a non invasive method of tumor detection by nuclear magnetic resonance. Biotelemetry 1: 337–350

Taylor J, Deutsch C (1988) ^{19}F-nuclear magnetic resonance: measurements of [O$_2$] and pH in biological systems. Biophys J 53: 227–233

Terroux KG, Sekelj P, Burgen ASV (1959) Oxygen consumption and blood flow in the submaxillary gland of the dog. Can J Biochem Physiol 37: 5–15

Tsukamoto K, Murakami M, Seo Y, Watari H, Hironaka T, Oka T (1988) Biliary secretion and energetics of the cold preserved liver measured by means of nuclear magnetic resonance. In: Wong PYD, Young JA (eds) Exocrine secretion. Hong Kong University Press, Hong Kong, pp 195–198

Young JA, Schögel E (1966) Micropuncture investigation of sodium and potassium excretion in rat submaxillary saliva. Pflügers Arch 291: 85–98

Young JA, Cook DI, Evans LAR, Pirani D (1987) Effects of ion transport inhibition on rat mandibular gland secretion. J Dent Res 66: 531–536

Graded Modelling of Exocrine Secretion Using Network Thermodynamics *

Y. Imai

Introduction

This paper outlines a study on the modelling of an exocrine secretion system. Oster et al. (1973) introduced network thermodynamics as a method for modelling physiological systems. Though network thermodynamics were expected to become a useful tool, only a few concrete uses have been reported, perhaps because the method was somewhat complicated and incomplete (Imai 1989).

The bond graphs (Oster et al. 1973; Karnopp and Rosenberg 1975; Thoma 1975) of network thermodynamics have been used in this paper. However, a new two-port capacitive element and an elemental coupling circuit have been introduced (Imai 1989). The two-port capacitor provides for the relation of the concentration change, the solute flow and the volume flow in solution. The elemental circuit with two one-port resistive elements and a transducer provides for the coupled flows across the membranes.

In order to reduce the complexity of the model, a technique of graded modelling has been adopted. Before beginning the modelling, the system is subdivided conceptually into the elemental thermodynamic processes that can be represented by bond graph elements. In the first step, modules that represent the functions of the structural subsystems of the membrane transport system are modelled by bond graphs. The resistive (R) module expresses the transport processes in the membrane or barrier in which a set of driving forces determines a set of flows. The capacitive (C) module expresses the charging or discharging process in the solution compartment in which a set of flows determines a set of force variable changes. In the second step, a topological combination of modules then permits development of a complete model of the membrane transport system.

Since each element of the bond graphs can be represented by an equation, the module, which is made up of bond graphs, can be represented by simultaneous equations. Then the complete model, which is made up of a set of modules, can be represented by a set of simultaneous equations which are

---

* The work was supported by a Grant-in-Aid for Scientific Research from the Ministry of Education, Science and Culture, Japan.

used for the computer simulation. These procedure allows some predictions to be made and suggests useful lines of experimental research.

Bond Graph Representation of Modules

In the membrane transport system, the membrane subsystem acts as a conductor or barrier for the transport components. Power dissipations and couplings result from flows taking place during the transport processes in the membrane. The solution compartment subsystem acts as a reservoir for the transport components. The reservoir is either a source or a sink for the various components, in which the free energy of every component decreases or increases due to flows occurring during the transport processes in the solution. These functions of the membrane and the solution subsystems can be modelled as modules with bond graphs.

The power balance in the system is held in the model made up of bond graphs. In a closed system, the rate of decrease of free energy is equal to the

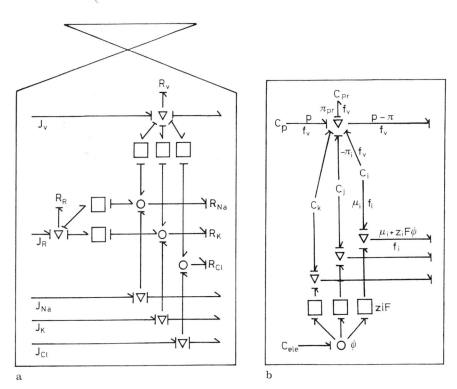

a   b

Fig. 1 a, b. Bond graph representation of modules. **a** A resistive (R) module expresses the membrane function. **b** A capacitive (C) module expresses the solution compartment function

power dissipation. In an open system, the input power equals the sum of the rate of increase of free energy and the power dissipation. As each module is assumed to be an open subsystem, the input power into an R module causes the power dissipation, and the output power from a C module causes the decrease of free energy.

In general, power is expressed as a product of a flow and its conjugate force variable. This expression make clear the power domain and the quantity. A bond graph element in a module corresponds to each power domain. The process of power dissipation is expressed by a resister, the process of free energy change by a capacitor, and the process of power coupling by a transducer.

The bond graphs of the modules represented in Fig. 1 have been described in detail elsewhere (Imai 1989; Imai et al. 1989). The bond graph of the R module (Fig. 1a) consists of some resisters and some transducers. This graph represents the Na^+, K^+ and Cl^- flows (J_i) and the volume flow (J_v) across the membrane. The volume flow circuit consists of a series circuit with hydraulic forces $(\Delta p - \Delta \pi)$ and coupled forces $(\Sigma (1 - \sigma_i) \bar{c}_i \Delta \tilde{\mu}_i)$ across the transducers, which have a transfer ratio of $(1 - \sigma_i) \bar{c}_i$. Each ionic circuit consists of a diffusive component driven by the electrochemical potential difference and a solvent drag component resulting from convection in parallel circuits. For the Na^+ and K^+ flows, active transport steps driven by the Na^+-, K^+-ATPase reaction are also represented. The reaction-transport coupling is represented by a transducer having a transfer ratio (stoichiometry), v_i, of 3 for Na^+ and -2 for K^+.

The R module is depicted by a 'bulb' to express the conductive function. The R module can be described by the following simultaneous transport-reaction equations,

$$J_v = L_p (\Delta p - \Delta \pi + \Sigma (1 - \sigma_i) \bar{c}_i \Delta \tilde{\mu}_i) \tag{1}$$

$$J_R = L_R (A_{ATP} - 3 \Delta \tilde{\mu}_{Na} + 2 \Delta \tilde{\mu}_K) \tag{2}$$

$$J_{Na} = \omega_{Na} \bar{c}_{Na} \Delta \tilde{\mu}_{Na} + (1 - \sigma_{Na}) \bar{c}_{Na} J_v - 3 J_R \tag{3}$$

$$J_K = \omega_K \bar{c}_K \Delta \tilde{\mu}_K + (1 - \sigma_K) \bar{c}_K J_v + 2 J_R \tag{4}$$

$$J_{Cl} = \omega_{Cl} \bar{c}_{Cl} \Delta \tilde{\mu}_{Cl} + (1 - \sigma_{Cl}) \bar{c}_{Cl} J_v \tag{5}$$

for which the nomenclature and bond graph notations are summarized in Table 1.

The bond graph of the C module (Fig. 1b) consists of one-port capacitors, two-port capacitors and transducers. The C module represents changes of hydrostatic pressure, of osmotic pressure and of electrochemical potential due to various flows. The two-port capacitor (C_i) in the module expresses ionic concentration change due both to ionic flow (f_i) and volume flow (f_v). One port of the two-port capacitor responds to the ionic power and the

Table 1. Bond graph notations and nomenclature

$\xrightarrow[J]{X}$ R	One-port resister	$R = X/J$
$\xleftarrow[f]{e}$ C	One-port capacitor	$de/dt = -f/C$
$\xleftarrow[f_v]{-\pi_i}$ C $\xrightarrow[f_i]{\mu_i}$	Two-port capacitor	$d\pi_i/dt = RT(c_if_v - f_i)/V$ $d\mu_i/dt = RT(c_if_v - f_i)/n_i$
$\xrightarrow[f_1]{e_1}$ |r| $\xrightarrow[f_2]{e_2}$	Transducer (Transformer type)	$e_2 = re_1$ $f_1 = rf_2$
∇	Series junction	$\Sigma\,\alpha_i e_i = 0$
$\bigcirc$	Parallel junction	$\Sigma\,\alpha_i f_i = 0$
A_{ATP}	Affinity of Na^+-, K^+-ATPase reaction	
c_i	Concentration of i	
$\bar{c}_i$	Logarithmic mean concentration $(:\Delta c_i/\Delta \ln c_i)$	
e	Force variable	
f	Flow variable	
F	Faraday constant	
G	Gibbs free energy	
i	Components	
J	Resistive flow	
k	Compliance	
L	Conductance (1/R)	
L_p	Hydraulic conductance	
L_R	Reaction conductance	
n_i	Moles of i	
p	Hydrostatic pressure	
R	Gas constant	
T	Temperature (Kelvin)	
V	Volume of compartment	
X	Driving force, potential difference of R	
z_i	Electric charge	
α_i	Bond graph direction 1 or -1	
Δ	Difference	
μ_i	Chemical potential	
$\tilde{\mu}_i$	Electrochemical potential $(:\mu_i + z_i F\psi)$	
σ_i	Reflection co-efficient	
π	Osmotic pressure	
ψ	Electric potential	
ω_i	Permeability, mobility	

other port responds to a part of the osmotic activity of the ion. The one-port capacitors (C_p, C_{pr} and C_{ele}) in the module express the force-variable change due to a conjugated flow, in other words, the hydrostatic and colloid osmotic pressure changes due only to volume flow, and the electrical potential changes due to the current. The electrochemical power coupling is represented by a transducer that has a transfer ratio of $z_i F$.

The C module is depicted by a rectangle to express its reservoir function. The C module can be described by the following simultaneous equations:

$$dV = -f_v\, dt \tag{6}$$

$$dp = -dV/k \tag{7}$$

$$dc_i = (c_i f_v - f_i)\, dt/V \tag{8}$$

$$d\psi = -\Sigma z_i F f_i\, dt/C_{ele} \tag{9}$$

$$d\pi_i = RT dc_i \tag{10}$$

$$d\mu_i = d\pi_i/c_i \tag{11}$$

The nomenclature for these equations is shown in Table 1. In this C module, a reaction capacitor is also shown that is assumed to have a constant reaction affinity, A_{ATP} ($dA_{ATP}=0$). A capacitor having constant force is an actual power source in the system. Thus, the R module determines the flows due to the driving forces across the R module, and the C module determines the force variable changes due to flows from the C module.

Whole-System Model with Modules

A simple membrane transport system can be modelled with an R module and two C modules (Fig. 2a) which correspond to rates (valve symbols) and levels (rectangles) as used in urban dynamics (Forrester 1969). This system model corresponds to a cell suspension system consisting of a membrane and an extra- and intracellular fluid compartment. When the volume of the extracellular fluid compartment (ECF) is assumed to be large, no concen-

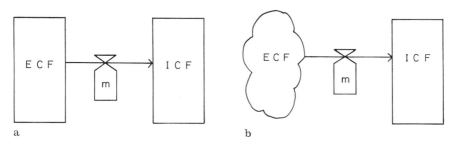

Fig. 2a, b. Whole-system model of a simple membrane (*m*) transport system. **a** A closed system expressed as an R module and two C modules. **b** An open system expressed as a source (*'cloud'* symbol), an R module and a C module. *ECF*, extracellular fluid; *ICF*, intracellular fluid

tration change is detected in the ECF. In this case, the C module of the ECF can be represented by a source or sink module ('cloud' symbol) which indicates that it lies outside the system and has constant potentials (Fig. 2b). In the simple system of Figs. 2a and 2b, the following relations exist between the resistive flow vector, $\mathbf{J}$ (J_v, J_R, J_{Na}, J_K, J_{Cl}), and the capacitive flow vector, $\mathbf{f}$ (f_v, f_R, f_{Na}, f_K, f_{Cl}):

$$\mathbf{f}_{ecf} = \mathbf{J}_m = -\mathbf{f}_{cell} \tag{12}$$

In addition, the following relations exist between the resistive driving force vector, $\mathbf{X}$ (Δp, $-\Delta \pi$, $\Delta \mu_{Na}$, $\Delta \mu_K$, $\Delta \mu_{Cl}$, $\Delta \psi$), and the capacitive potential vector, $\mathbf{e}$ (p, $-\pi$, μ_{Na}, μ_K, μ_{Cl}, ψ):

$$\mathbf{X}_m = \mathbf{e}_{ecf} - \mathbf{e}_{cell} \tag{13}$$

For the chemical reaction of ATP hydrolysis, a reaction capacitor having constant affinity, A_{ATP}, is assumed to be present in one of the C modules.

Power balance as a closed system (Fig. 2a) is given as follows:

$$\begin{aligned}
\left(\frac{dG}{dt}\right)_{C\text{-module}} &= \mathbf{f}_{ecf}^T \mathbf{e}_{ecf} + \mathbf{f}_{cell}^T \mathbf{e}_{cell} \\
&= \mathbf{J}_m^T (\mathbf{e}_{ecf} - \mathbf{e}_{cell}) \\
&= \mathbf{J}_m^T \mathbf{X}_m \\
&= \Phi_{R\text{-module}}
\end{aligned} \tag{14}$$

where dG/dt is the rate of free energy change in the C modules and Φ is the dissipation in the R module.

Power balance as an open system (Fig. 2b) can be represented as follows:

$$\begin{aligned}
\text{Input Power} &= \mathbf{f}_{ecf}^T \mathbf{e}_{ecf} \\
&= -\mathbf{f}_{cell}^T \mathbf{e}_{cell} + \mathbf{J}_m^T \mathbf{X}_m \\
&= \left(\frac{dG}{dt}\right)_{cell} + \Phi_m
\end{aligned} \tag{15}$$

Using the whole system model made up of the modules with known parameters and initial values, some responses of the system can be simulated because the model determines the flows, and potential changes continuously. Here we discuss the relation between the membrane potential, $\Delta \psi$, and the intracellular K^+ activity, a_K^i (γc_K^i; γ = activity coefficient), for a cell in steady-state conditions. Mori et al. (1984) reported the $\Delta \psi - a_K^i$ relation in their experiment on superfused canine mandibular gland slices using double-barrelled K^+-selective microelectrodes. Their results are shown in Fig. 3a.

For computer simulation, the step-by-step method of Von Euler was adopted using Eqs. (1) to (13) which were deduced from the model of Figs. 1a, 1b and 2b. The system model then achieves a steady state in simulation, that is, all final variables in the model become constant for any given parameters and initial values. One simulation study gave a $\Delta\psi - a_K^i$ relation in the steady state. These simulation data were plotted in various condition

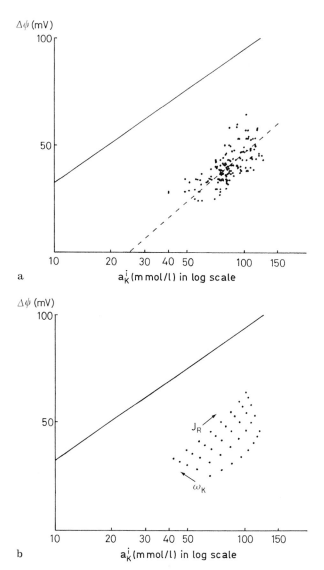

Fig. 3a, b. Relation between $\Delta\psi$ and a_K^i acinar cells. **a** Experimental data obtained by double-barrelled K^+ electrodes (Mori et al. 1983). **b** Simulated data changing J_R and ω_K. *Dots*, individual experimental data; *solid lines*, relation of the Nernst equilibrium potential to intracellular K^+ activity; *dotted line*, regression line of experimental data

to change J_R and ω_K, but other parameters and initial values were fixed (Fig. 3b). When J_R rises, $\Delta\psi$ and a_K^i increase. And when ω_K rises, $\Delta\psi$ increases, but a_K^i decreases.

Through the above simulation (Fig. 3b), a hypothesis arises that the dispersed data of the $\Delta\psi - a_K^i$ relation in the experiment may be due to different reaction rates and K^+ permeabilities in each cell condition.

Model of Acinar Secretion

Topological combinations of modules allow us to describe various membrane transport systems. A model of the acinar epithelial transport system is shown in Fig. 4b, which consists of three R modules and three C modules. The R modules represent the basolateral membrane, the luminal membrane and the intercellular route across the tight junction. The C modules represent the ECF, the intracellular fluid (ICF) and the luminal fluid (LF).

The $Na^+ - K^+$ active transport, $Na^+ - K^+ - 2Cl^-$ co-transport, ionic diffusion and volume flow mechanisms have been placed in the R module of the basolateral membrane. Circuits for ionic and volume flow have been placed in the R modules of the luminal membrane and the intercellular route. The power source for the ATP reaction coupled with the $Na^+ - K^+$ pump has been placed in the C module of the ICF.

Using this model, we simulated two steady states, resting and secreting. In order to establish the secreting state in this simulation, the K^+ permeability pathway and the $Na^+ - K^+ - 2Cl^-$ co-transport pathway in the R module of the basolateral membrane, and the Cl^- permeability pathway in the R module of the luminal membrane must increase about 20 times, although other parameters and initial values remain constant. Metabolism, which can be evaluated by the reaction rate of ATP in the simulation, increases several times. Thus, the unidirectional volume flow from ECF to ICF and from ICF to LF can be observed in the simulation. Hyperpolarization of the membrane potential appears also in the simulation (Fig. 4a). Although the values of the parameters used in this simulation were selected to mimic the known system behaviour, we checked the validity of the selected parameters to ensure that they were of similar numerical order to known values. We also checked the validity of the parameters by comparing the total power dissipation in simulation with the rate of metabolism in an experiment because the total power dissipation depended sensitively on the choice of system parameters.

Using module expression, the salivary secretion system was also modelled as shown in Fig. 5. This model allows us to deduce a set of simultaneous equations for simulation. However, little information on the numerical values of the parameters of the R elements and C elements in the modules of Fig. 5 is available. That is, the permeability, the reflection co-efficients, the concentrations, the volumes etc. have yet to be determined experimentally.

Consequently, the model simulation give only a qualitative and partial description as shown in Fig. 4.

Nakahari et al. (1986), using methods based both on morphological and impedance analysis, reported that the volume of the ECF, especially the interlobular space, decreases remarkably during secretion in the canine

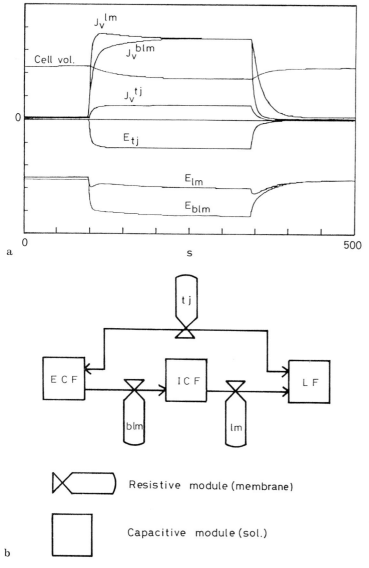

Fig. 4a. The resting and secreting steady states simulated with the acinar model. **b** The acinar model is expressed as three R modules and three C modules in series and parallel. *blm*, basolateral membrane; *lm*, luminal membrane; *tj*, tight junctions; *ECF*, extracellular fluid; *ICF*, intracellular fluid; *LF*, luminal fluid; *sol*, solution compartment

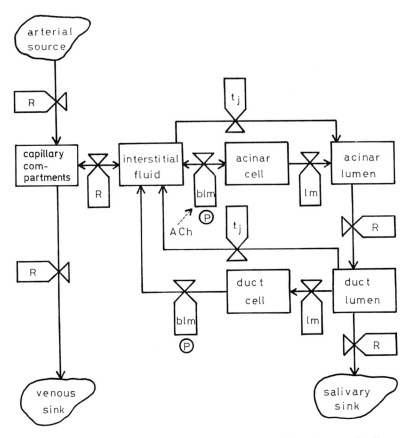

Fig. 5. Salivary secretion model with modules. Artery, vein and excreted saliva are expressed as a source or sink (*'cloud' symbols*). C modules express solution compartments of capillary, interstitial fluid (ECF), cells and duct lumens. R modules (*R*) express resistances of vessels, ducts, capillary wall, cell membranes and tight junctions. *blm*, basolateral membrane; *lm*, luminal membrane; *tj*, tight junction; *P*, active pump

mandibular gland. This decrease in ECF volume during secretion can be simulated using the model shown in Fig. 5. Similarly, the increasing osmotic pressure in the ECF is also predicted by the simulation.

Acknowledgement. I thank Professor J.A. Young, University of Sydney, Australia, for his helpful suggestions and discussions while editing and correcting this paper and also my colleagues for informative discussions.

References

Forrester JW (1969) Urban dynamics. MIT Press, Cambridge

Imai Y (1989) Membrane transport system modeled by network thermodynamics. J Membr Sci 41: 3–21

Imai Y, Yoshida H, Miyamoto M, Nakahari T, Fujiwara H (1989) Network synthesis of epithelial transport system. J Membr Sci 41: 393–403

Karnopp D, Rosenberg R (1975) System dynamics: A unified approach. Wiley, New York

Mori H, Nakahari T, Imai Y (1984) Intracellular K^+ activity in canine submandibular gland cells in resting and its change during stimulation. Jpn J Physiol 34: 1077–1088

Nakahari T, Yoshida H, Miyamoto M, Imai Y (1986) Measurement of extracellular fluid change in salivary gland using an impedance method. Jpn J Physiol 36: 565–583

Oster GF, Perelson AS, Katchalsky A (1973) Network thermodynamics: dynamic modeling of biophysical systems. Rev Biophys 6: 1–134

Thoma JV (1975) Introduction to bond graphs and their applications. Pergamon, Oxford

B Secretion in Individual Tissues

1 Salivary Glands

Role of Anion Transport in Secretion of Primary Saliva *

J. H. Poulsen and B. Nauntofte

Introduction

As suggested by Thaysen et al. (1954) and shown by Young and Schögel (1966) the primary saliva produced by the secretory endpieces (acini) of mammalian salivary glands is "plasmalike" and has a high concentration of chloride. Since the transepithelial potential difference is lumen negative in the secreting state (Lundberg 1957), the transport of Cl^- across the secretory epithelium evidently occurs against an electrochemical gradient and has to be active. It is interesting that a model based on transcellular, active transport of Cl^- was proposed by Lundberg as early as 1957. Subsequently, Lundberg's "chloride pump" model was criticized (Yoshimura and Imai 1967; Petersen and Poulsen 1968, 1969; Petersen 1970, 1972) and the concept of a Cl^- pump, i.e., transport of Cl^- directly linked to cell metabolism, was abandoned. In many subsequent studies, attention was paid mainly to the role of cations in the secretion of primary saliva. However, Poulsen and Kristensen (1982) demonstrated that addition of a cholinergic agonist to a preparation of collagenase-isolated rat parotid acini preequilibrated with $^{36}Cl^-$ caused a reduction in the cellular content of the isotope by approximately 50% within 7s, thus indicating an impressive stimulation-induced net efflux of Cl^-. This caused a renewed interest in the role of Cl^- in secretion of saliva and prompted a number of studies (Nauntofte and Poulsen 1984, 1986; Martinez and Cassity 1985a, 1986; Kawaguchi et al. 1986; Turner et al. 1986).

* The work was supported by grants from the Danish Medical Research Foundation (No. 126968) and the NOVO Foundation.

Uptake of Cl^-

The intracellular Cl^- concentration has been measured with a number of different techniques: chemical titration (Lundberg 1958; Schneyer and Schneyer 1960), isotope equilibration (Martinez and Cassity 1985a; Nauntofte and Poulsen 1986), ion-selective microelectrodes (Mori et al. 1983; Lau and Case 1988), and X-ray spectroscopy (Izutsu et al. 1987). Depending on the glands, species, and methods employed, values in the range 27 (activity) to 75 (concentration) mmol/l cell water have been reported. It is important to notice, however, that all results indicate that the intracellular Cl^- concentration is higher than that corresponding to electrochemical equilibrium. Consequently, the uptake of Cl^- via transport systems in the basolateral acinar cell membrane must be active.

Unstimulated Cells

The unidirectional uptake of chloride by isolated acini or acinar cells has been measured in several studies using $^{36}Cl^-$ (Martinez and Cassity 1985a; Nauntofte and Poulsen 1986; Kawaguchi et al. 1986). It is agreed that the turnover is substantial and that apparent isotope equilibrium is typically obtained in 3–5 min in the unstimulated state. In general, the schedule of sampling has not allowed a precise characterization of the initial rate of uptake, and due to difficulties in making good estimates of the surface area of the appropriate parts of the acinar cell membrane, proper influx data are not available. In a study by Nauntofte and Poulsen (1986), however, the initial rate of uptake of $^{36}Cl^-$ was found to be 3.5 μmol/s per g dry weight (corresponding to 2.2 mmol/s per l cell water) and an influx rate constant of 1.04 min^{-1}. It should be mentioned that in order to reduce trapping of extracellular $^{36}Cl^-$, the separation of acini loaded with $^{36}Cl^-$ from their incubation medium included a 16-fold dilution of the acinar suspension immediately before rapid centrifugation through silicone oil. Should it have happened that substantial reequilibration took place during the short time the acini spent in the diluted state before being separated from the medium by passing through the silicone oil, the method would tend to underestimate the real values. Because of this, the experimental procedure was refined, and recent experiments performed in our laboratory without the aforementioned dilution step indicate that the influx rate constant is as high as 3.3 min^{-1}, (SEM $= 0.18$; $n = 6$; Fig. 1). In principle, the dilution step used by Nauntofte and Poulsen (1986) might also tend to underestimate the cellular Cl^- concentration under isotope steady-state conditions, although this possibility seems to be unlikely because the steady-state cellular Cl^- concentration was found to be as high as 75 mmol/l cell water.

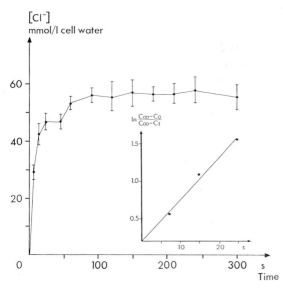

Fig. 1. Time course of uptake of $^{36}Cl^-$ by unstimulated, collagenase-isolated rat parotid acini. Values are means $\pm$ SEM, $n=6$. The isotope was added at time 0. Samples of 200 µl acinar suspension were centrifuged through silicone oil without dilution, but otherwise treated as described by Nautofte and Poulsen (1986). Intracellular water space was determined by use of ^3H_2O and $[^{14}C]$ inulin. The *insert* is a semilogarithmic plot illustrating the time course of the initial uptake from a representative experiment. The regression line was calculated by use of a linearized least squares fit. The influx rate constant calculated from six experiments was 3.3 min^{-1}, SEM $= 0.18$

Stimulated Cells

Measurement of unidirectional uptake of $^{36}Cl^-$ by cholinergically stimulated acinar cells were attempted with limited success by Poulsen and Kristensen (1982), Martinez and Cassity (1985a) and Nauntofte and Poulsen (1986). Because the intracellular amount of $^{36}Cl^-$ was reduced to approximately 50% and isotope equilibration took place very rapidly (typically within less than 15 s), it was not possible to obtain meaningfull values concerning the uptake of Cl^-. However, some observations do lend support to the view that the influx of Cl^- is indeed enhanced by stimulation. Thus, Poulsen and Kristensen (1982) found that the uptake of Na^+ was increased by cholinergic stimulation. If the uptake of Na^+ happens exclusively, or predominantly via a cotransporter with Cl^- (and K^+; see below) the uptake of Cl^- must also be increased upon stimulation.

Effect of Loop Diurectics

Furosemide has been found to inhibit uptake of $^{36}Cl^-$ (Martinez and Cassity 1985a; Nauntofte and Poulsen 1986; Kawaguchi et al. 1986) as well as secondary reuptake after cholinergically induced release of acinar chloride (Nauntofte and Poulsen 1984, 1986). Furthermore, the more specific blocker, bumetanide, was found to inhibit uptake (Kawaguchi et al. 1986) and secondary reuptake of $^{36}Cl^-$ (Melvin et al. 1987). It should be noted that secondary reuptake of Cl^- in the continuous presence of agonist, as shown in Fig. 2, was observed neither by Poulsen and Kristensen (1982) nor by Martinez and Cassity (1985a). However, semiquantitative measurements of stimulation-induced volume changes monitored by use of light scatter give independent support to the existance of secondary reuptake of Cl^- (Poulsen et al. 1988). Thus, it cannot be ruled out that the failure to demonstrate reuptake of Cl^- may reflect less than optimal function of the acinar preparation.

In the study by Martinez and Cassity (1985a) the steady-state chloride concentration was reduced to about one half of the control value in the presence of furosemide, while the time course of uptake of $^{36}Cl^-$ was uninfluenced. In contrast, Nauntofte and Poulsen (1986) found that the influx rate constant was reduced by furosemide to one third of the control value, while the steady-state value was uninfluenced by this diuretic. The latter finding represents a paradox since a reduction in the intracellular Cl^- concentration would be expected in response to inhibition of the uptake step. Similarly, we found in a recent series of experiments performed without a dilution step that the intracellular steady-state concentration of Cl^- in unstimulated acini was 62.2 mmol/l cell water, (SEM = 0.9 mmol/l, $n = 4$) in

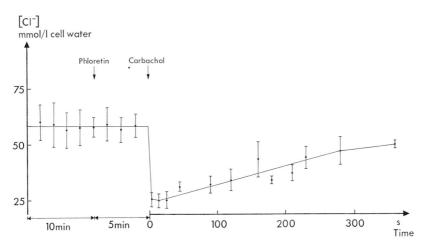

Fig. 2. The effect of carbachol (20 µmol/l) on the intracellular Cl^- concentration after apparent isotope equilibrium was established. Phloretin (250 µmol/l) was present as indicated. Number of experiments = 3

Table 1. Calculation of the ion products determining the gradient for a cotransporter with a stoichiometry of: $1\,Na^+:1\,K^+:2\,Cl^-$

Ion	Extracellular (mmol/l)	Intracellular (mmol/l)
Na^+	145	15^a
K^+	4.8	135^b
Cl^-	118	63^c
$[Na^+][K^+][Cl^-]^2$	9.7×10^6	8.0×10^6

The intracellular concentrations are from:
[a] Poulsen and Kristensen (1982)
[b] Nauntofte and Dissing (1988 b)
[c] Present study

the presence of bumetanide (50 µmol/l, a concentration which is sufficient to inhibit influx of K^+ as shown by Nauntofte and Dissing 1988 b), while the corresponding control value was 63.3 mmol/l cell water.

The data shown in Table 1 indicate that in unstimulated acinar cells having a high Cl^- concentration, a cotransport system with a stoichiometry of $1\,Na^+:1\,K^+:2\,Cl^-$ operates very close to equilibrium conditions. Consequently, even a severe inhibition of such a cotransport system would not lead to significant reduction in the intracellular Cl^- concentration unless, in addition to the cotransporter, other transport systems such as Cl^- channels contributed to a significant extent in the unstimulated state.

Uptake Mechanisms

The uptake of Cl^- against an electrochemical gradient must represent an important step in the transcellular transport of Cl^- underlying the secretion of primary saliva. Since loop diuretics like furosemide and bumetanide are established inhibitors of $Na^+-Cl^--(K^+)$ cotransporters (Palfrey et al. 1980), such drugs have been used as experimental tools. In experiments on perfused salivary glands it has been demonstrated that furosemide is able to inhibit secretion of saliva (Poulsen et al. 1982; Martinez and Cassity 1985b; Novak and Young 1986). With the aid of preparations of isolated acini as well as acinar cells, a number of important observations have been made: (1) Uptake of $^{22}Na^+$ is dependent on the presence of extracellular Cl^- (Poulsen and Kristensen 1982); (2) uptake of $^{22}Na^+$ can be inhibited by furosemide (Poulsen and Kristensen 1982); (3) uptake of $^{36}Cl^-$ can be inhibited by furosemide and bumetanide (Martinez and Cassity 1985a; Nauntofte and Poulsen 1986; Kawaguchi et al. 1986); (4) poststimulatory reuptake of Cl^- can be abolished by furosemide and bumetanide (Nauntofte and Poulsen 1984, 1986; Melvin et al. 1987). Accordingly, it was concluded that cotransport of Cl^- and Na^+ is responsible for the uptake of Cl^- against the electrochemical gradient across the basolateral membrane of the acinar cell.

In the earlier of the studies quoted it was assumed that the stoichiometry of the cotransport system was $1\,Na^+:1\,Cl^-$. Later it was suggested that the stoichiometry was $1\,Na^+:1\,K^+:2\,Cl^-$ as originally found in a study on Ehrlich ascites tumor cells by Geck et al. (1980). That the stoichiometry of the cotransporter in salivary glands is $1\,Na^+:1\,K^+:2\,Cl^-$ was demonstrated in an elegant vesicle study by Turner et al. (1986). The same conclusion was reached by the indirect approach of relating Cl^- transport to oxygen consumption (Smaje et al. 1986; Poulsen and Nauntofte 1987).

Evidence obtained from studies on perfused salivary glands (Case et al. 1984; Novak and Young 1986; Pirani et al. 1987), on isolated acini (Nauntofte and Dissing 1988a), and on membrane vesicles (Turner and George 1988) indicates that in addition to the cotransporter, a $Cl^- - HCO_3^-$ exchanger, indirectly coupled to a $Na^+ - H^+$ exchanger, contributes to the transport of Cl^- across the basolateral acinar cell membrane.

Relase of Cl^-

As early as 1956, Burgen demonstrated that stimulation of salivary glands leads to a spectacular release of cellular K^+. The mechanism of the K^+ release, i.e., opening of Ca^{2+}-activated K^+ channels, has been extensively studied (for review see Petersen 1986). Furthermore, Burgen (1967) stated as an "unpublished observation" based on measurements on excised segments of intact, autoperfused glands that salivary gland cells shrink in response to stimulation. This observation has recently been confirmed by Nauntofte and Poulsen (1986) and Poulsen et al. (1988) who found that cholinergic stimulation is able to cause a significant reduction in the volume of intracellular water in a preparation of isolated acini. Accordingly, the information required to make it possible to infer that a net efflux of anions must happen together with the well-established net efflux of K^+ has in principle been available for a long time.

Cholinergically Induced Net Efflux of Cl^-

A number of studies using isolated salivary gland acini or acinar cells and $^{36}Cl^-$ have confirmed that stimulation causes a dramatic net efflux of Cl^- (Nauntofte and Poulsen 1984, 1986; Martinez and Cassity 1985a, 1986; Melvin et al. 1987). The experiments performed with the best temporal resolution have revealed that the net release is completed during the initial 7–10s of stimulation. Similar results have been observed with adrenergic stimulation (Ambudkar et al. 1988; Poulsen et al. 1988). These observations have been supported by results obtained with chloride-selective microelectrodes (Mori et al. 1983; Lau and Case 1988). In the microelectrode studies both the absolute and the relative stimulation-induced reduction in

Table 2. Rate constant of $^{36}Cl^-$ transport across the membranes of rat parotid acinar cells incubated in KRB buffer

State	Method	Direction	Rate constant (s^{-1})[a]	SEM	n
Resting	Centrifuged, undiluted[b]	Influx	0.055	0.0032	6
Resting	Centrifuged, stop[c]	Efflux	0.039	0.0025	3
Resting	Filtration, undiluted[d]	Efflux	0.049	0.0023	20
Stimulation[e]	Filtration, undiluted	Efflux	0.192	0.0178	13
Stimulation, furosemide[f]	Filtration, undiluted	Efflux	0.204	0.0354	4

[a] Influx rate constants were calculated as described in Fig. 1. Efflux rate constants (k_{Cl}) were calculated from measurements of radioactivity in the medium according to:

$$k_{Cl} = \ln(C_\infty - C_0) \times (C_\infty - C_t)^{-1} t^{-1}$$

k_{Cl} was determined by use of a linearized least squares fit.
[b] Centrifuged, undiluted refers to separation of acini from medium by centrifugation through silicone oil as described in Fig. 1. Influx rate constant represents slope of line through three time points obtained within 25 s.
[c] Centrifuged, stop refers to centrifugation through silicone oil preceeded by dilution into an ice-cold stop solution containing the blocker 2-cyclooctylamino-5-nitro-benzoic acid in a concentration of 100 μmol/l. Samples were treated as described by Nauntofte and Dissing (1988 b). Efflux rate constant represent slope of line through six time points obtained within 25 s.
[d] Filtration, undiluted refers to separation of acini from medium by a rapid filtration method based upon a method originally developed by Dalmark and Wieth (1972). Efflux rate constant represent slope of line through six time points obtained within 15 s in the unstimulated state and within 8 s in the stimulated state.
[e] Stimulation indicates stimulation by carbachol (20 μmol/l).
[f] Stimulation, furosemide indicates stimulation as above but in the presence of furosemide (0.7 mmol/l).

intracellular Cl^- activity was less than in the isotope studies. This apparent discrepancy is at least in part due to the loss of intracellular water that accompanies the release of Cl^- (and K^+). In the isotope experiments, cellular chloride is generally related to dry weight, protein, or DNA. Therefore, it is evident that the stimulation-induced reduction in chloride content exceeds the reduction in activity (concentration). In Table 2, data from experiments based on the use of very rapid filtration methods for the separation of cells from incubation medium (J. Brahm, S. Dissing, B. Nauntofte and J. Hedemark Poulsen, unpublished) indicate that under stimulated steady-state conditions the efflux rate constant for Cl^- is increased 4-fold in comparison with unstimated conditions. Accordingly, the uptake must have been increased as well. However, this is difficult to demonstrate directly, partly because the acini lose Cl^- on stimulation. In principle it is possible to estimate the stimulated Cl^- influx by correcting for the rapid efflux as has been done for K^+ (Nauntofte and Dissing 1988 b).

Effect of Diuretics and Cl^- Channel Blockers

Data presented in Table 2 indicate that furosemide does not influence the rate constant for the stimulated efflux of Cl^-. Similarly, furosemide and bumetanide were found to be without effect on the stimulation-induced net efflux of Cl^- in other studies (Nauntofte and Poulsen 1984, 1986; Martinez and Cassity 1985a; Melvin et al. 1987). In agreement with these observations, it is shown in Fig. 2 that phloretin (250 µmol/l), which is a potent inhibitor of chloride transport in erythrocytes (Wieth et al. 1974), is unable to inhibit carbachol-induced net efflux of Cl^-. On the other hand, a Cl^- channel blocker (Wangemann et al. 1986) such as 2-cylcooctylamino-5-nitrobenzoic acid, in a concentration of 100 µmol/l (Poulsen et al. 1988), was able to inhibit net efflux of Cl^- induced by carbachol by 100%. Partial inhibition was obtained by use of diphenylamine-2-carboxylate (DPC), which inhibited by 60% in a concentration of 1 mmol/l (Melvin et al. 1987). In a series of unpublished experiments by B. Nauntofte and J. Hedemark Poulsen it was found that DPC in a concentration of 100 µmol/l inhibited carbachol-induced net efflux of Cl^- from rat parotid acini by 51%.

Mechanism of Cl^- Release

The quoted studies based on use of isotopes and of ion-selective microelectrodes have clearly demonstrated that the stimulation-induced net efflux of Cl^- takes place in the direction of the electrochemical gradient and is thus mediated by passive transport mechanisms. However, these studies do not allow firm conclusions to be drawn concerning the transport mechanisms involved or whether the efflux occurs across the luminal and/or the basolateral acinar cell membrane. Fortunately, patch-clamp studies using the whole-cell configuration have revealed that in acinar cells of lacrimal glands (Marty et al. 1984; Findlay and Petersen 1985) and salivary glands (Cook et al. 1988) calcium-dependent chloride channels are activated upon stimulation. Even though a quantitative comparison of single-channel chloride currents in patch-clamp experiments and net efflux of chloride in isotope experiments has not as yet been carried out, it seems very likely that the reported stimulation-induced release of Cl^- is due to electrodiffusion through Cl^- channels.

The whole-cell clamp experiments referred to above cannot give information about the location of channels in the luminal and/or the basolateral cell membranes, however. A luminal location is obvious if the chloride channels are related to secretion of primary saliva. It is therefore comforting that a luminal location of Cl^- channels has been demonstrated directly in patches from the rectal gland of the shark, which in many respects is similar to salivary glands (Greger et al. 1985).

Control of Secretion of Primary Saliva

It has been concluded in a number of studies that more or less modified versions of the model originally proposed by Silva et al. (1977) to account for secretion by the rectal gland of the shark are able to account for secretion of primary saliva (e.g., Poulsen and Kristensen 1982; Poulsen et al. 1982; Petersen and Maruyama 1984; Nauntofte and Poulsen 1984, 1986; Martinez and Cassity 1985a, 1985b; Turner et al. 1986; Kawaguchi et al. 1986; Melvin et al. 1987; Cook et al. 1988). According to the simplest version of the model, control of secretion can theoretically be exerted at any of the four principal components: (1) the basolaterally located Na^+-, K^+-ATPase, (2) the basolateral cotransporter, (3) the basolateral K^+ channel, (4) the luminally located Cl^- channel. In addition, the more elaborated versions of the model (Case et al. 1984; Novak and Young 1986; Pirani et al. 1987; Turner and George 1988; Nauntofte and Dissing 1988a) allows for further control via: (5) the basolateral Na^+-H^+ exchanger and (6) a $Cl^--HCO_3^-$ exchanger. Finally, (7) the permeability of the tight junctions might be subject to control.

It is well established that stimulation-induced regulation via inositol phosphates and Ca^{2+} of the open-state probability of the basolaterally localized K^+ channels plays a major role in the control of secretion (for a recent review see Petersen and Gallacher 1988). Similarly, direct evidence from whole-cell clamp experiments (Cook et al. 1988) as well as indirect evident based on $^{36}Cl^-$ flux experiments (Poulsen and Kristensen 1982; Nauntofte and Poulsen 1984, 1986; Martinez and Cassity 1985a, 1986; Melvin et al. 1986; Ambudkar et al. 1988) and on experiments with ion-selective microelectrodes (Mori et al. 1983; Lau and Case 1988) indicates that luminal Cl^- channels are activated upon stimulation and that a stimulation-induced increase in intacellular free calcium concentration may be involved.

That activation of both Cl^- (and K^+) channels are necessary to obtain stimulation-induced release of Cl^- (and K^+), and thereby secretion of primary saliva, is illustrated by the experiments shown in Fig. 3. The normal stimulation-induced release of Cl^- shown in Fig. 2 can be prevented by blocking the K^+ channels with quinine. However, addition of the K^+ ionophore, valinomycin, to acini preincubated with quinine compensates in part for the inhibition of K^+ channels by quinine and allows carbachol, which probably activates Cl^- channels under both conditions, to cause a net release of Cl^-, together with K^+ (Nauntofte and Dissing 1988b) and water.

The simple, unifying view that a stimulation-induced rise in the cellular free calcium concentration leads to parallel activation of both basolateral K^+ channels and luminal Cl^- channels has been questioned by Nauntofte and Dissing (1987, 1988b), who found that in the presence of valinomycin, a normal efflux of Cl^- could be obtained in response to carbachol, while the stimulation-induced rise in free intracellular calcium concentration was

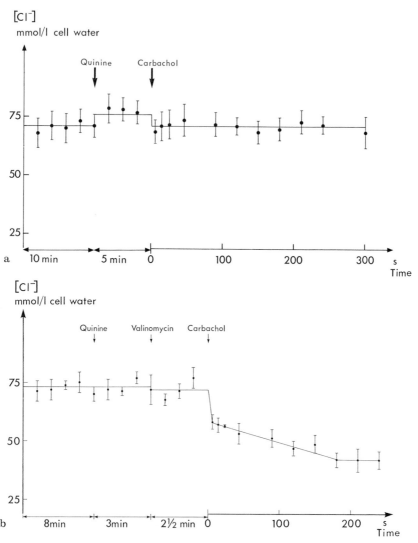

Fig. 3a. Effect of carbachol (20 µmol/l) on the intracellular Cl⁻ concentration in the presence of quinine (500 µmol/l). Number of experiments=6. **b** Effect of carbachol in the presence of quinine and valinomycin (10 µmol/l). Number of experiments=6

abolished. It has been suggested (Poulsen et al. 1988) that opening of luminal Cl⁻ channels might require simultaneous stimulation via intracellular free calcium and the diacylglycerol-protein kinase C system. However, no experimental evidence supporting this idea is available.

Information about a direct activation of other components of the secretion model has not been presented. Even though activation of basolateral K⁺ channels and luminal Cl⁻ channels would in principle allow not only for a transient net efflux of K^+ and Cl^-, but also for a maintained indirect activation of the basolateral cotransporter (due to reductions in cellular K^+ and Cl^- concentrations presumably establishing an inwardly directed gradient), it is questionable whether such an effect would be sufficient. The observation (Fig. 2) that a partial, net reuptake of Cl^- can occur in the continous presence of carbachol (Nauntofte and Poulsen 1986; Melvin et al. 1987) seems difficult to reconcile with a simple gradient-determined behavior of the cotransporter. Thus it seems probable that at the least the cotransporter might be directly controlled by stimulation, presumably mediated via intracellular messengers.

Conclusion

Transport of chloride by salivary gland acinar cells is a very rapid process both in the resting and in the stimulated state. It is now well established that secretomotor agonists cause a substantial release of chloride from salivary gland acinar cells. This efflux, which seems to be meadiated by chloride channels in the luminal cell membrane, is likely to be one of the key steps in secretion of primary saliva. The maintenance of a high intracellular chloride concentration in the unstimulated state and its partial recovery established during prolonged stimulation is supposed to take place via a cotransport system operating with a stoichiometry of $1\,Na^+:1\,K^+:2\,Cl^-$. As a result, the secondary active uptake of chloride is coupled to active sodium transport by the Na^+-, K^+-ATPase. In addition, a $Cl^- - HCO_3^-$ exchanger coupled to a $Na^+ - H^+$ exchanger may contribute.

The control of chloride channels seems in part to be mediated via the cytosolic concentration of free calcium, but other messengers are also likely to contribute. As far as the cotransporter is concerned, theoretical considerations indicate that it might be subject to control, but no direct experimental evidence is available. Finally, it can be concluded that a substantial number of studies has provided qualitative support for the applicability of extented versions of the model by Silva et al. (1977) to secretion of primary saliva.

References

Ambudkar IS, Melvin JE, Baum BJ (1988) Alpha$_1$-adrenergic regulation of Cl^- and Ca^{2+} movements in rat parotid acinar cells. Pflügers Arch 412: 75–79

Burgen ASV (1956) The secretion of potassium in saliva. J Physiol (Lond) 132: 20–39

Burgen ASV (1967) Secretory processes in salivary glands. In: Code CF (ed) Alimentary canal. American Physiological Society, Washington DC, pp 561–579 (Handbook of physiology, vol 2)

Case RM, Hunter M, Novak I, Young JA (1984) The anionic basis of fluid secretion by the rabbit mandibular gland. J Physiol (Lond) 349: 619–630

Cook DI, Gard GB, Champion M, Young JA (1988) Patch-clamp studies of the electrolyte secretory mechanism of rat mandibular gland cells stimulated with acetylcholine or isoproterenol. In: Thorn NA, Treiman M, Petersen OH (eds) Molecular mechanisms in secretion. Munksgaard, Copenhagen, pp 133–145 (Alfred Benzon Symposium 25)

Dalmark M, Wieth JO (1972) Temperature dependence of chloride, bromide, iodide, thiocyanate and salicylate transport in human red cells. J Physiol (Lond) 224: 583–610

Findlay I, Petersen OH (1985) Acetylcholine stimulates a Ca^{2+}-dependent Cl^- conductance in mouse lacrimal acinar cells. Pflügers Arch 403: 328–330

Geck P, Pietrzyk C, Burckhard BC, Pfeiffer B, Heinz E (1980) Electrically silent cotransport of Na^+, K^+ and Cl^- in Ehrlich cells. Biochim Biophys Acta 600: 342–477

Greger R, Schlatter E, Gögelein H (1985) Cl^--channels in the apical membrane of the rectal gland "induced" by cAMP. Pflügers Arch 403: 446–448

Izutsu KT, Johnson DE, Goddard M (1987) Intracellular element concentrations in resting and secreting rat parotid glands. J Dent Res 66: 537–540

Kawaguchi M, Turner RJ, Baum B (1986) $^{36}Cl^-$ and $^{86}Rb^+$ uptake in rat parotid acinar cells. Arch Oral Biol 31: 679–683

Lau KR, Case RM (1988) Evidence for apical chloride channels in rabbit mandibular salivary glands. A chloride-selective microelectrode study. Pflügers Arch 411: 670–675

Lundberg A (1957) Secretory potentials in the sublingual gland of the cat. Acta Physiol Scand 40: 21–34

Lundberg A (1958) Electrophysiology of salivary glands. Physiol Rev 38: 21–40

Martinez JR, Cassity N (1985a) ^{36}Cl fluxes in dispersed rat submandibular acini: effects of acetylcholine and transport inhibitors. Pflügers Arch 403: 50–54

Martinez JR, Cassity N (1985b) Cl^- requirement for saliva secretion in the isolated, perfused rat submandibular gland. Am J Physiol 249: G464–G469

Martinez JR, Cassity N (1986) ^{36}Cl fluxes in dispersed rat submandibular acini: effects of Ca^{2+} omission and of the ionophore A23187. Pflügers Arch 407: 615–619

Marty A, Tan YP, Trautmann A (1984) Three types of calcium-dependent channel in rat lacrimal glands. J Physiol (Lond) 357: 293–325

Melvin JE, Kawaguchi M, Baum BJ, Turner RJ (1987) A muscarinic agonists-stimulated chloride efflux pathway is associated with fluid secretion in rat parotid acinar cells. Biochem Biophys Res Commun 145: 754–759

Mori H, Murakami M, Nakahari T, Imai Y (1983) Intracellular Cl^- activity of canine submandibular gland cells: an in vitro observation. Jpn J Physiol 33: 869–873

Nauntofte B, Dissing S (1987) Stimulation-induced changes in cytosolic calcium in rat parotid acini. Am J Physiol 253: G290–G297

Nauntofte B, Dissing S (1988a) Cholinergic-induced electrolyte transport in rat parotid acini. Comp Biochem Physiol [A] 90: 739–746

Nauntofte B, Dissing S (1988b) K^+ transport and membrane potentials in isolated rat parotid acini. Am J Physiol 255: C508–C518

Nauntofte B, Poulsen JH (1984) Chloride transport in rat parotid acini: furosemide-sensitive uptake and calcium-dependent release. J Physiol (Lond) 357: 61P

Nauntofte B, Poulsen JH (1986) Effects of Ca^{2+} and furosemide on Cl^- transport and O_2 uptake in rat parotid acini. Am J Physiol 251: C175–C185

Novak I, Young JA (1986) Two independent anion transport systems in rabbit mandibular salivary glands. Pflügers Arch 407: 649–656

Palfrey HC, Feit PW, Greengard P (1980) cAMP-stimulated cation cotransport in avian erythrocytes: inhibition by "loop" diuretics. Am J Physiol 238: C139–C148

Petersen OH (1970) Some factors influencing stimulation-induced release of potassium from the cat submandibular gland to fluid perfused through the gland. J Physiol (Lond) 208: 431–447

Petersen OH (1972) Acetylcholine-induced ion transport involved in the formation of saliva. Acta Physiol Scand [Suppl] 381: 1–57

Petersen OH (1986) Calcium-activated potassium channels and fluid secretion by exocrine glands. Am J Physiol 251: G1–G13

Petersen OH, Gallacher DV (1988) Electrophysiology of pancreatic and salivary acinar cells. Annu Rev Physiol 50: 65–80

Petersen OH, Maruyama Y (1984) Calcium-activated potassium channels and their role in secretion. Nature 307: 693–696

Petersen OH, Poulsen JH (1968) Secretory potentials, potassium transport and secretion in the cat submandibular gland during perfusion with sulphate Locke's solution. Experientia 24: 919–920

Petersen OH, Poulsen JH (1969) Secretory transmembrane potentials and electrolyte transients in salivary glands. In: Botelho SY, Brooks FP, Shelley WB (eds) Exocrine glands. University of Pennsylvania Press, Philadelphia, pp 3–20

Pirani DC, Evans LAR, Cook DI, Young JA (1987) Intracellular pH in the rat mandibular gland: the role of $Na-H$ and $Cl-HCO_3$ antiports in secretion. Pflügers Arch 408: 178–184

Poulsen JH, Kristensen LØ (1982) Is stimulation-induced uptake of sodium in rat parotid acinar cells mediated by a sodium/chloride co-transport system? In: Case RM, Garner A, Turnberg LA, Young JA (eds) Electrolyte and water transport across gastrointestinal epithelia. Raven, New York, pp 199–208

Poulsen JH, Nauntofte B (1987) Is the stoichiometry of the parotid co-transporter $1 Na : 1 K : 2 Cl$? J Dent Res 66: 608–609

Poulsen JH, Laugesen LP, Nielsen JOD (1982) Evidence supporting that basolaterally located Na^+-K^+-ATPase and a co-transport system for sodium and chloride are key elements in secretion of primary saliva. In: Case RM, Garner A, Turnberg LA, Young JA (eds) Electrolyte and water transport across gastrointestinal epithelia. Raven, New York, pp 157–159

Poulsen JH, Dissing S, Nauntofte B (1988) Is receptor-activated chloride transport in parotid acini controlled by the cytosolic, free calcium concentration? In: Thorn NA, Treiman M, Petersen OH (eds) Molecular mechanisms in secretion. Munksgaard, Copenhagen, pp 152–164 (Alfred Benzon Symposium 25)

Schneyer LH, Scheyer CA (1960) Electrolyte and inulin spaces of rat salivary glands and pancreas. Am J Physiol 199: 649–652

Silva P, Stoff J, Field M, Fine L, Forrest JN, Epstein FH (1977) Mechanism of active chloride secretion by shark rectal gland: role of Na–K-ATPase in chloride transport. Am J Physiol 233: F298–F306

Smaje LH, Poulsen JH, Ussing HH (1986) Evidence from O_2 uptake measurements for $Na^+-K^+-2Cl^-$ co-transport in the rabbit submandibular gland. Pflügers Arch 406: 492–496

Thaysen JH, Thorn NA, Schwartz IL (1954) Excretion of sodium, potassium, chloride and carbon dioxide in human parotid saliva. Am J Physiol 178: 155–159

Turner RJ, George JN (1988) $Cl^--HCO_3^-$ exchange is present with $Na^+-K^+-Cl^-$ cotransport in rabbit parotid acinar basolateral membranes. Am J Physiol 254: C391–C396

Turner RJ, George JN, Baum BJ (1986) Evidence for a $Na^+/K^+/Cl^-$ cotransport system in basolateral membrane vesicles from the rabbit parotid. J Membr Biol 94: 143–152

Wangemann P, Wittner M, Di Stefano A, Englert HC, Lang HJ, Schlatter E, Greger R (1986) Cl^--channel blockers in the thick ascending limb of the loop of Henle. Structure activity relationship. Pflügers Arch [Suppl 2] 407: 128–141

Wieth JO, Funder J, Gunn RB, Brahm J (1974) Passive transport pathways for chloride and urea through the red cell membrane. In: Bolis L, Bloch K, Luria SE, Lynen F (eds) Comparative biochemistry and physiology of transport. North Holland, Amsterdam, pp. 319–337

Yoshimura H, Imai Y (1967) Studies on the secretory potential of acinar cells of dog's submaxillary gland and the ionic dependency of it. Jpn J Physiol 17: 280–293

Young JA, Schögel E (1966) Micropuncture investigation of sodium and potassium excretion in rat submaxillary saliva. Pflügers Arch 291: 85–98

The Role of Transcellular Chloride Transport in Exocrine Secretion

J. R. Martinez

Introduction

An upsurge of interest in transepithelial Cl^- transport has occurred over the last decade, as a result of the recognition that epithelia exhibit Na-linked, secondary active transport of this ion, which is now generally recognized as the most important ionic movement in the formation of several exocrine gland secretions (Frizzell and Duffey 1980; Widdicombe and Welsh 1980; Martinez and Cassity 1983; Shorofsky et al. 1984; Case et al. 1984; Gaginella 1984; Martinez and Cassity 1985b; Marin 1986; Sato 1986; Smaje et al. 1986; Martinez 1987). Although suggestions of the Cl^- dependency of exocrine secretions had been made before (Lundberg 1958), it was not until 1977 that a model was proposed that could more accurately explain transcellular Cl^- transport (Ernst and Mills 1977; Silva et al. 1977). This model recognized that the direction of Cl^- transport was determined by the membrane localization of a transport protein carrying Cl^- in a coupled fashion with cations, so that the presence of this carrier in the basolateral cell membrane, coupled with a Cl^- conductance pathway in the apical cell membrane, would lead to Cl^- secretion. This cotransport-conductance model has now been applied to a number of secretory epithelia (Greger and Burkhardt 1986). Our purpose here is to review some aspects of transcellular Cl^- transport in secretory epithelia by selecting representative examples of two types of Cl^--transporting tissues, glandular structures that produce a Cl^--rich primary secretion, and tissues that transport Cl^- across the surface linings of some major organ systems. Other comprehensive reviews provide information about Cl^- transport in other epithelia or epithelial cell lines (Simmons 1981; Forte and Wolosin 1987; Schulz 1987; Klyce 1982).

Basic Model of Transcellular Cl^- Transport in Secretory Epithelia

The basic model originally proposed for the shark rectal gland (Silva et al. 1977) and now for a variety of secretory epithelia is illustrated in Fig. 1. Cl^- enters the cell by way of a loop diuretic-sensitive symport located in the

Young · Wong, Epithelial Secretion of Water and Electrolytes
© Springer-Verlag Berlin · Heidelberg 1990

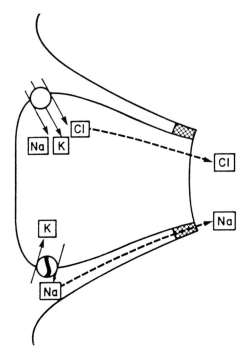

Fig. 1. Basic model of transcellular Cl^- transport in secretory epithelia. Cl^- enters the cell by way of a loop diuretic-sensitive Na^+-K^+-$2Cl^-$ cotransport system in the basolateral cell membrane. A Na^+-, K^+-ATPase present in the same membrane maintains a favorable Na^+ gradient for downhill Na^+ movement into the cell, and some of the energy of the pump is used, therefore, to concentrate Cl^- in the cytosol above electrochemical equilibrium. Cl^- moves out of the cell through anion selective channels in the apical cell membrane and provides a driving force for Na^+ (extruded by the pump into the intercellular space) to move across the tight junction. The work of the pump is therefore translated into a transcellular flow of Cl^-

basolateral membrane, which is energized by the Na^+ gradient maintained by the ouabain-sensitive Na^+-,K^+-ATPase (or Na^+ pump) present in the same membrane. As Na^+ runs down its gradient into the cell, some of the energy of the pump is used to concentrate Cl^- in the cytosol above electrochemical equilibrium. Cl^- then enters the lumen through anion selective channels present in the apical cell membrane, while Na^+ is actively extruded into the intercellular space by the Na^+-,K^+-ATPase. Luminal Cl^- provides a driving force for the movement of Na^+ across the tight junction and the two ions then generate the necessary osmotic gradient for the movement of water across the epithelium. The work of the Na^+-,K^+-ATPase is therefore translated into a transcellular flow of Cl^- in the secretory direction. It has been calculated that with this system, 10 µmol of NaCl will be secreted for each 1.7 µmol of ATP hydrolyzed (Young and Cook 1986).

This model gives rise to a number of predictions that can be tested experimentally. The first is that substances or conditions that inhibit the cotransporter will lead to reduction in both Cl^- uptake and secretion. Results with different preparations (Dartt et al. 1981; Heintze et al. 1983; Dharmsathoporn et al. 1985; Welsh 1983; Young et al. 1987; Martinez 1987), fulfill this prediction, as loop diuretics or removal of external Na^+ or K^+ inhibit one or the other of these responses. The interdependence of the transported ions and the sensitivity of transport to loop diuretics argues in favour of the cotransporter. A second prediction of the model is that intracellular Cl^- activity should be above electrochemical equilibrium. Measurements in resting and stimulated cells have shown this to be the case in several of the epithelial cells being considered (Saito et al. 1985; Lau and Case 1986; Shorofsky et al. 1984). A third prediction is that stimulation should increase the Cl^- conductance of the apical cell membrane. Studies in salivary cells (Lundberg 1958) and in tracheal cells (Welsh 1986b) have shown that this is indeed the case. Other mechanisms for Cl^- entry appear to be present, however, in some secretory epithelia such as salivary acini, where a stilbene sulfonic-sensitive Cl^--HCO_3^- exchange has been documented (Martinez and Cassity 1985c; Novak and Young 1986; Turner and George 1988). Furthermore, the model does not seem to apply strictly to another Cl^--secreting epithelium, the acinar segment of the exocrine pancreas, in which Cl^- entry appears to occur by anion exchange and not by the cotransport system (Seow et al. 1986).

The basic model of Fig. 1 suggests that control of the Cl^- secretory rate and, thus, of overall secretion may be exerted at the level of Cl^- entry or Cl^- efflux in opposite cell membranes. Some recent evidence in this area will now be reviewed. Regulation of other transport mechanisms present in secretory epithelia is discussed in additional contributions to this volume.

Regulation of Transcellular Cl^- Transport

Autonomic Regulation

The relative efficacy of cholinergic and adrenergic stimuli to enhance transcellular Cl^- transport varies in different epithelia and seems to correlate with the relative densities of individual receptors or with their role in fluid/electrolyte secretion. Thus, in airway surface epithelium, where β-adrenergic receptors are abundant (Marin 1986), Cl^- secretion is enhanced by β-agonists. Sweat gland coils respond to both cholinergic and β-adrenergic agonists, which enhance fluid secretion and induce transepithelial PD changes compatible with Cl^- secretion, although the responses are quantitatively different (Sato 1984). A negative luminal PD of about 10 mV developed across isolated segments of the secretory coil during stimulation with methacholine. Isoproterenol stimulation generated a negative luminal

PD of 1.9 mv. In salivary and lacrimal cells, which have both cholinergic and β-adrenergic receptors (Bylund et al. 1982; Stolze and Sommer 1985), fluid secretion and transcellular Cl^- transport are enhanced primarily by cholinergic stimuli (Martinez et al. 1988a; Saito et al. 1985) and by α-adrenergic agonists (Martinez and Reed 1988).

Information about the regulation of Cl^- entry is indirect as not enough is known about the transport carrier or carriers to allow a more direct analysis of its physiological regulation. In acini isolated from the rat mandibular gland, for example, uptake of the isotopic tracer, $^{36}Cl^-$, is enhanced by β-adrenergic agonists and this effect is inhibited by furosemide (Martinez et al. 1988a). In contrast, tracer content is reduced by exposure to acetylcholine as a result of a rapid increase in Cl^- efflux (Martinez and Cassity 1985a). The initial efflux is followed in parotid acini (Nauntofte and Poulsen 1984, 1986) and, to a lesser extent, in mandibular cells (Martinez and Cassity 1986) by Cl^- reuptake, which is sensitive to furosemide (Nauntofte and Poulsen 1984, 1986). In lacrimal glands and sweat glands, furosemide inhibits Cl^- secretion induced by cholinergic stimuli (Dartt et al. 1981; Sato and Sato 1987), which suggests that stimulation activates the basolateral symport. Similar observations have been made in tracheal epithelium stimulated by β-adrenergic agonists (Welsh 1983, 1986a; Widdicombe et al. 1983) and in mammalian intestine, where agonist-induced Cl^- secretion is sensitive to Na^+ replacement and to addition of furosemide to the serosal solution (Heintze et al. 1983).

A primary target of autonomic stimuli seems to be the Cl^- conductance pathway (Findlay and Petersen 1985). Agonist-activated Cl^- channels have been directly demonstrated by patch clamping in salivary (Young et al. 1988), lacrimal (Evans and Marty 1986a) and tracheal epithelial cells (Welsh 1986b). More indirect evidence also suggests activation of anion conductances in some tissues. Thus, N-phenyl anthranilic acid, a Cl^- channel blocker, inhibits vasoactive intestinal peptide (VIP)-induced Cl^- secretion in T_{84} cells (Donowitz and Welsh 1986); in rat mandibular acini, acetylcholine increases net efflux of $^{36}Cl^-$ from tracer-preloaded cells and diphenylcarboxylic acid (DPC) inhibits this response (Martinez et al. 1987).

The findings summarized above suggest that Cl^--transporting epithelia belong to two classes with respect to the autonomic regulation of apical Cl^- conductance pathways. The first includes tissues such as the shark rectal gland and the trachea, in which this regulation is primarily by β-adrenergic stimuli. The second includes salivary and lacrimal cells, in which regulation is by cholinergic stimuli. In the sweat gland, on the other hand, Cl^- conductance appears to be regulated, albeit to a different extent, by both types of stimuli (Sato and Sato, 1981), and, in tracheal epithelium cholinergic stimuli also enhance Cl^- secretion by stimulating the serosa to mucosa flux of Cl^- (Widdicombe and Welsh 1980).

As predicted by the model of Fig. 1, the ratio of the observed intracellular Cl^- activity to the expected equilibrium activity will change with stimulation, depending on the extent to which the stimulus increases Cl^- entry or efflux. This ratio was found to be greater than unity in resting salivary cells (4.95 ± 0.33) and fell 50% after stimulation, suggesting the activation of an Cl^- exit pathway (Lau and Case 1986). Similar results were observed in canine tracheal cells, in which epinephrine reduced the difference between measured Cl^- and equilibrium Cl^- concentrations from 30 to 11 mmol/l (Shorofsky et al. 1984). Stimulation with acetylcholine also reduces the Cl^- content of lacrimal cells (Saito et al. 1985) and of cells of the secretory coil of sweat glands of the monkey palm (Saga and Sato 1986).

Role of Intracellular Mediators

Two major signal transduction mechanisms (Putney 1986; Donowitz and Welsh 1986) have been implicated in the regulation of Cl^- transport in secretory epithelia. In tissues such as canine and human trachea, exogenous derivatives of cyclic AMP or exposure to substances that increase formation of this nucleotide enhance Cl^- secretion or Cl^- conductance pathways (Marin 1986; Welsh 1986a). In tissues such as salivary and lacrimal cells where Cl^- transport is regulated primarily by cholinergic receptors, Cl^- secretion (efflux) or Cl^- channels can be modified by changes in cell Ca^{2+} (Martinez and Cassity 1986; Nauntofte and Poulsen 1986; Evans and Marty 1986a, b). Such a strict distinction between the two signal-transducing mechanisms is not as clear in other secretory epithelia. Thus, both signaling systems may be involved in the regulation of Cl^- transport in the sweat gland coil (Sato and Sato 1983) and in the intestine (Fondacaro 1986). Likewise, in tracheal epithelium, changes in cell Ca^{2+} induced by α agonists or by A23187 appear to participate in the modulation of Cl^- channels through the activation of basolateral K^+ channels (Welsh and McCann 1985).

Relatively little information is available regarding the role of intracellular messenges in regulating Cl^- entry by way of the Na^+-K^+-$2Cl^-$ symport, but cyclic AMP may be involved in activation of the symport in rat mandibular acini (Martinez et al. 1988a). Indirect evidence supports the view that in cases where Ca^{2+} seems to control the putative apical Cl^- conductances, both internal and external Ca^{2+} are involved. In rat mandibular acini, for example, efflux of $^{36}Cl^-$ in the presence of acetylcholine is of small magnitude and transient in the absence of Ca^{2+}, but becomes sustained when Ca^{2+} is present (Martinez and Cassity 1986). Inhibition of internal Ca^{2+} release with 3,4,5-trimethoxybenzoic acid 8-(diethyllamino)octyl ester (TMB-8) reduced the transient efflux of $^{36}Cl^-$ observed in Ca^{2+}-free medium (Martinez et al. 1988b). The divalent cation ionophore, A23187, only causes the second phase of K^+ release from salivary fragments (Putney 1976). In contrast to the first phase of release, this phase is dependent on external Ca^{2+} and is probably due, therefore, to Ca^+ influx across the cell membrane. These observations suggest that A23187 does not enhance internal Ca^{2+} release to any significant extent. Similarly, A23187 fails to induce $^{36}Cl^-$ efflux in the absence of external Ca^{2+} (Martinez and Cassity 1986), which also suggests that it causes Cl^- efflux by enhancing external Ca^{2+} influx. Recent studies in our laboratory using fluorescence spectroscopy of Fura-2 have shown that acetylcholine causes a sustained increase in cytosolic Ca^{2+} of rat mandibular cells incubated in a Ca^{2+}-containing medium, but a more transient change in a Ca^{2+}-free medium (Martinez and Camden, 1989). Other recent studies have shown that, as in other cells, release of internal Ca^{2+} in salivary acini seems to depend on the formation of inositol trisphosphate (IP_3), because 1,4,5 and 1,3,4 IP_3 enhances the release of $^{45}Ca^{2+}$ from an ATP-dependent, nonmitochondrial pool in permeabilized acini (Camden and Martinez 1988). In lacrimal gland cells, internal application of IP_3 elicited Ca^{2+}-dependent Cl^- (and K^+) currents similar to those observed with acetylcholine (Evans and Marty 1986b), and the effect was inhibited by sustained depolarization and by removal of external Ca^{2+} (Llano et al. 1987). Similar effects were observed after internal exposure to the guanosine triphosphate (GTP) analogue, GTP-γ-S, and it was suggested that a GTP-binding protein was activated by receptor stimulation and that this, in turn, activated phospholipase C and the production of IP_3 (Evans and Marty 1986b).

Involvement of Protein Kinase C

Recent evidence in three Cl^--secreting epithelia indicates that protein kinase C (PK_C) may be involved in the regulation of transcellular Cl^- transport. PK_C is activated by tumor-promoting phorbol esters (Nishizuka 1984), and Llano and Marty (1987) have recently shown that preincubation with 12-0-tetradecanocyl-phorbol-13-acetate (TPA) inhibited acetylcholine-induced, Ca^{2+}-dependent Cl^- (and K^+) currents in rat lacrimal cells. Cl^- currents induced by IP_3 were not modified by TPA, while those induced by GTP-γ-S were inhibited by the phorbol derivative. In cultured canine tracheal epithelial cells, TPA and synthetic diacylglycerol 1-oleolyl-2-acetylglycerol (OAG) stimulated short-circuit current, an effect abolished in Cl^--free solutions, and transepithelial $^{36}Cl^-$ flux (Barthelson et al. 1987). The authors speculate that PK_C may directly interact with Cl^- channels or with other transport proteins involved in Cl^- secretion, blocking their activation by cyclic AMP (Barthelson et al. 1987).

Welsh has also reported (1987) that another phorbol ester (PMA) stimulates Cl^- secretion in both native and cultured monolayers of canine tracheal epithelium, and that this effect was not dependent on prostaglandin or cyclic AMP production. However, at higher concentrations, PMA inhibited cyclic AMP-induced secretion, and at submaximal concentrations it amplified the response to forskolin (Welsh 1987). Thus, PK_C may modulate the response to agents that increase cyclic AMP or stimulate secretion directly.

Similar results have been documented in intestinal epithelia, where phorbol esters have been shown to stimulate Cl^- secretion in porcine jejunum (Weikel et al. 1985), in rat small intestine (Fondacaro and Henderson 1985) and in rabbit and chicken distal ileum (Chang et al. 1985). In the latter tissues the response was inhibited by indomethacin, suggesting that it was mediated by prostaglandins.

Effects of Other Biologically Active Substances

Cl^- secretion induced by A 23187 in tracheal epithelium (Welsh 1987) or by cholinergic agents in rabbit or chicken ileum (Chang et al. 1985) was inhibited by indomethacin, which suggests a role for prostaglandins (PG) as modulators of transcellular Cl^- transport. Likewise, in rabbit colonic mucosa, A 23187 and arachidonic acid increased Cl^- secretion, and the effect was abolished by indomethacin (Smith and McCabe 1984). Leukotrienes increased short circuit current and net $^{36}Cl^-$ flux toward the mucosa in canine tracheal epithelium, and the former effect was reduced by indomethacin, suggesting that lipooxygenase products modulated Cl^- secretion through the release of PG (Leirkaug et al. 1986). By contrast, PG did not modify uptake or net efflux or $^{36}Cl^-$ in rat mandibular acini (Martinez and Barker 1987).

VIP increases net Cl^- secretion and short-circuit current in T_{84} cells, an effect inhibited by bumetanide and by the omission of Na^+, K^+ or Cl^- from the serosal medium, suggesting the involvement of a Na^+-K^+-$2Cl^-$ cotransport system (Dharmsathaphorn et al. 1985). Histamine caused a rapid and transient increase in Cl^- secretion in these cells, an effect associated with an increased free cytostolic Ca^{2+} concentration (Wasserman et al. 1988).

Interaction of Cl^- Transport with the Transport of Other Ions

Ca^{2+}-dependent K^+ channels have been described in several of the tissues under discussion (Petersen and Maruyama 1984). The K^+ lost by passive efflux upon stimulation is recycled back into the cells by way of the Na^+-, K^+-ATPase and the Na^+-K^+-$2Cl^-$ cotransport system. K^+ efflux is therefore thought to be in some manner associated with subsequent activation of these mechanisms. K^+ efflux also appears to be functionally linked to Cl^- efflux in rat mandibular acini, as net efflux of $^{36}Cl^-$ is induced by the K^+ ionophore valinomycin and inhibited by the K^+ channel blocker, quinidine (Martinez et al. 1987). A similar link has been demonstrated in canine tracheal epithelium, in which Ca^{2+}-regulated basolateral K^+ channels functionally linked to Cl^- secretion have been described (Welsh and McCann 1985). K^+ efflux is also prominent in lacrimal cells (Trautmann

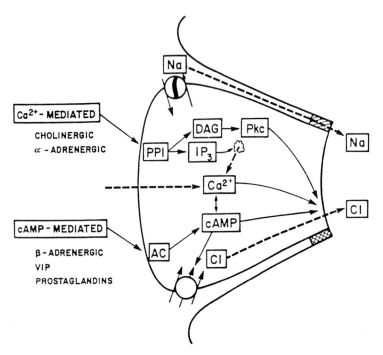

Fig. 2. Expanded model of trancellular Cl^- transport in secretory epithelia, including some important regulatory phenomena. Cl^- exit from the cell can be influenced, depending on the tissue and the receptors being stimulated, by an increased cell Ca^{2+} or an increased cyclic AMP. The increase in cell Ca^{2+} is the result of release of internal Ca^{2+} and influx of external Ca^{2+}. The first of these movements is dependent on an increased turnover of membrane phosphoinositides and the formation of inositol trisphosphate (IP_3). Another product of this turnover, diacylglycerol (DAG), activates protein kinase C (PKc), which in some exocrine tissues appears to affect apical Cl^- channels directly. PKc can also modulate the response to substances that increase cyclic AMP in some tissues, such as tracheal and intestinal epithelium. In the rodent mandibular salivary gland cyclic AMP may regulate the activity of the Na^+-K^+-$2Cl^-$ symport in the basolateral membrane

and Marty 1984), although a potential link with Cl^- transport has not been directly investigated.

Cl^- Transport and Secretion: An Expanded Model

Based on the evidence summarized above, the basic model shown in Fig. 1 can now be expanded (Fig. 2) to include the following additional elements: (a) Stimulation-induced K^+ efflux through Ca^{2+}- and voltage-regulated channels in the basolateral cell membrane is prominent in some of the tissues under discussion and may be functionally linked to activation of both the Na^+-K^+-$2Cl^-$ symport and the apical Cl^- channels; (b) two types of regulatory influences may affect transcellular Cl^- transport. The first involves the hydrolysis of membrane phosphoinositides and the production of IP_3 and diacylglycerol. These products then influence Cl^- transport, respectively, by inducing release of Ca^{2+} from internal stores and by activating PK_C. The increase in cystosolic Ca^{2+} that results in the first case regulates the opening of apical Cl^- channels and, thus, movement of Cl^- into the lumen. PK_C may directly modulate these channels or modify the activation of the basolateral symport by cyclic AMP. The second regulatory pathway of Cl^- transport involves the production of cyclic AMP and the activation of protein kinase A. In some of the tissues under discussion, these appear to influence both Cl^- entry and Cl^- efflux by effects on the basolateral symport and the apical anion channels. In tissues such as the intestine, cyclic AMP may also influence internal Ca^{2+} release and in both tracheal and intestinal epithelium changes in cell Ca^{2+} may affect Cl^- transport by enhancing PG formation and, thus, the formation of cyclic AMP.

Clearly, additional extensive research is necessary to elucidate further what are undoubtedly complex interactions in the regulation of transcellular Cl^- transport. These interactions are likely to vary in different Cl^--secreting epithelia, and caution must be exercised in extrapolating from one to the others.

Abnormalities of Cl^- Transport: Cystic Fibrosis

The importance of transcellular Cl^- transport in exocrine tissues is highlighted by mounting evidence that a primary alteration in the hereditary human disease cystic fibrosis involves epithelial Cl^- transport. Quinton (1983) first demonstrated that the reabsorptive ducts of the sweat glands of affected individuals have alterations in transepithelial PD compatible with Cl^- impermeability. Subsequently, electrophysiological studies in nasal and airway epithelium indicated a defective secretion of Cl^- (Knowles et al. 1983). More recent evidence has shown that this defect is associated with abnormal regulation of apical Cl^- channels at a step beyond the generation of cyclic AMP (Frizzell et al. 1986; Welsh and Liedtke 1986). A similar lack of response to isoproterenol has been demonstrated in the sweat gland, which fails to show secretory or electrophysiological responses to this agonist (Sato and Sato 1984). Bijman et al. (1988) have also reported a defective Cl^- secretion in stripped ileal mucosa of cystic fibrosis patients which involves significantly reduced responses to cyclic nucleotides and to Ca^{2+}-mediated agonists.

References

Barthelson RA, Jacoby DB, Widdicombe JH (1987) Regulation of chloride secretion in dog tracheal epithelium by protein kinase C. Am J Physiol 253: C802–C808

Bijman J, Kansen M, Hoogeveen AH, Scholte B, Van der Kamp A, de Jong H (1988) Electrolyte transport in normal and CF epithelia. In: Wong PYF, Young JA (eds) Exocrine secretion. Hong Kong University Press, Hong Kong, pp 17–20

Bylund DB, Martinez JR, Pierce DL (1982) Regulation of autonomic receptors in rat submandibular gland. Mol Pharmacol 21: 27–35

Camden J, Martinez JR (1988) Effect of inositol triphosphate (IP$_3$) on ATP-dependent ^{45}Ca uptake in permeabilized rat submandibular acini. In: Wong PYD, Young JA (eds) Exocrine secretion. Hong Kong University Press, Hong Kong, pp 37–38

Case RM, Hunter M, Novak I, Young JA (1984) The anionic basis of fluid secretion by the rabbit mandibular gland. J Physiol (Lond) 349: 619–630

Chang EB, Wang N, Rao MC (1985) Phorbol ester stimulation of active anion secretion in intestine. Am J Physiol 249: C356–C361

Dartt DA, Möller M, Poulsen JH (1981) Lacrimal gland electrolyte and water secretion in the rabbit: localization and role of Na$^+$ and K$^+$ activated ATP-ase. J Physiol (Lond) 321: 557–569

Dharmsathaphorn K, Mandel KG, Masui H, McRoberts JA (1985) Vasoactive intestinal polypeptide-induced chloride secretion by a colonic epithelial cell line. J Clin Invest 75: 462–471

Donowitz M, Welsh MJ (1986) Ca^{2+} and cyclic AMP in regulation of intestinal Na, K, and Cl transport. Annu Rev Physiol 48: 135–150

Ernst SA, Mills JW (1977) Basolateral plasma membrane localization of ouabain-sensitive sodium transport sites in the secretory epithelium of the avian salt gland. J Cell Biol 75: 74–94

Evans MG, Marty A (1986a) Calcium dependent chloride currents in isolated cells from rat lacrimal glands. J Physiol (Lond) 378: 437–460

Evans MG, Marty A (1986b) Potentiation of muscarinic and adrenergic responses by an analogue of guanosine 5' triphosphate. Proc Natl Acad Sci USA 83: 4099–4103

Findlay I, Petersen OH (1985) ACh stimulates a Ca^{2+} dependent Cl$^-$ conductance in mouse lacrimal acinar cells. Pflügers Arch 403: 328–330

Fondacaro JD (1986) Intestinal ion transport and diarrheal disease. Am J Physiol 250: G1–G8

Fondacaro JD, Henderson LS (1985) Evidence for protein kinase C as a regulator of intestinal electrolyte transport. Am J Physiol 249: G422–G426

Forte JG, Wolosin JM (1987) HCl secretion by the gastric oxyntic cell. In: Johnson LR (ed) Physiology of the gastrointestinal tract, 2nd edn. Raven, New York, pp 853–864

Frizzell RA, Duffey ME (1980) Chloride activities in epithelia. Fed Proc 39: 2860–2864

Frizzell RA, Rechkemmer G, Shoemaker RL (1986) Altered regulation of airway epithelial cell chloride channels in cystic fibrosis. Science 233: 558–560

Gaginella TS (1984) Neuromodulation of intestinal ion transport. Fed Proc 43: 2929–2934

Greger R, Burkhardt G (1986) Epithelial anion transport – hormonal regulation. Pflügers Arch 407 (Suppl 2): S59–S186

Heintze K, Stewart CP, Frizzell RA (1983) Sodium dependent chloride secretion across rabbit descending colon. Am J Physiol 244: G357–G365

Klyce SD (1982) Cl transport in rabbit cornea. In: Zadunaisky JA (ed) Chloride transport in biological membranes. Academic, New York, pp 199–222

Knowles MR, Stutts MJ, Spock A, Fischer NL, Gatzy JT, Boucher RC (1983) Abnormal ion permeation through cystic fibrosis respiratory epithelium. Science 221: 1067–1070

Lau KR, Case RM (1986) Chloride activity in mandibular salivary gland cells during secretion. Biomed Res 7 (Suppl 2): 181–184

Leirkaug GD, Ueki IF, Widdicombe JH, Nadel JA (1986) Alterations of chloride secretion across canine tracheal epithelium by lipoxygenase products of arachidonic acid. Am J Physiol 250: F47–F53

Llano I, Marty A (1987) Protein kinase C activators inhibit the inositol triphosphate-mediated muscarinic current responses in rat lacrimal cells. J Physiol (Lond) 394: 239–248

Llano I, Marty A, Tanguy J (1987) Dependence of intracellular effects of GTPγS and inositol triphosphate on cell membrane potential and on external calcium ions. Pflügers Arch 409: 499–506

Lundberg A (1958) Electrophysiology of salivary glands. Physiol Rev 38: 21–40

Marin MG (1986) Pharmacology of airway secretion. Pharmacol Rev 38: 273–289

Martinez JR (1987) Ion transport and water movement. J Dent Res 66: 638–647

Martinez JR, Barker S (1987) Effect of prostaglandins on Cl and K transport in rat submandibular acini. Arch Oral Biol 32: 843–847

Martinez JR, Cassity N (1983) Effect of transport inhibitors on secretion by perfused rat submandibular glands. Am J Physiol 245: G711–G716

Martinez JR, Cassity N (1985a) ^{36}Cl fluxes in dispersed rat submandibular acini: effects of acetylcholine and transport inhibitors. Pflügers Arch 403: 50–54

Martinez JR, Cassity N (1985b) Cl requirement for saliva secretion in the isolated perfused rat submandibular gland. Am J Physiol 249: G464–G469

Martinez JR, Cassity N (1985c) Effects of 4,4′-diisothiocyano-2,2′-stilbene disulphonic acid and amiloride on saliva secretion by isolated, perfused rat submandibular glands. Arch Oral Biol 30: 797–803

Martinez JR, Cassity N (1986) ^{36}Cl fluxes in dispersed rat submandibular acini: effects of Ca^{2+} omission and of the ionophore A23187. Pflügers Arch 407: 615–619

Martinez JR, Reed P (1988) Selective effects of α and β-adrenergic receptor stimulation on ^{36}Cl fluxes in rat submandibular acini. J Dent Res 67: 561–564

Martinez JR, Cassity N, Reed P (1987) Apparent functional linkage between K^+ efflux and ^{36}Cl efflux in rat submandibular acini. Arch Oral Biol 32: 891–895

Martinez JR, Cassity N, Reed R (1988a) Effects of isoproterenol on Cl transport in rat submandibular salivary gland acini. Arch Oral Biol 32: 891–895

Martinez JR, Cassity N, Reed P (1988b) Effects of two types of Ca^{2+} antagonists on ^{36}Cl efflux in rat submandibular acini. In: Wong PYD, Young JA (eds) Exocrine secretion. Hong Kong University Press, Hong Kong, pp 115–118

Martinez JR, Camden J (1989) Ca^{2+} mobilization and Cl^- efflux in submandibular salivary cells of adult and newborn rats. Arch Oral Biol 34: 147–152

Nauntofte B, Poulsen JH (1984) Chloride transport in rat parotid acini: furosemide-sensitive uptake and calcium-dependent release (Abstract). J Physiol (Lond) 357: 61P

Nauntofte B, Poulsen JH (1986) Effects of Ca^{2+} and furosemide on Cl^- transport and O_2 uptake in rat parotid acini. Am J Physiol 251: C175–C185

Nishizuka Y (1984) The role of protein kinase C in cell surface signal transduction and tumor production. Nature 308: 693–698

Novak I, Young JA (1986) Two independent anion transport systems in rabbit mandibular salivary glands. Pflügers Arch 407: 649–656

Petersen OH, Maruyama Y (1984) Calcium-activated potassium channels and their role in secretion. Nature 301: 693–696

Putney JW (1976) Biphasic modulation of potassium release in rat parotid gland by carbachol and phenylephrine. J Pharmacol Exp. Ther 198: 375–384

Putney JW (1985) Identification of cellular activation mechanisms associated with salivary secretion. Annu Rev Physiol 48: 75–88

Quinton PM (1983) Chloride impermeability in cystic fibrosis. Nature 301: 421–422

Saga K, Sato K (1986) Effects of inhibitors of sweat secretion on intracellular Na^+, K^+, and Cl^- levels in the eccrine sweat gland during cholinergic stimulation as studied by x-ray microanalysis. Clin Res 34: 421–422

Saito Y, Ozawa T, Hazasaki H, Nishiyama A (1985) Acetylcholine-induced changes in intracellular Cl activity of the mouse lacrimal acinar cells. Pflügers Arch 405: 108–111

Sato K (1984) Differing luminal potential difference of cystic fibrosis and control sweat secretory coils in vitro. Am J Physiol 247: R646–R649

Sato K (1986) Effect of methacholine on ionic permeability of basal membrane of the eccrine secretory cell. Pflügers Arch 407 (Suppl 2): S100–S106

Sato K, Sato F (1981) Cholinergic potentiation of isoproterenol-induced cyclic AMP level in the sweat gland. Am J Physiol 240: R55–R51

Sato K, Sato F (1983) Cholinergic potentiation of isoproterenol-induced cAMP level in the sweat gland. Am J Physiol 245: C189–C195

Sato K, Sato F (1984) Defective beta adrenergic response of cystic fibrosis sweat glands in vivo and in vitro. J Clin Invest 73: 1763–1771

Sato K, Sato F (1987) Non-isotonicity of simian eccrine primary sweat induced in vitro. Am J Physiol 252: R1099–R1105

Schulz I (1987) Electrolyte and fluid secretion in the exocrine pancreas. In: Johnson LR (ed) Physiology of the gastrointestinal tract, 2nd edn. Raven, New York, pp 1147–1172

Seow KTF, Lingard JM, Young JA (1986) Anionic basis of fluid secretion by rat pancreatic acini in vitro. Am J Physiol 250: G140–G148

Shorofsky SR, Field M, Fozzard HA (1984) Mechanism of Cl secretion in canine trachea: changes in intracellular chloride activity with secretion. J Membr Biol 81: 1–8

Silva R, Stoff J, Field M, Fine L, Forrest JN, Epstein FH (1977) Mechanism of active chloride secretion by shark rectal gland: role of Na-K-ATPase in Cl transport. Am J Physiol 233: F298–F306

Simmons NL (1981) Ion transport in tight epithelial monolayer of MDCK cells. J Membr Biol 59: 105–114

Smaje LH, Poulsen JH, Ussing HH (1986) Evidence from O_2 uptake measurements for Na^+-K^+-$2Cl^-$ co-transport in the rat submandibular gland. Pflügers Arch 406: 492–496

Smith PL, McCabe RD (1984) A23187-induced changes in colonic K and Cl transport are mediated by separate mechanisms. Am J Physiol 247: G695–G702

Stolze HH, Sommer HJ (1985) Influence of secretagogues on volume and protein pattern in rabbit lacrimal fluid. Curr Eye Res 4: 489–492

Trautman A, Marty A (1984) Activation of Ca dependent K channels by carbamylcholine in rat lacrimal glands. Proc Natl Acad Sci USA 81: 611–615

Turner RJ, George HN (1988) Cl^-/HCO_3^- exchange is present with Na^+-K^+-Cl^- transport in rabbit parotid acinar basolateral membranes. Am J Physiol 254: C391–C396

Wasserman SI, Barrett KE, Huott PA, Beurlein G, Kagnoff MF, Dharmsathaphorn K (1988) Immune-related intestinal Cl^- secretion. I. Effect of histamine on the T84 cell line. Am J Physiol 254: C53–C62

Weikel CS, Sando JJ, Geurrant RL (1985) Stimulation of porcine jejunal ion secretion in vivo by protein kinase C activators. J Clin Invest 76: 2430–2435

Welsh MJ (1983) Inhibition of chloride secretion by furosemide in canine tracheal epithelium. J Membr Biol 71: 219–226

Welsh MJ (1986a) Adrenergic regulation of ion transport by primary cultures of canine tracheal epithelium: cellular physiology. J Membr Biol 91: 121–128

Welsh MJ (1986b) An apical membrane chloride channel in human tracheal epithelium. Science 232: 1648–1650

Welsh MJ (1987) Effect of phorbol ester and Ca ionophore on chloride secretion in canine tracheal epithelium. Am J Physiol 253: C828–C834

Welsh MJ, Liedtke CM (1986) Chloride and potassium channels in cystic fibrosis airway epithelia. Nature 322: 467–470

Welsh MJ, McCann JD (1985) Intracellular Ca regulates basolateral K channels in a chloride secreting epithelium. Proc Natl Acad Sci USA 82: 8823–8826

Widdicombe JH, Welsh MJ (1980) Ion transport by dog tracheal epithelium. Fed Proc 39: 3062–3066

Widdicombe JH, Nathanson IT, Highland E (1983) Effects of "loop" diuretics on ion transport by dog tracheal epithelium. Am J Physiol 245: C388–C396

Young JA, Cook DI (1986) Secretion of salt and water by glandular epithelia. Biomed Res 7 (Suppl 2): 165–176

Young JA, Cook DI, Evans LAR, Pirani D (1987) Effects of ion transport inhibition on rat mandibular gland secretion. J Dent Res 66: 531–536
Young JA, Gard GB, Champion MP, Cook DI (1988) Patch-clamp studies on muscarinic stimulus-secretion coupling in rat mandibular gland endpiece cells. In: Wong PYD, Young JA (eds) Exocrine secretion. Hong Kong University Press, Hong Kong, pp 219–222

Bicarbonate Transport by Salivary Gland Acinar Cells*

K. R. Lau, A. C. Elliott, P. D. Brown, and R. M. Case

Introduction

Saliva Bicarbonate Concentration

In human saliva collected from the openings of the main salivary gland ducts, HCO_3^- concentration is about 5 mmol/l during spontaneous secretion, but increases dramatically to 40–60 mmol/l when salivation is stimulated (e.g. by the application of citric acid to the tongue; Ferguson 1975). This increased HCO_3^- output has a beneficial effect in the mouth. Oral bacteria rapidly produce acid from dietary sugars, causing an immediate drop in plaque pH in the mouth (Stephan 1940). In subjects where salivation is inhibited this drop in pH is large and sustained, whereas in normal subjects, salivation attenuates the fall in pH and reduces the duration of lowered plaque pH (Englander et al. 1959). Low plaque pH is associated with dental caries as it causes dissolution of tooth enamel (Hillam 1975; Jenkins 1978). Thus, salivary HCO_3^- appears to have a protective role, and secretion of HCO_3^- can be considered an important function of the salivary glands in man.

The transport mechanisms responsible for this increase in HCO_3^- output are not easy to elucidate in human volunteers. In other species, patterns of salivary HCO_3^- secretion vary greatly. Young and his co-workers have described at least 5 different patterns in 10 different mammalian species and have emphasized not only the differences between species, but also the differences among different types of salivary glands in the same species (Young and Schneyer 1981; Young et al. 1980). It is a moot point whether a single mechanism could be responsible for all these patterns of HCO_3^- secretion. Nonetheless, recent studies that we have carried out suggest a possible mechanism that could account for the variety of HCO_3^- secretory patterns observed.

---

* Work in the authors' laboratory has been supported by the Wellcome Trust, the Cystic Fibrosis Research Trust (UK) and the Science and Engineering Research Council (UK)

Ductal Regulation of Bicarbonate Output

The two-stage hypothesis of salivary secretion (Thaysen 1960) suggests that a primary secretion, similar in composition to an ultrafiltrate of plasma, is first elaborated by the endpiece (or acinar) portions of the glands and is then modified by transport processes in the ducts. As ductal transport is principally absorptive and the ducts are highly impermeable to water, this results in a saliva that is hypo-osmotic to the primary secretion.

The composition of the primary secretion in a number of glands has been studied using micropuncture techniques (Table 1). The limitations of these techniques when applied to salivary glands have been well rehearsed (Schneyer et al. 1972), the principal difficulty being that samples can only be collected from regions of the ductal tree below the acini. Nonetheless, the composition of fluid sampled in this way has generally been similar to that predicted by the two-stage hypothesis. Although HCO_3^- concentration has generally not been measured directly in these micropuncture samples (because of technical difficulties), the available data suggest that it is not likely to exceed 30 mmol/l (Young and Schneyer 1981; Young and Van Lennep 1979) and that it does not change with stimulation (Schneyer et al. 1972). This has led to the view that changes in saliva HCO_3^- concentration are brought about wholly or largely by ductal transport mechanisms. Ductal perfusion studies *in vitro* and *in vivo* (Grant et al. 1974; Young et al. 1970, 1980; Martin et al. 1973; Martin and Young 1971; Knauf et al. 1982; Denniss and Young 1978; Jirakulsomchok and Schneyer 1979) and recent whole-gland perfusion studies (Martinez and Cassity 1986; Case et al. 1988a) confirm that in rat and rabbit mandibular glands, at least, the ducts are able to secrete HCO_3^- in a regulated way. In the rat mandibular gland this has been attributed to $K^+ - H^+$ exchange in the luminal membrane of duct cells (Knauf et al. 1982), whereas in the rabbit mandibular gland it is thought that $Cl^- - HCO_3^-$ exchange may be responsible (Young and Van Lennep 1979). These data therefore suggest that the acini secrete saliva containing HCO_3^- at a fixed concentration, to which the ducts may add a further, variable amount of HCO_3^-.

Acinar Bicarbonate Transport

Electroneutral Co-Transport

The elaboration of primary saliva is usually explained in terms of the neutral co-transport model of secretion (Silva et al. 1977; Greger et al. 1984), in which transport of Cl^- is the primary secretory process (Fig. 4). Considerable evidence has been adduced in support of this model in salivary acini (Case et al. 1984; Lau and Case 1988; Martinez and Cassity 1985; Smaje

Table 1. Anion deficits and HCO_3^- concentrations in primary secretion collected by micropuncture

Gland	Agonist	Anion deficit (mequiv/l)	$[HCO_3^-]$ (mmol/l)	Source
Rabbit				
Parotid	Pilocarpine/ Carbachol	31.2	27.8 ± 3.7^a	Mangos et al. 1973a
Mandibular	Pilocarpine/ Carbachol	36.4	26.3 ± 4.1^a	
Rat				
Sublingual	Resting	38.4	—	Martin and Young 1971
	Carbachol	45.1		
Neonatal rat				
Terminal-tubule	Resting	40.0	—	Holzgreve et al. 1966
Rat				
Mandibular	Resting	25.0	—	Martinez et al. 1966
Rat				
Mandibular	Resting	39.3	—	Young and Martin 1971
	Carbachol	43.3	—	
	Isoproterenol	50.2	—	
Mouse				
Parotid	Resting	34.6	—	Mangos et al. 1973b
	Pilocarpine	—	34.5 ± 4.9^a	
Mandibular	Resting	32.1	—	
	Pilocarpine	39.2	—	
Cat				
Mandibular	Resting	42.1	—	Kaladelfos and Young 1974
	Carbachol	52.5	—	
	Resting	35.9	—	
	Isoproterenol	30.7	—	
Ferret				
Parotid	Resting	41.8	21.8 ± 4.5	Mangos et al. 1981
	Pilocarpine	56.5	63.5 ± 6.5	
Mandibular	Resting	41.5	24.0 ± 3.8	
	Pilocarpine	10.8	11.5 ± 3.3	
Sheep				
Parotid^b	Sodium replete:			
	Resting	52.0	$\sim 35^c$	Compton et al. 1980
	Stimulated	67.3	35	
	Sodium depleted:			
	Resting	13.6	35	
	Stimulated	17.3	35	

^{a} Estimated from retrograde injection of poly-L-lysine.
^{b} Residual anions include phosphate contribution.
^{c} Calculated from pH determination of primary fluid.

et al. 1986; Turner et al. 1986; Petersen and Maruyama 1984). However, the model takes no account of HCO_3^- transport and in the perfused rabbit mandibular gland does not explain how, provided HCO_3^- is present, fluid

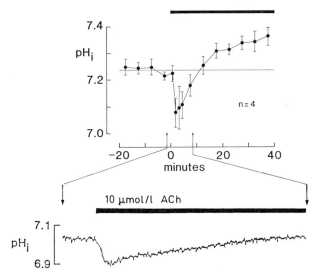

Fig. 1. The effect of 1 µmol/l ACh (*bar, upper trace*) and 10 µmol/l ACh (*bar, lower trace*) on pH_i in rabbit mandibular gland acinar cells measured by nuclear magnetic resonance (NMR) spectroscopy (*upper trace*) and BCECF fluorescence (*lower trace*). NMR data adapted from Steward et al. 1989. The NMR measurements extend to 40 min, whereas the fluorescence measurements to only 10 min. Calibration of the ^{31}PNMR signal was carried out as described by Murakami et al. (this volume, pp 97–139). Calibration of the BCECF fluorescence was carried out as described in Lau et al. (1989)

secretion continues either (a) in the complete absence of Cl^- or (b) when $Na^+-K^+-2Cl^-$ co-transport is inhibited by loop diuretics such as bumetanide (Case et al. 1982, 1984, 1986, 1988a). In order to investigate the mechanism of this HCO_3^--supported secretion, we have been studying intracellular pH (pH_i) in the rabbit mandibular gland with the aim of characterizing acinar HCO_3^- transport pathways.

Studies on Intracellular pH

pH_i has been measured in perfused glands using NMR spectroscopy (Steward et al. 1989; further details are given by Steward et al. in this volume) and in suspensions of dissociated acini using the pH-sensitive fluorescent dye, 2',7'-bis(carboxyethyl)-5(6')-carboxyfluorescein (BCECF) (Lau et al. 1989). Both techniques showed that stimulation with 1 µmol/l acetylcholine (ACh) caused pH_i to decrease by about 0.1 pH units, after which it returned towards control values (BCECF fluorescence) and eventually became more alkaline (NMR spectroscopy; Fig. 1).

The process of acidification induced by ACh could be inhibited by atropine and was dose dependent with maximal and half-maximal doses of approximately 1 µmol/l and 0.2 µmol/l, respectively (Lau et al. 1989). These values compare favourably with those established by Case et al. (1980) for fluid secretion in the whole gland. Changes in pH_i do not necessarily indicate changes in HCO_3^- activity. However, if the experiments were repeated in HCO_3^--free hydroxylethylpiperazine ethanesulphonic acid (HEPES)-buffered solutions, the same concentration of ACh failed to elicit the acidosis measured either by NMR spectroscopy or BCECF fluorescence (Steward et al. 1989; Lau et al. 1989). Together, these data imply that ACh-evoked secretion is accompanied by a HCO_3^- efflux from the acinar cells.

Classical mechanisms for the movement of acid equivalents (including HCO_3^-) across cell membranes are $Cl^- - HCO_3^-$ exchange and $Na^+ - H^+$ exchange. When dissociated acini were suspended in a Cl^--free solution, the resting pH_i was significantly higher than in normal media (compare Fig. 2a with Fig. 1). However, inclusion of the anion exchange inhibitor DIDS (0.1 mmol/l) in the Cl^--free media prevented the increase in pH_i (Lau et al. 1989). These data suggest that acinar cells accumulate HCO_3^- when bathed in Cl^--free medium through a $Cl^- - HCO_3^-$ exchange mechanism. However, in Cl^--free solutions, the addition of ACh was still able to elicit an acidosis whose magnitude was not significantly different from that elicited in normal

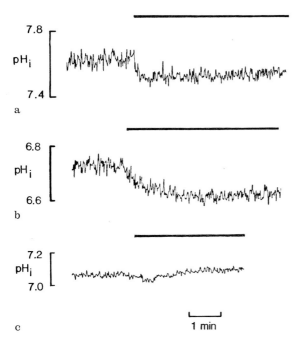

Fig. 2a–c. The effect of 1 μmmol/l ACh on isolated acini suspended in a Cl^--free solution (glucuronate substitution). b Na^+-free solution (N-methyl-D-glucamine substitution). c acini incubated in HCO_3^--buffered solution containing 1 mmol/l diphenylamine-2-caboxylic acid (DPC). The lack of a recovery phase in a and b is probably due to inhibition of $Na^+ - H^+$ exchange by the elevated pH_i in a (>7.1, see Lau et al. 1989) and by the absence of Na^+ in b. The *bars* over the *traces* indicate the presence of ACh

solutions (Fig. 2). An acidosis could also be elicited in normal and Cl^--free solutions containing DIDS (0.1 mmol/l). These experiments demonstrate that a DIDS-sensitive, Cl^--dependent mechanism (probably $Cl^- - HCO_3^-$ exchange) capable of alkalinising the cell is present in mandibular gland acinar cells, but that such a mechanism is not involved in the acidosis evoked by ACh.

In a similar way, $Na^+ - H^+$ exchange, and indeed all forms of Na^+-dependent HCO_3^- co-transport processes such as those described in corneal endothelium and renal tubules (Boron and Boulpaep 1983; Jentsch et al. 1984; Yoshito et al. 1985) could be eliminated as mechanisms responsible for the acidosis. For example, Fig. 2 shows that when acini were suspended in Na^+-free media, ACh was able to elicit an acidosis even though cellular pH had fallen to 6.7 (Brown et al. 1989a).

Acinar Anion Channels

Since the HCO_3^- efflux pathway does not appear to be an exchanger or a co-transporter, the simplest alternative is a channel permeable to HCO_3^-. Very few reports of HCO_3^- channels exist. In the choroid plexus, a HCO_3^- channel has been proposed, but has not been verified (Saito and Wright 1983, 1984). However, Cl^- channels that are also permeable to HCO_3^- have been reported in cultured mouse spinal neurones (Bormann et al. 1987), in crayfish muscle (Kaila and Voipio 1987) and in rat colonic cells (Reinhardt et al. 1987). To seek evidence for such channels in the rabbit mandibular gland, dissociated acini were preincubated with the Cl^- channel blocker diphenylamine-2-carboxylate (DPC). Under these conditions ACh failed to

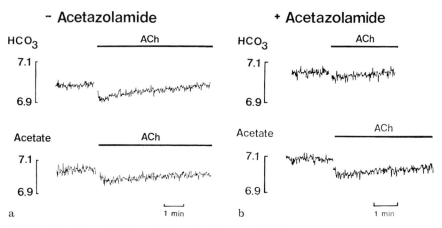

Fig. 3a. The effect of ACh on isolated acini suspended in HCO_3^-- or acetate-containing solutions. **b** The effect of ACh in the presence of 1 mmol/l acetazolamide on acini suspended in HCO_3^-- or acetate-containing solutions; 25 mmol/l HEPES was present as buffer in acetate-containing soutions

induce an acidosis (Fig. 2). Other Cl^- channel blockers (5-nitro-2-(3-phenylpropylamino)-benzoate, NPPB, and compound 131; Wangemann et al. 1986, also blocked the ACh-induced acidosis (Brown et al. 1989b). These results are consistent with the idea that the acidosis induced by ACh is due to HCO_3^- efflux through the apical Cl^--channels proposed by the neutral co-transport model of secretion.

The selectivity of the proposed channel was investigated by substituting HCO_3^- in the incubation medium with other weak acid anions. Propionate, butyrate and acetate were all able to support the ACh-evoked acidosis equally as well as HCO_3^-. Lactate supported a reduced acidosis, while salicylate, formate, and pyruvate failed to support an acidosis (Brown et al. 1989b).

The mechanism by which these anions may accumulate within the cell is illuminated by the experiment shown in Fig. 3. Here, the presence of the carbonic anhydrase inhibitor acetazolamide (1 mmol/l) almost completely inhibited the ACh-induced acidosis in HCO_3^--containing solutions, but not in acetate-containing solutions. This suggests that the effect of acetazolamide is due only to inhibition of carbonic anhydrase activity. Thus, accumulation of HCO_3^- probably involves permeation of lipophilic CO_2 across the membrane and its subsequent hydration by carbonic anhydrase. In a similar way, acetate presumably enters the cell as the lipophilic acetic acid molecule, dissociates, and subsequently leaves the cell as the anion during stimulation, causing the transient acidosis (Fig. 4).

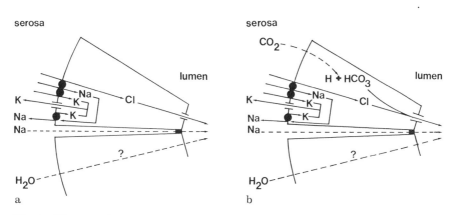

Fig. 4a. The neutral co-transport model of secretion. Cl^- is accumulated within the cell by the action of electroneutral $Na^+ - K^+ - 2Cl^-$ co-transporters in the basolateral membrane. The energy for this co-transport is provided by the Na^+ gradient generated by Na^+-, K^+-ATPases. The excess K^+ by the co-transport is refluxed via basolateral K^+ channels. Secretion is evoked when ACh activates apical Cl^- channels allowing Cl^- to flow into the acinar lumen. Na^+ and water follow passively. The route of water flow is unknown at present. **b** Modification of the neutral co-transport model to account for the role of HCO_3^- in secretion. HCO_3^- and other weak acid anions enter the cell by non-ionic diffusion. They compete with Cl^- for a common channel in the apical pathway during secretion

In separate studies we have also monitored changes in acinar cell Cl^- activity in rabbit mandibular gland pieces using Cl^--selective microelectrodes (Lau and Case 1986, 1988). Resting Cl^- activity is 44 mmol/l. During stimulation with 10 μmol/l ACh it falls to 32 mmol/l. By measuring the initial rates of change of Cl^- and by calculating the initial rates of change of HCO_3^- activity from the observed changes in pH_i (Lau et al. 1989; see Table 2) it is possible to estimate the selectivity of the presumed anion channel for Cl^- over HCO_3^- using the Goldman-Hodgkin-Katz flux equation:

$$J = \frac{-PzF\phi\,[c^o - c^i \exp(zF\phi/RT)]}{RT\,[1 - \exp(zF\phi/RT)]} \tag{1}$$

Table 2. Permeability ratio calculated from initial rates on stimulation

	Initial rates (mmol l^{-1} s^{-1})	c_0 (mmol/l)	c_i (mmol/l)	ϕ (mV)	P_{HCO}/P_{Cl}
Cl^-	1.66 ± 0.39	88	44	-60	0.65
HCO_3^-	0.21 ± 0.06	17.5	9.4	-60^a	

c_0 and c_i, activities in the extracellular and intracellular solutions respectively; ϕ membrane potential; P_{HCO} and P_{Cl}, permeabilities of HCO_3^- and Cl^-, respectively
^{a} Assumed value

Taking the ratio of initial rates for Cl^- and HCO_3^- allows us to write

$$\frac{J_{HCO}}{J_{Cl}} = \frac{P_{HCO}\,[c^o_{HCO} - c^i_{HCO}\exp(z_{HCO}F\phi/RT)]}{P_{Cl}\,[c^o_{Cl} - c^i_{Cl}\exp(z_{Cl}F\phi/RT)]} \tag{2}$$

J represents the ionic flux, the ratio of which is equal to the ratio of observed initial rates, P represents the permeability, c represents the activities of the ions in the outside (^{o}) and intracellular (^{i}) solutions and ϕ represents the membrane potential. The other symbols have their usual meanings.

Inserting the values of Table 2 into the equation gives a $P_{HCO}:P_{Cl}$ selectivity ratio of about 0.6 for the putative channel. This compares with ratios ranging from 0.2 to 0.5 reported for other tissues (Bormann et al. 1987; Kaila and Voipio 1987; Reinhardt et al. 1987).

The picture that emerges from these studies is one which includes relatively unselective anion channels in the apical membrane of the acinar cell which are activated following stimulation with ACh. From the pH_i data, it can be calculated that intracellular HCO_3^- activity in mandibular gland acinar cells is about 9 mmol/l (Lau et al. 1989). Assuming that the potential across the apical membrane is similar to that across the basolateral membrane (i.e. about -50 mV in stimulated glands; Lau and Case 1986, 1988), this means that there is an outwardly directed electrochemical gradient for HCO_3^- (as has also been found for Cl^-; Lau and Case 1986, 1988). Activation of acinar cells by ACh thus allows both HCO_3^- and Cl^- to flow through the channels into the lumen, resulting in the secretion of saliva. The two ions compete for access to the channels so that under normal circumstances there is a much greater secretion of Cl^- than HCO_3^- (Fig. 4).

This mechanism explains the seemingly paradoxical observations made in perfused whole glands that whereas complete replacement of perfusate Cl^- by impermeant ions (e.g. isethionate) results in a reduced secretion supported by HCO_3^-, complete replacement of HCO_3^- has no effect on secretory rate (Case et al. 1982, 1984). Replacement of HCO_3^- merely allows Cl^- free access to the apical channels so that secretory rate is sustained. The reduced flow rate observed when Cl^- is replaced by a non-transported anion simply reflects the lower concentration of HCO_3^- present in the cell.

Acinar Bicarbonate Secretion—A Model Prediction

When the isolated perfused rabbit mandibular gland is stimulated with ACh, the rate of salivary secretion is initially very brisk and then declines to reach a plateau over a period of about 20 min (Case et al. 1980; Steward et al. 1989). By making the assumption that the permeability ratio calculated above (i.e. 0.6) does not change during prolonged stimulation or with changing concentration of HCO_3^- or Cl^-, and knowing the flux ratio and the intracellular activities of HCO_3^- and Cl^- in this phase, Eq. 2 can be used to predict the HCO_3^- composition of the primary saliva in the plateau phase of secretion. The intracellular HCO_3^- activity in this phase is known from our NMR studies (Steward et al. 1989) and the intracellular Cl^- activity from our Cl^- microelectrode studies (Lau and Case 1986). We have studied the dependence of the acidosis on HCO_3^- activity (Brown et al. 1989) and from this can plot the initial rate of change of HCO_3^- activity as a function

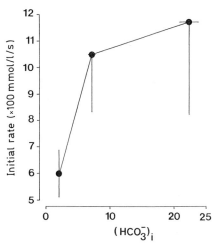

Fig. 5. The dependence of the initial rate of change of intracellular HCO_3^- activity on intracellular HCO_3^- (mmol/l) when isolated acini are stimulated with ACh. The intracellular HCO_3^- activity was calculated from the external pH, measured resting pH_i and measured extracellular HCO_3^- concentration (see Lau et al. 1989; the activity coefficient for HCO_3^- was taken as 0.7). Each point is the mean $\pm$ SEM of 3 experiments for both initial rate and HCO_3^- activity

Table 3. Prediction of primary secretion saliva HCO_3^- activity

	Initial rates	c_i	ϕ	c_{saliva}
HCO_3^-	0.28	17.5^b	-50^c	27.3
Cl^-	1.66	32	-50^c	91^a

c_{saliva}, activity in the primary secretion; ϕ, in this instance apical membrane potential; other symbols as in Table 1

[a] This value is calculated from Mangos et al. 1973.
[b] This value is calculated from NMR data of Steward et al. 1989.
[c] Apical membrane potential is assumed to equal basolateral potential.

of intracellular HCO_3^- activity (Fig. 5). Thus, knowing the intracellular HCO_3^- activity, we can estimate the initial rate of change of HCO_3^- activity during the plateau phase of secretion. Although intracellular Cl^- activity during this phase is known, we cannot estimate the initial rate of change of Cl^- activity from our data. We therefore assume that it does not change. This is not altogether unreasonable since the initial rate of change of HCO_3^- activity begins to saturate at intracellular activities approaching those of Cl^-; we would therefore predict that the change in Cl^- activity would not produce a significant change in Cl^- efflux rate. With these values (Table 3), Eq. 2 can be solved to give the predicted HCO_3^- activity of the primary secretion. This is 27 mmol/l, equivalent to a concentration of 39 mmol/l.

In the rabbit mandibular gland, indirect estimates of HCO_3^- concentration in primary saliva are about half this predicted value (Mangos et al. 1973). However, anion deficit calculation of the HCO_3^- concentration in micropuncture samples of primary saliva is in close agreement with our prediction (Table 1). Similarly, the anion deficits that can be calculated from the literature for other salivary glands are close to, or higher than the concentration of HCO_3^- that we have calculated (Table 1). The only notable exception is the ferret mandibular gland studied by Mangos et al. (1981).

Perfusion studies on whole glands also provide some evidence that HCO_3^- output in the primary secretion may be greater than is often supposed. During perfusion with a HEPES-buffered, HCO_3^--free solution, the resulting saliva has elevated concentrations of Cl^- and Na^+ compared with saliva secreted during perfusion with HCO_3^--containing solutions (Case et al. 1980). Table 4 shows the data from a recent set of experiments (Case et al. 1989). In the absence of HCO_3^-, the concentrations of Cl^- and Na^+ in saliva are approximately twice those during perfusion with HCO_3^--buffered solutions. The simplest way of interpreting these data is to assume that the increased Cl^- concentration is the result of Cl^- taking the place of HCO_3^- in the primary secretion. If this is true, the HCO_3^- concentration of primary saliva secreted during perfusion with more physiological HCO_3^--buffered solutions must be about 40–45 mmol/l, close to the concentration predicted above. These separate pieces of evidence thus present a consistent picture of a primary secretion in the rabbit mandibular gland with a HCO_3^- concentra-

Table 4. Effect of HCO_3^--free perfusate on final saliva composition

	J_v	Cl^- (mmol/l)	K^+ (mmol/l)	Na^+ (mmol/l)
$+HCO_3^-$	51.4 ± 6.1	43.0 ± 5.3	15.8 ± 1.4	37.1 ± 5.3
$-HCO_3^-$	52.6 ± 7.9	85.4 ± 3.7	16.3 ± 1.9	75.8 ± 5.8

Values are means $\pm$ SEM for 12 experiments ($+HCO_3^-$) and for 4 experiments ($-HCO_3^-$). J_v, secretory rate in μl/min

tion rather higher than is usually thought, and higher than that observed in the final saliva (Table 4). This implies that absorption of HCO_3^- takes place in the ducts.

Models of Bicarbonate Transport — Weak Acid Studies

Weak acids such as bicarbonate, propionate, acetate, butyrate, lactate, pyruvate, and valerate have been observed to stimulate fluid and electrolyte transport in a variety of epithelia, including toad urinary bladder (Singer et al. 1969), gastric and duodenal mucosa (Flemström and Garner 1982), gall bladder (Petersen et al. 1981; Heintze et al. 1981), kidney proximal tubule (Bidet et al. 1988; Ullrich et al. 1971), pancreatic ducts (Case et al. 1979) and rabbit mandibular gland (Case et al. 1982; Novak and Young 1989). A number of different models have been proposed to explain this effect. These include general surface charge effects at the cell membranes (Singer et al. 1969), anion exchange (Case et al. 1979), coupled Na^+-H^+ and Cl^--anion exchange (Petersen et al. 1981) and Na^+-anion co-transport (Bidet et al. 1988). Could any of these mechanisms be invoked to explain our results with rabbit mandibular gland acinar cells?

In kidney proximal tubule cells, both recovery of pH_i from acid loading and fluid and electrolyte absorption are stimulated by weak acids in the sequence butyrate > propionate > acetate (Bidet et al. 1988; Ullrich et al. 1971). pH_i recovery from acid loading has been attributed to an inwardly directed Na^+-monocarboxylate co-transport by Bidet et al. (1988). The ability of HCO_3^- to enhance electrolyte and fluid absorption by the proximal tubule is now thought to be due to a basolaterally sited electrogenic Na^+ $-HCO_3^-$ co-transport, promoting HCO_3^- efflux from the cell (Boron and Boulpaep 1983). In bovine corneal endothelium, an electrogenic Na^+ $-HCO_3^-$ co-transport mechanism appears to be involved in pH_i regulation (Jentsch et al. 1984). In both tissues, the co-transport is inhibited by DIDS and is insensitive to amiloride (Jentsch et al. 1988). These data suggest that the Na^+-monocarboxylate co-transporter is the same as the electrogenic $Na^+-HCO_3^-$ co-transporter. $Na^+-HCO_3^-$ co-transport could mediate

HCO_3^- efflux or influx depending on the stoichiometry (Jentsch et al. 1988). However, mechanisms involving Na^+ seem unlikely as explanations for our data because removal of Na^+ from the extracellular solution does not prevent ACh from eliciting an acidosis in the presence of HCO_3^-.

In the guinea-pig gall bladder, HCO_3^- is normally secreted and is accompanied by Na^+ and K^+ (Heintze et al. 1979, 1981). In contrast, HCO_3^- is absorbed in the rabbit gall bladder (Diamond 1964). In both tissues, Na^+ absorption is stimulated by HCO_3^- and other weak acids in the sequence butyrate > propionate > acetate. This has been explained by the coupling of Na^+-H^+ and Cl^--anion exchange through intracellular pH (Petersen et al. 1981). However, in *Necturus* gall bladder, there is evidence for a basolateral Cl^- conductance that can be stimulated by HCO_3^-/CO_2 (Stoddard and Reuss 1988). This could also account for the observed enhancement of Na^+ transport. The involvment of a Cl^- conductance represents a mechanism closer to the one we have describes for the mandibular gland. However, stimulation of a Cl^- conductance by HCO_3^- is not the same as permeation by HCO_3^- of a Cl^- channel.

In the pancreas, HCO_3^- is necessary for secretion by the ducts (Case and Argent 1986), but not the acini (Seow et al. 1986). The extent to which weak acids are able to substitute for HCO_3^- in supporting ductal secretion follows the sequence acetate > propionate > butyrate (Case et al. 1979)—the reverse of that observed in the kidney proximal tubule and gall bladder already discussed. On the basis of this work it was suggested that pancreatic ductal secretion may involve the action of anion exchangers. In recent studies on isolated rat pancreatic ducts, (Arkle et al. 1986; Novak and Greger 1988a), the stimulatory effect of HCO_3^- has been shown to be electrogenic, causing a depolarization of the membrane potential (Gray et al. 1988a; Novak and Greger 1988a). Acetate has been shown to depolarize the membrane potential. The effect of HCO_3^- was independent of Na^+ and so unlikely to involve electrogenic $Na^+-HCO_3^-$ co-transport. Further study suggested that HCO_3^- stimulation was due to activation of Cl^- channels coupled to anion exchange (Gray et al. 1988b; Novak and Greger 1988b). The nature of this coupling is, however, unknown and there is at yet no clear evidence that an anion exchanger is present in the same membrane as the channel.

Apart from the reversed order of effectiveness of the weak acids, the obvious similarities between these data for pancreas and for gall bladder makes it tempting to suggest that the same underlying mechanism is involved. The significance of the reversed order is difficult to assess since the sequences probably refect both the lipid: water partition co-efficients as well as the selectivities of the transport processes.

In the isolated perfused rabbit mandibular gland, low concentrations of acetate or butyrate (Novak and Young 1989) stimulate secretion. Acetate is certainly secreted by the gland (Case et al. 1982) and can sustain a reduced rate of secretion in the absence of Cl^- (Novak and Young 1989). These last two observations are readily explained by permeation of acetate through non-specific apical anion channels.

In summary, it seems that, although weak acids have similar stimulatory effects in these tissues, at least two classes of mechanism must be invoked to explain the data. One class involves Na^+ anion co-transport, which may or may not be electrogenic: the other involves Cl^- channels. We have proposed that in rabbit mandibular gland acinar cells, the ability of weak acids to sustain an acidosis, and to sustain secretion, is due entirely to the presence of anion channels in the luminal membrane. An alternative suggestion, arising from studies of pancreatic ducts, is that Cl^- channels closely coupled to anion exchangers account for the stimulation and dependence of secretion on the presence of weak acids. The attraction of our proposal is its simplicity and consistency with the pH_i data. However, it does not readily explain the stimulatory effects of acetate and other weak acids. The coupled Cl^- channel and anion exchanger model successfully explains the stimulatory effects of the weak acids, but the evidence for the role of the anion exchanger in either the mandibular gland or the pancreatic duct is not strong. It is also difficult, at present, to understand how a population of channels could be tightly coupled to a population of anion exchangers in the way proposed.

Conclusion

The mechanism of acinar HCO_3^- transport that we have described (Fig. 4a) enables us to explain data that at present are inconsistent with the standard, neutral co-transport model of acinar secretion (Fig. 4b). Simple analysis suggests that the model is capable of generating high concentrations of HCO_3^- in saliva. It could thus be generally applied to tissues secreting HCO_3^- as the major anion. In particular, it could explain how HCO_3^- is secreted in human saliva where HCO_3^- appears in high concentrations and is thought to have a protective function against tooth decay.

In the rabbit mandibular gland, our studies suggest that acinar cells may contribute all of the HCO_3^- secreted by the gland. This would imply that the ducts modulate the net HCO_3^- output by absorbing HCO_3^-. It is not inconceivable that acinar cells are also able to regulate the HCO_3^- concentration of the saliva without the intervention of ductal transport processes. One way of achieving this would be with separate, regulated HCO_3^- and Cl^- efflux pathways (e.g. channels) rather than the common pathway that we have suggested. Another way would be to vary the HCO_3^- concentration in the cell. As HCO_3^- concentration rises in the cell, so it forms a greater proportion of secreted anion in the primary saliva. NMR studies in our laboratory raise the possibility that HCO_3^- entry into the acinar cell may be mediated by $Na^+ - HCO_3^-$ co-transport which could be regulated (Steward et al. 1989). Even if acinar secretion of HCO_3^- is regulated, further adjustment of the HCO_3^- concentration could be made by ductal transport processes. The net result would be close control of HCO_3^- concentration at all flow rates. The involvement of both acinar and ductal transport processes in the secretion of HCO_3^- could be the explanation for the complex variety of HCO_3^- secretory patterns observed in salivary glands. However, further progress in understanding the transport and control of HCO_3^- in salivary glands depends upon reaching a clearer understanding of the identities and regulation of both acinar and ductal transport processes for HCO_3^-.

Acknowledgements. We would like to acknowledge helpful discussions with Drs D. B. Ferguson and M. C. Steward.

References

Arkle, S, Lee CM, Cullen MJ, Argent BE (1986) Isolation of ducts from pancreas of copper-deficient rats. Q J Exp Physiol 71:249–265

Bidet M, Merst J, Tauc MR, Poujeol P (1988) Role of monocarboxylic acid transport in intracellular pH regulation of isolated proximal cells. Biochim Biophys Acta 938:257–269

Bormann J, Hamill OP, Sakmann B (1987) Mechanism of anion permeation through channels gated by glycine and γ-aminobutric acid in mouse cultured spinal neurones. J Physiol (Lond) 385:243–286

Boron WF, Boulpaep EL (1983) Intracellular pH regulation in the renal proximal tubule of the salamander: basolateral HCO_3^- transport. J Gen Physiol 81:53–94

Brown PD, Donohue M, Elliott AC, Lau KR (1989a) $Na^+ - HCO_3^-$ co-transport is not involved in the acetylcholine-induced acidosis in acini isolated from rabbit mandibular salivary gland. J Physiol (Lond) 410:44P

Brown PD, Elliott AC, Lau KR (1989b) Evidence for the presence of non-specific anion channels in rabbit mandibular salivary gland acinar cells. J Physiol (Lond) 414:415–431

Case RM, Argent BE (1986) Bicarbonate secretion by pancreatic duct cells: mechanisms and control. In: Go VLW et al. (eds) The exocrine pancreas: biology, pathobiology, and diseases. Raven, New York, pp 213–243

Case, RM, Hotz J, Hutson D, Scratched T, Wynne RDA (1979) Electrolyte secretion by the isolated cat pancreas during replacement of extracellular bicarbonate by organic anions and chloride by inorganic anions. J Physiol (Lond) 286:563–576

Case RM, Conigrave AD, Novak I, Young JA (1980) Electrolyte and protein secretion by the perfused mandibular gland stimulated with acetylcholine or catecholamines. J Physiol (Lond) 300:467–487

Case RM, Conigrave AD, Favaloro EJ, Novak I, Thomson CH, Young JA (1982) The role of buffer anions and protons in secretion by the rabbit mandibular salivary gland. J Physiol (Lond) 322:273–286

Case RM, Hunter M, Novak I, Young JA (1984) The anionic basis of fluid secretion by the rabbit mandibular salivary gland. J Physiol (Lond) 349:619–630

Case RM, Howorth AJ, Lau KR (1986) The effects of bumetanide on the stimulated rabbit mandibular salivary gland. J Physiol (Lond) 378:103P

Case RM, Howorth AJ, Padfield PJ (1988a) Effects of acetylcholine, isoprenaline and forskolin on electrolyte and protein composition of rabbit mandibular saliva. J Physiol (Lond) 406:411–430

Case RM, Lau KR, Steward MC, Brown PD (1988b) Perspectives on epithelial ion transport. In: Mastella G, Quinton PM (eds) Cellular and molecular basis of cystic fibrosis. San Francisco Press, San Francisco, pp 8–25

Compton JS, Nelson J, Wright RD, Young JA (1980) A micropuncture investigation of electrolyte transport in the parotid glands of sodium-replete and sodium-depleted sheep. J Physiol (Lond) 309:429–446

Denniss AR, Young JA (1978) Modification of salivary duct electrolyte transport in rat and rabbit by physalaemin, VIP, GIP and other enterohormones. Pflügers Arch 376:73–80

Diamond, JM (1964) The mechanism of isotonic water transport. J Gen Physiol 48:14–42

Englander HR, Shklair IL, Fosdick LS (1959) The effects of saliva on the pH and lactate concentration in dental plaques. J Dent Res 38:848–853

Ferguson DB (1975) In: Lavelle CLB (ed) Applied physiology of the mouth. Bristol, pp 145–179

Flemström G, Garner A (1982) Gastroduodenal HCO_3^- transport: characteristics and proposed role in acidity regulation and mucosal protection. Am J Physiol 242:G183–G193

Grant SBJ, Endre ZH, Young JA (1974) Steady-state electrolyte concentrations and transepithelial electrical potential differences in the rabbit submaxillary main duct perfused in vivo. Proc Aust Physiol Pharmacol Soc 5:206–208 P

Gray MA, Greenwell JR, Argent BE (1988a) Ion channels in pancreatic duct cells: characterization and role in bicarbonate secretion. In: Mastella G, Quinton PM (eds) Cellular and molecular basis of cystic fibrosis. San Francisco Press, San Francisco, pp 205–221

Gray MA, Greenwell JA, Argent BE (1988b) Secretin-regulated chloride channel on the apical plasma membrane of pancreatic duct cells. J Membr Biol 105:131–142

Greger R, Schlatter R, Wang F, Forrest JN (1984) Mechanism of NaCl secretion in rectal gland tubules of spiny dogfish (Squalus acanthias). III. Effect of stimulation of secretion by cyclic AMP. Pflügers Arch 402:376–384

Heintze K, Petersen K-U, Olles P, Saverymuttu SH, Wood JR (1979) Effects of bicarbonate on fluid and electrolyte transport by the guinea pig gall-bladder: a bicarbonate-chloride exchange. J Membr Biol 45:43–59

Heintze J, Petersen K-U, Wood JR (1981) Effects of bicarbonate on fluid and electrolyte transport by guinea pig and rabbit gall-bladder: stimulation of absorption. J Membr Biol 62:175–181

Hilliam DG (1975) Dental plaque and associated deposits on the teeth. In: Lavelle CLB (ed) Applied physiology of the mouth. Bristol, pp 124–144

Holzgreve H, Martinez JR, Vogel A (1966) Micropunture and histologic study of submaxillary glands of young rats. Pflügers Arch 290:134–143

Jenkins GN (1978) The physiology and biochemistry of the mouth. Blackwell, Oxford

Jentsch TJ, Keller SK, Koch M, Wiederholt M (1984) Evidence for coupled transport of bicarbonate and sodium in cultured bovine corneal endothelial cells. J Membr Biol 81:189–204

Jentsch TJ, Korbmacher C, Janicke I, Fischer DG, Stahl F, Helbig H, Cragoe EJ, Keller SK, Wiederholt M (1988) Regulation of cytoplasmic pH of cultured bovine corneal endothelial cells in the absence and presence of bicarbonate. J Membr Biol 103:29–40

Jirakulsomchok D, Schneyer CA (1979) α- and β-adrenergic effects on Na, K, Cl, and HCO_3 transport in perfused salivary duct during sympathetic nerve stimulation. Proc Soc Exp Biol Med 161:479–483

Kalla K, Voipio J (1987) Postsynaptic fall in intracellular pH induced by GABA-activated bicarbonate conductance. Nature 330:163–165

Kaladelfos G, Young JA (1974) Water and electrolyte excretion in the cat submaxillary gland studied using micropuncture and duct cannulation techniques. Aust J Exp Biol Med Sci 52:67–79

Knauf H, Kubcke R, Kreutz W, Sachs G (1982) Interrelationships of ion transport in rat submaxillary duct epithelium. Am J. Physiol 242:F132–F139

Lau KR, Case RM (1986) Chloride activity in mandibular salivary gland cells during secretion. Biomed Res 7 (Suppl 2):181–184

Lau KR, Case RM (1988) Evidence for apical chloride channels in rabbit mandibular salivary glands: a chloride-selective microelectrode study. Pflügers Archiv 411:670–675

Lau KR, Elliott AC, Brown PD (1989) Acetylcholine-induced intracellular acidosis in rabbit salivary gland acinar cells. Am J Physiol 256:C288–C295

Lau KR, Howorth AJ, Case RM (1990) The effect of bumetanide, amiloride and Ba^{2+} on fluid and electrolyte secretion in the rabbit mandibular salivary gland. J Physiol (Lond) (in press)

Mangos JA, McSherry NR, Irwin K, Hong R (1973a) Handling of water and electrolytes by rabbit parotid and submaxillary glands. Am J Physiol 225:450–455

Mangos JA, McSherry NR, Nousia-Arvanitakis S, Irvin K (1973b) Secretion and transductal fluxes of ions in exocrine glands of the mouse. Am J Physiol 225:18–24

Mangos JA, Boyd RL, Loughlin GM, Cockrell A, Fucci R (1981) Secretion of monovalent ions and water in ferret salivary glands: a micropuncture study. J Dent Res 60:733–737

Martin CJ, Young JA (1971) Electrolyte concentrations in primary and final saliva of the rat sublingual gland studied by micropuncture and catheterization techniques. Pflügers Arch 324:344–360

Martin CJ, Frömter E, Gebler B, Knauf H, Young JA (1973) The effects of carbachol on water and electrolyte fluxes and transepithelial electrical potential differences of the rabbit submaxillary main duct perfused in vitro. Pflügers Arch 341:131–142

Martinez JR, Cassity N (1985) ^{36}Cl fluxes in dispersed rat submandibular acini: effects of acetylcholine and transport inhibitors. Pflügers Arch 403:50–54

Martinez JR, Cassity N (1986) Effects of cyclic nucleotide derivatives on acetylcholine-induced secretion from isolated, perfused rat submandibular salivary glands. Arch Oral Biol 31:483–487

Martinez JR, Holzgreve H, Frick A (1966) Micropuncture study of submaxillary glands of adult rats. Pflügers Arch 290:124–133

Novak I, Greger R (1988a) Electrophysiological study of transport systems in isolated perfused pancreatic ducts: properties of the basolateral membrane. Pflügers Arch 411:58–68

Novak I, Greger R (1988b) Properties of the luminal membrane of isolated perfused rat pancreatic ducts. Effect of cyclic AMP and blockers of chloride transport. Pflügers Arch 411:546–553

Novak, I, Young JA (1989) Acetate stimulates secretion in the rabbit mandibular gland. Pflügers Arch 414:68–72

Petersen, K-U, Wood JR, Schulze G, Heintze K (1981) Stimulation of gallbladder fluid and electrolyte absorption by butyrate. J Membr Biol 62:183–193

Petersen OH, Maruyama Y (1984) Calcium-activated potassium channels and their role in secretion. Nature 307:693–696

Reinhardt R, Bridges RJ, Rummel W, Lindemann B (1987) Properties of an anion-selective channel from rat colonic enterocyte plasma membranes reconstituted into planar phospholipid bilayers. J Membr Biol 95:47–54

Saito Y, Wright EM (1984a) Bicarbonate transport across the frog choroid plexus and its control by cyclic nucleotides. J Physiol (Lond) 336:635–648

Saito Y, Wright EM (1984b) Regulation of bicarbonate transport across the brush border membrane of the bull-frog choroid plexus. J Physiol (Lond) 350:327–342

Schneyer LH, Young JA, Schneyer CA (1972) Salivary secretion of electrolytes. Physiol Rev 52:720–777

Seow, KTF, Lingard JM, Young JA (1986) Anionic basis of fluid secretion by rat pancreatic acini in vitro. Am J Physiol 250:G140–G148

Silva P, Stoff J, Field M, Fine L, Forrest JN, Epstein, FH (1977) Mechanism of active chloride secretion by shark rectal gland: role of Na-K-ATPase in chloride transport. Am J Physiol 233:F298–F306

Singer I, Sharp GWG, Civan MM (1969) The effect of propionate and other organic anions on sodium transport across toad bladder. Biochim Biophys Acta 193:430–443

Smaje LH, Poulsen JH, Ussing HH (1986) Evidence from O_2 uptake measrements for $Na^+ - K^+ - 2Cl^-$ co-transport in the rabbit submandibular gland. Pflügers Arch 406:492–496

Stephan RM (1940) Changes in the hydrogen-ion concentration on tooth surfaces and in carious lesions. J Am Dent Assoc 27:718–723

Steward MC, Seo Y, Case RM (1989) Intracellular pH during secretion in the perfused rabbit mandibular salivary gland measured by ^{31}P NMR spectroscopy. Pflügers Arch 414:200–207

Stoddard JS, Reuss L (1988) Dependence of cell membrane conductances on bathing solution HCO_3^-/CO_2 in Necturus gallbladder. J Membr Biol 102:163–174

Thaysen JH (1960) Handling of alkali metals by exocrine glands other than the kidney. In: Ussing HH (ed) The alkali metal ions in biology. Springer, Berlin Heidelberg New York, chap 5 pp 424–507 (Handbuch der experimentellen Pharmakologie, part II, vol 13)

Turner RJ, George JN, Baum BJ (1986) Evidence for a $Na^+/K^+/Cl^-$ co-transport system in basolateral membrane vesicles from the rabbit parotid. J Membr Biol 94:143–152

Ullrich KJ, Radtke HW, Rumrich G (1971) The role of bicarbonate and other buffers on isotonic fluid absorption in the proximal convolution of the rat kidney. Pflügers Arch 330:149–161

Wangemann P, Wittner M, di Stephano A, Englert HC, Lang HJ, Schlatter E, Greger R (1986) Cl^--channel blockers in the thick ascending limb of the loop of Henle: structure activity relationships. Pflügers Arch 407(S2):128–141

Yoshitomi K, Burckhardt B-Ch, Frömter E (1985) Rheogenic sodium-bicarbonate co-transport in the pertibular cell membrane of rat renal proximal tubule. Pflügers Arch 405:360–366

Young JA, Martin CJ (1971) The effect of a sympatho- and a parasympathomimetic drug on the electrolyte concentrations of primary and final saliva of the rat submaxillary gland. Pflügers Arch 327:285–302

Young JA, Schneyer CA (1981) Composition of saliva in mammalia. Aust J Exp Biol Med Sci 59:1–53

Young JA, van Lennep EW (1979) Transport in salivary and salt glands. In: Giebisch G (ed) Transport organs. Springer, Berlin Heidelberg New York, pp 563–674 (Membrane transport in biology, vol 4/A)

Young JA, Martin CJ, Asz M, Weber FD (1970) A microperfusion investigation of bicarbonate secretion by the rat submaxillary gland. The action of a parasympathomimetic drug on electrolyte transport. Pflügers Arch 319:185–199

Young JA, Case RM, Congrave AD, Novak I (1980) Transport of bicarbonate and other anions in salivary secretion. Ann N.Y. Acad Sci 341:172–189

Electrophysiology of Salivary Acinar Cells: Microelectrode Studies

A. Nishiyama, H. Hayashi, H. Takahashi, and Y. Saito

Introduction

In 1955 Lundberg, using conventional Ling-Gerard microelectrodes, first recorded the intracellular membrane potential from acinar cells in the cat mandibular gland in vivo. Either parasympathetic or sympathetic nerve stimulation caused membrane hyperpolarization, which he termed the "secretory potential". From subsequent studies (Lundberg 1957a, b, c) on the cat sublingual gland, he postulated that the stimulus-evoked secretory potentials were due to activation of an inwardly directed active transport mechanism for Cl^-. Since subsequent microelectrode studies on stimulus-evoked potential responses in many salivary glands could not be explained by Lundberg's proposition, however, it was postulated instead that the stimulus-evoked membrane response was due to activations of conductive pathways permeable to K^+ and Na^+ and of the electrogenic Na^+ pump, located in the basolateral membrane (see Petersen 1980; Gallacher and Petersen 1983). Recently, Suzuki and Petersen (1985) suggested instead that the stimulus-evoked potential response might be due to activation of a K^+-conductive pathway and the electrogenic Na^+ pump in the basolateral membrane plus activation of a Cl^--conductive pathway in the luminal membrane (see also Petersen and Gallacher 1988). This model was derived from one first postulated for the rectal gland of the dogfish (Hannafin et al. 1983).

Electrical Equivalent Circuit

Microelectrode studies on exocrine glands normally involve measurement of the membrane potential and input resistance across the basolateral plasma membrane between the cell interior and interstitium. However, the electrical properties measured across the basolateral membrane do not reflect the properties of the basolateral membrane alone, unless the luminal or paracellular shunt resistance is infinitely large. A low paracellular shunt resistance will result in coupling of electrical events at the basolateral and luminal membranes. Lundberg (1957b) presented direct evidence for a low

Young · Wong, Epithelial Secretion of Water and Electrolytes
© Springer-Verlag Berlin · Heidelberg 1990

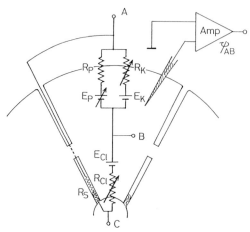

Fig. 1. Equivalent electrical circuit model for salivary acini. E_K and R_K, and E_P and R_P denote the K^+ equilibrium potential and its resistance and the driving force arising from the electrogenic pump and its resistance across the basolateral membrane, respectively. E_{Cl} and R_{Cl} denote the Cl^- equilibrium potential and its resistance across the luminal membrane

transcellular resistance in the cat sublingual gland, and a recent morphological study (Simon and Bank 1984) on rat parotid acini has also suggested that the tight junctions are leaky. Previous microelectrode studies on acinar cells had been made on the assumption that the membrane potential events recorded across the basolateral membrane predominantly related to the event at the basolateral membrane. Patch-clamp whole-cell recording from the lacrimal (Trautmann and Marty 1984; Findlay and Petersen 1985) and parotid (Iwatsuki et al. 1985) acinar cells, however, demonstrated the presence of a high-conductance pathway for Cl^- presumed to be located in the luminal membrane. Figure 1 shows the equivalent electrical circuit model for ion transport in lacrimal and salivary acini as proposed by Suzuki and Petersen (1985).

Resting Membrane Potential and Input Resistance

Values of the potential differences that have been recorded across the basolateral membranes of unstimulated salivary acinar cells are shown in Table 1. Different species and glands seem to have different resting membrane potentials, although some of the variability may reflect differences in the recording methods used. Petersen (1973), using isolated superfused segments of mouse parotid and mandibular glands, demonstrated that the resting membrane potentials were higher than those previously reported in vivo. Since that time, isolated superfused gland segments have been utilized extensively for microelectrode studies on exocrine acinar cells. The resting membrane potentials of both rat and mouse salivary acinar cells lie between -50 and $-70\,mV$.

Table 1. Resting membrane potentials and input resistances in salivary acini

Cells	RMP (mV)	RIR (MΩ)	Reference
Cat mandibular gland	-20		Lundberg (1955)
Cat parotid gland	-36	5.0	Emmelin et al. (1980)
Cat sublingual gland	-33	2.0	Lundberg (1957a, b)
Rabbit mandibular gland	-50	$6-8$	Kagayama and Nishiyama (1974)
Dog mandibular gland	-42	18.0	Imai (1965a)
Rat mandibular gland	-28		Schneyer and Yoshida (1969)
Rat mandibular gland[a]	-57	4.8	Roberts and Petersen (1978)
Mouse mandibular gland[a]	-57	5.2	Nishiyama and Petersen (1974)
Mouse parotid gland[a]	-69		Pedersen and Petersen (1973)
Mouse sublingual gland[a]	-55		Nishiyama et al. (1980)

RMP, resting membrane potential; RIP, resting input resistance
[a] Measurements from superfused gland segments

The Na^+, K^+, and Cl^- equilibrium potentials of acinar cells as determined by flame photometry or ion-sensitive microelectrodes are shown in Table 2. None of the ions is in equilibrium with the resting membrane potential across the basolateral membrane, although it seems more closely to reflect the extracellular K^+ concentration (Petersen and Petersen 1973; Nishiyama and Petersen 1974). Gallacher and Morris (1986), measuring the reversal potential for single channel K^+ currents from cell-attached membrane patches of isolated mouse mandibular acini, found the resting membrane potential across the basolateral membrane to be -45 mV, a value close to that reported by conventional microelectrode studies. They speculated that the value of -45 mV was due to the balance between the resting permeability to K^+ at the basolateral membrane and to Cl^- at the luminal membrane. The electrogenic Na^+-K^+ pump contributes slightly to the resting membrane potential, however, since application of ouabain causes an immediate depolarization of a few mV (Nishiyama and Petersen 1974; Roberts et al. 1978).

Table 2. Equilibrium potentials for K^+, Na^+ and Cl^- in salivary acini

Cells	E_{K^+} (mV)	E_{Na^+} (mV)	E_{Cl^+} (mV)	Reference
Cat sublingual gland	-97	$+29$	-12	Lundberg (1958)
Dog mandibular gland	-87	$+103$	-17	Imai (1965b)
Rabbit mandibular gland[a]			-41	Lau and Case (1986)
Rat mandibular gland	-94	$+71$	-31	Schneyer and Schneyer (1969)
Rat parotid gland	-91	$+50$	-23	Schneyer and Schneyer (1969)
Mouse mandibular gland[a]	-95			Poulsen and Oakley (1979)

[a] Values calculated from determinations of intra- and extracellular ionic activities

Neighbouring cells within an acinus are electrically coupled (Roberts et al. 1978) so that intracellularly placed microelectrodes record the membrane potential and input resistance of the electrically coupled unit. In exocrine glands, the resting input resistances of such a unit is of the order of several $M\Omega$.

Effects of Stimulation

Effects of Cholinergic Stimulation

Lundberg (1955) observed the parasympathetic nerve stimulation in cat mandibular acinar cells in vivo resulted in a change in membrane potential across the basolateral membrane as a monophasic hyperpolarization of about 20 mV and subsequently recorded a similar hyperpolarizing response evoked by parasympathetic nerve stimulation in the cat sublingual gland in vivo (Lundberg 1957a, b). Using double-barreled microelectrodes, he found that the size of the hyperpolarizing responses was not dependent on the membrane potential level when it was set between -30 mV and -100 mV by passing current through the one barrel of the electrode (Lundberg 1957b). He found that replacement of Cl^- by NO_3^- in the perfusing solution severely reduced the hyperpolarization and the fluid secretory responce evoked by direct stimulation with acetylcholine (ACh) (Lundberg 1957c). During the period of about 30 years after Lundberg's studies, numerous microelectrode studies on the stimulus-evoked potential response in salivary glands in vivo and in vitro have provided evidence that is not in agreement with his findings, however.

Evidence for the Stimulus-Evoked Depolarization

In the mandibular glands of cat, rabbit (Kagayama and Nishiyama 1974) and rat (Schneyer and Yoshida 1969), parasympathetic nerve stimulation in vivo evokes different patterns of potential response. Kagayama and Nishiyama (1974) found that the form of the stimulus-evoked potential change was dependent on the spontaneous transmembrane potential (Fig. 2). At lower resting potentials, the cells exhibited a hyperpolarizing response, but those cells with higher resting potentials responded with a biphasic potential change with an initial depolarization and a delayed hyperpolarization. Petersen (1973), using isolated superfused segments of mouse parotid and mandibular glands, found a similar, but more definite dependence of the ACh-evoked potential response on the spontaneous resting potential. Nishiyama and Petersen (1974) demonstrated that the ACh-evoked potential change in mouse mandibular acinar cells was associated with a pronounced reduction in input resistance. Roberts et al. (1978) demonstrated more

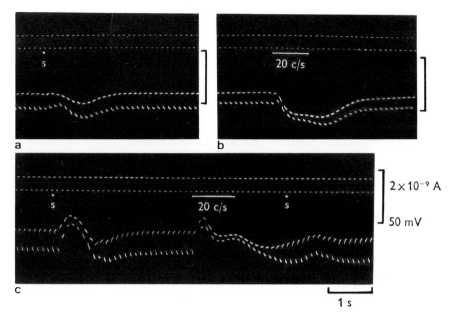

Fig. 2a – c. Effects of chordalingual nerve stimulation on membrane potential and resistance in acinar cells. The upper two records show a hyperpolarizing response after **a** single or **b** repetitive stimulations. **c** Biphasic responses after single and repetitive stimulations are seen. Rabbit mandibular gland in vivo (from Kagayama and Nishiyama 1974)

directly that the potential change evoked by ionophoretically applied ACh depended on the transmembrane potential gradient in superfused isolated segments of mouse parotid. The resting potential of these cells was $-65\,mV$ and stimulation with ACh normally evoked a biphasic potential change consisting of an initial depolarization associated with a reduction in input resistance followed by a delayed hyperpolarization, during which the input resistance returned to the pre-stimulus level. Passing direct current through one of the two intracellular electrodes, they obtained reversal of the potential response evoked by ACh stimulation. The reversal potential, E_{ACh}, was $-60\,mV$. Gallacher and Petersen (1980) made an analysis of the field stimulation-evoked potential response in the mouse parotid gland. They obtained similar responses to those evoked by ionophoretic application of ACh. Again, the reversal potential was $-60\,mV$.

Evidence for Existence of Two Separate Conductive Pathways

The findings that the reversal potential evoked by externally applied ACh or by release of ACh from nerve endings was $-60\,mV$, a less negative value than E_K ($-90\,mV$) across the basolateral membrane, could be explained by postulating that ACh opened up a conductive pathway permeable to both K^+ and Na^+ (Roberts et al. 1978; Petersen 1980). Wakui and Nishiyama

(1980a, b) analysed the initial presponse evoked by ionophoretically applied ACh in the mouse mandibular gland. They applied small doses of ACh, which did not induce the delayed hyperpolarization (which is due to activation of the electrogenic Na^+ pump), and found that the initial response to ACh could be explained by the asynchronous activation of two conductive pathways. The direction and size of the potential responses were not only dependent on the transmembrane potential, but also on the doses of ACh applied. As shown in Fig. 3, small doses of ACh evoked simple depolarization, whilst medium doses induced biphasic potential changes (depolarization followed by hyperpolarization). Both depolarization and hyperpolarization were associated with a marked reduction in input resistance (Fig. 4).

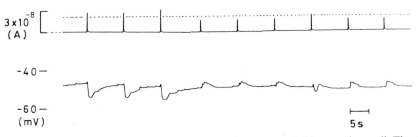

Fig. 3. Effects of different doses of ACh on membrane potential in an acinar cell. The dose of ACh was changed by ejecting current pulses of varying strength with constant pulse duration (50 ms) and retaining current (20 nA). The *lower trace* shows ACh-evoked potential changes. Mouse mandibular gland in vitro (from Wakui and Nishiyama 1980a)

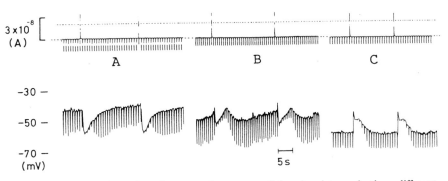

Fig. 4. Effect of ACh ionophoresis on membrane potential and resistance in three different acini. *A*, Simple hyperpolarization type; *B*, biphasic response type; *C*, simple depolarization type. *Upper trace* shows current pulses for ACh ejection presented as upward deflections (duration, 50 ms) and for measurement of resistance as downward deflections (duration, 100 ms). *Lower trace* shows membrane potential changes. Mouse mandibular gland in vitro (from Wakui and Nishiyama 1980a)

Evidence That the Stimulus-Induced Hyperpolarization Is Due to Activation of a K^+ Conductive Pathway in the Basolateral Membrane and That the Depolarization Is Due to Activation of a Cl^- Conductive Pathway in the Luminal Membrane

In the perfused mandibular glands of dog (Imai 1965b) and cat (Petersen and Poulsen 1968; Petersen 1970b, 1971), the stimulus-evoked hyperpolarization was not abolished by omission of Cl^- from the perfusing solution, but was dependent on the presence of extracellular K^+ and Na^+. A similar dependency of the ACh-evoked potential response on extracellular K^+ and Na^+ concentrations was found in the superfused segment preparations of mouse parotid (Roberts et al. 1978) and mandibular glands (Nishiyama and Petersen 1974; Wakui and Nishiyama 1980a, b). These findings again had suggested that ACh increased the K^+ and Na^+ conductance of acinar cell membranes. Roberts et al. (1978) found that replacement of Cl^- in the superfusion solution by SO_4^{2-} increased the size of the ACh-evoked hyperpolarization and shifted E_{ACh} to $-78\,mV$, a value close to E_k. Nishiyama and Petersen (1974) also found that ACh caused membrane hyperpolarization to a value close to E_k during exposure to a Cl^--free SO_4^{2-} solution. Roberts et al. (1978) postulated that omission of Cl^- from the extracellular solution might reduce the ACh-evoked Na^+ conductance. In patch-clamp studies on mouse and rat salivary glands, Maruyama et al. (1983) demonstrated the presence of Ca^{2+}-activated K^+ channels. These channels, which were localized to the basolateral membrane, are impermeable to Na^+ and anions. They also found the presence of Ca^{2+}-activated nonselective cation channels permeable to Na^+ in a few patch membranes from the basolateral membranes, but these channels conduct equally well in the absence or presence of Cl^-. Since a Cl^--dependent Na^+-conductive pathway causing the stimulus-evoked depolarization has not been found in the basolateral membrane, Suzuki and Petersen (1985) proposed that the depolarization must be associated with a Ca^{2+}-activated Cl^- conductance in the luminal membrane as had already postulated in lacrimal acinar cells (Trautmann and Marty 1984; Findlay and Petersen 1985). This implies that the two plasma membranes, basolateral and luminal, are electrically coupled through a low-resistance paracellular shunt pathway.

Evidence that ACh-Evoked Na^+ or Cl^- Influx is Mediated Via the Cotransporter

Ionophoretic application of ACh can evoke a delayed hyperpolarization following the initial potential change in the acinar cells as already described. Roberts et al. (1978) found that the delayed hyperpolarization could not be. reversed at potential levels between -17 and $-150\,mV$. This hyperpolarization was abolished in Na^+- or K^+-free media or by addition of ouabain. Suzuki and Petersen (1985) proposed that ACh evoked the Na^+ influx via a $Na^+-K^+-2Cl^-$ cotransporter. Our recent microelectrode studies (Nis-

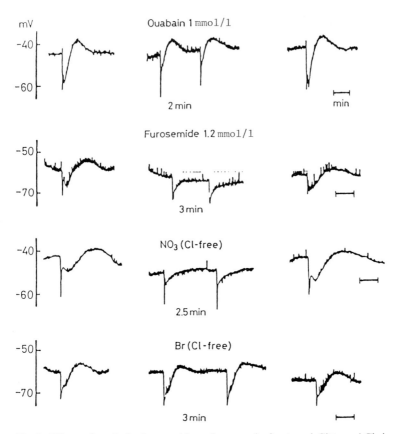

Fig. 5. Effects of ouabain, furosemide and removal of external Cl^- on ACh ionophoresis-evoked potential response (ejecting current 100 nA for 100 ms, retaining current 20 nA). *Left side*, records in control solution; *middle traces*, records at the times after shift to test solution as indicated; *right traces*, records after return to control solution. Mouse mandibular gland in vitro (from Nishiyama et al. 1988a)

hiyama et al. 1988a) have confirmed that ACh-evoked Na^+ influx could be interpreted as the result of stimulation of the $Na^+ - K^+ - 2Cl^-$ cotransporter. The electrogenic Na^+ pump activation evoked by ACh in the mouse mandibular acinar cells was little affected by replacement of Cl^- by Br^- in the superfusion solution, but it was severely reduced in Cl^--free NO_3^-- or SO_4^{2-}-containing solutions and by the addition of the sulfamoylanthranilic acid diuretic, furosemide (Fig. 5). Furthermore, Nishiyama et al. (1988b) provided electrophysiological evidence in the superfused mouse parotid gland that Cl^- was taken up together with Na^+ into the cell via the cotransporter. As shown in Fig. 6, prolonged stimulation with ACh (5×10^{-8} mol/l) for 2–5 min evoked a sustained hyperpolarization of about 20 mV. In the presence of ouabain, ACh evoked only a transient hyperpolarization. Within 1 min after starting the stimulation, the ACh-evoked hyperpolariza-

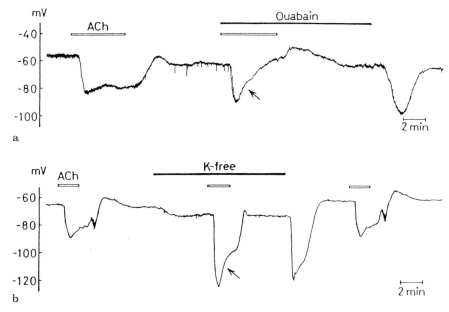

Fig. 6a. Effects of ouabain and **b** omission of extracellular K^+ on membrane potential responses to prolonged stimulations with ACh (5×10^{-8} mol/l). *Arrows* in each record show the depolarizing component that seems to be associated with an activation of the Cl^--conductive pathway at the luminal membrane. Mouse parotid gland in vitro (from Nishiyama et al. 1988 b)

tion gradually decreased, and within 2–3 min the membrane potential depolarized close to the resting potential. Withdrawal of ACh stimulation transiently caused a further slight depolarization and the membrane potential then returned to the prestimulated level. In Cl^--free NO_3^-- or gluconate$^-$-containing solutions, or in the presence of furosemide, ACh stimulation evoked a sustained hyperpolarization that was little affected by addition of ouabain. In a K^+-free solution, ACh evoked a large hyperpolarization that was, however, quickly and markedly attenuated following the onset of stimulation (Fig. 6b). In a Cl^-- and K^+-free, or furosemide-containing K^+-free solution, ACh also evoked a sustained hyperpolarization. These results indicate that the depolarizing responses that appear in the presence of ouabain or in a K^+-free solution are associated with activation of a Cl^- conductive pathway in the luminal membrane. Under conditions where $Na^+ - K^+ - 2Cl^-$ cotransport is inhibited by removal of Na^+ or Cl^- or by addition of furosemide, Na^+ and Cl^- influx decrease and the resultant fall in intracellular Cl^- concentration could be expected to result in a shift of the Cl^- equilibrium potential to a more negative value and might lead to a decrease in the permeability of the Cl^- conductive pathway. Consequently, both the hyperpolarization due to activation of the electrogenic $Na^+ - K^+$ pump and the depolarization associated with activation of the Cl^-

conductive pathway were simultaneously reduced. In this way, in a similar study on lacrimal acinar cells, Suzuki and Petersen (1985) explained the shift of E_{ACh} to more negative values than the control.

Effects of Adrenergic Stimulation

α-Adrenergic Receptor Stimulation

Lundberg (1955) recorded a hyperpolarizing potential change in the cat mandibular gland in vivo following sympathetic nerve stimulation similar to the parasympathetically evoked response. The resemblance between these two responses has also been reported in the rat mandibular glands in vivo (Schneyer and Yoshida 1969) and in superfused segments of mouse parotid glands (Pedersen and Petersen 1973; Petersen and Pedersen 1974; Roberts and Petersen 1978; Roberts et al. 1978; Gallacher and Petersen 1980). The effect of adrenaline on the acinar cell membrane is identical to that of ACh, i.e., an initial potential change associated with an increase in membrane conductance followed by a delayed ouabain-sensitive hyperpolarization. The initial potential change evoked by α-adrenergic agonists could be either a depolarization or a hyperpolarization, depending on the level of the resting potential (Roberts and Petersen 1978; Roberts et al. 1978). The reversal potential (E_{Adr}) for the adrenaline-evoked potential response was identical to E_{ACh} in the mouse parotid gland (Gallacher and Petersen 1980).

β-Adrenergic Receptor Stimulation

Petersen and Pedersen (1974) found that the β-receptor agonist isoproterenol evoked a membrane depolarization in the acinar cells in the superfused segments of mouse parotid. Emmelin et al. (1980) recorded a depolarizing potential response in the cat parotid gland in vivo following sympathetic nerve stimulation. The potential response was accompanied by a reduction in input resistance and the reversal potential for the potential response was -20 mV.

Katoh et al. (1983) found in the superfused mouse and rat mandibular glands that direct application of small doses of isoproterenol or noradrenalin in the presence of the α-adrenergic blocker, phentolamine, evoked a membrane hyperpolarization, whereas these agonists at higher doses evoked depolarization. The hyperpolarization evoked by small doses of β-agonists was not associated with a reduction in input resistance and was abolished in the presence of ouabain or in Na^+- or K^+-free solutions. These findings indicate that β-agonists activated an electrogenic $Na^+ - K^+$ pump. Recently, Nishiyama et al. (1988a) showed that β-agonists activate the Cl^- conductive pathway at the luminal membrane resulting in membrane depolarization and an increase in the Na^+ influx via the $Na^+ - K^+ - 2Cl^-$ cotransporter, resulting in activation of the electrogenic $Na^+ - K^+$ pump. Ionophoretic application of the weak β_1-agonist salbutamol evoked a biphasic potential change, consisting of an initial hyperpolarization followed by a delayed depolarization. The initial hyperpolarization was abolished in the presence of ouabain or in a Na^+- or K^+-free solution. The hyperpolarization was also inhibited in Cl^--free NO_3^-- or SO_4^{2-}-containing solutions, or in solutions

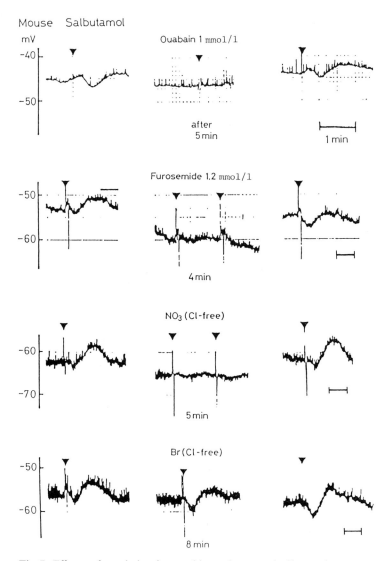

Fig. 7. Effects of ouabain, furosemide and external Cl^- replacements on salbutamol ionophoresis-evoked response (ejecting current 600 nA for 1.0 s, retaining current 40 nA). *Left side*, records in control solution; *middle traces*, times after shift to test solution as indicated; *right traces*, after return to control solution. Mouse mandibular gland in vitro (from Nishiyama et al. 1988a)

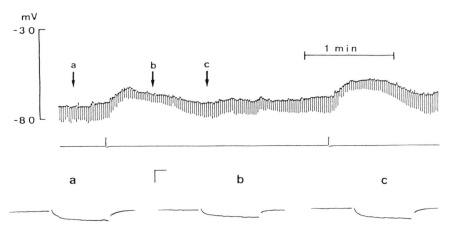

Fig. 8. Effect of isoproterenol ionophoresis on membrane potential and resistance in an acinar cell. The *upper traces* show the pen recordings. At the marker signals isoproterenol was ejected (ejecting current pulses, 100 nA for 5 s, retaining current 20 nA). Rectangular hyperpolarizing current pulses (6 nA for 100 ms) were injected through the electrode impaled into an electrically coupled neighbouring cell. The *lower traces* show oscilloscope photographs at the times *a, b* and *c* indicated in the pen recording. Calibration: horizontal 20 ms; vertical 10 ms. Mouse parotid gland in vitro (from Iwatsuki and Nishiyama 1982)

containing furosemide (Fig. 7). The hyperpolarization was not inhibited in a Cl^--free, Br^--containing solution. Iwatsuki and Nishiyama (1982) demonstrated that the depolarization evoked by isoproterenol was associated with reduction in input resistance (Fig. 8). The reversal potential for the depolarizing response was about -25 mV. The depolarization evoked by isoproterenol was severely reduced not only in a Na^+-free, but also in a Cl^--free, SO_4^{2-}-containing solution. Our recent studies have shown that the depolarization is markedly reduced in Cl^--free NO_3^-- or gluconate$^-$-containing solutions, or in the presence of furosemide, but not in Cl^--free, Br^--containing solutions (Nishiyama et al., unpublished data).

Microlelectrode Studies and Mechanisms of Electrolyte Secretion

The Cholinergic Mechanism

The intracellular membrane potential response evoked by ACh in salivary gland acini is well explained by the transport model for NaCl secretion proposed by Hannafin et al. (1983) and by Suzuki and Petersen (1985). All the machinery necessary for the transport model, i.e. the Ca^{2+}-activated K^+ channels (Maruyama et al. 1983), the Na^+-K^+ pump (Bundgaard et al.

1977), the $Na^+ - K^+ - 2Cl^-$ cotransporter (Hannafin et al. 1983; Turner et al. 1986) at the basolateral membrane and Ca^{2+}-activated Cl^- channels presumably located in the luminal membrane (Iwatsuki et al. 1985), has been demonstrated in salivary gland acini. ACh acts on the acinar membrane receptor, resulting in elevation of the intracellular Ca^{2+} concentration, which in turn opens the Ca^{2+}-activated K^+-conductive pathway at the basolateral membrane and the Ca^{2+}-activated Cl^--conductive pathway at the luminal membrane. Since the basolateral and luminal membranes are electrically coupled, stimulation with ACh changes the transmembrane potential across the basolateral membrane to a level between E_K and E_{Cl} that is determined by the balance between the K^+ and Cl^- conductance changes. The decreases in intracellular K^+ and Cl^- concentrations associated with activation of the two conductive pathways promote the uptake of Na^+ and Cl^- via the cotransporter. The increase in intracellular Na^+ activates the electrogenic Na^+ pump, which participates in the stimulus- evoked potential response.

We emphasize here that microelectrode studies could provide important information about the electrically neutral transport system as well as the conductive pathways. Our microelectrode studies (Nishiyama et al. 1988a) on mouse salivary acini have demonstrated that the ACh-activated electrogenic Na^+ pump activity, which results from the Na^+ influx, shows a characteristic dependency on extracellular Cl^- and a high sensitivity to furosemide. These two characteristics seem to be sufficient to distinguish the cotransport system from the other modes of cation permeation (Palfrey and Rao 1983). Our microelectrode studies (Nishiyama et al. 1988b) also provided indirect, but clear evidence for Cl^- uptake via the cotransporter. The importance of the cotransporter in ACh-evoked fluid secretion has been demonstrated in perfused mandibular glands (Case et al. 1984; Novak and Young 1986), and ^{22}Na uptake (Poulsen and Kristensen 1982) and ^{36}Cl uptake (Martinez and Cassity 1985; Nauntofte and Poulsen 1986) via the cotransporter have been demonstrated in intact mandibular and parotid acini. The Cl^--dependent K^+ reuptake following ACh-evoked K^+ release found by Petersen (Petersen 1970a) was confirmed to be mediated via the $Na^+ - K^+ - 2Cl^-$ cotransporter (Exley et al. 1986; Nishiyama et al. 1988a). The $1 Na^+$, $1 K^+$, $2 Cl^-$ stoichiometry has been demonstrated in basolateral membrane vesicles from rabbit parotid gland (Turner et al. 1986).

Recently, evidence for the presence of two antiporters, $Na^+ - H^+$ and $Cl^- - HCO_3^-$, has been obtained from measurements of fluid secretion (Novak and Young 1986) and intracellular pH (Pirani et al. 1987) in perfused mandibular glands and in flux measurements from parotid basolateral membrane vesicles (Manganel and Turner 1988; Turner and George 1988), so it appears that these two antiporters may also participate in the ACh-evoked NaCl influx. However, our microelectrode studies on mouse parotid acini (Nishiyama et al. 1988b) could not find clear evidence that ACh stimulation caused Na^+ influx via the $Na^+ - H^+$ antiporter. Consequently, we have speculated that the Na^+ influx via this antiporter must be too small to detect electrophysiologically in this gland. There is evidence that ACh causes NaCl influx via these two antiporters in mouse lacrimal acini, which possess Ca^{2+}-activated K^+ channels (Findlay 1984) and Ca^{2+}-activated Cl^- channels (Trautmann and Marty 1984; Findlay and Petersen 1985). Measurements (Saito et al. 1987a, b; Ozawa et al. 1988a, b) of intracellular Cl^- and Na^+ activities in the mouse lacrimal acini support the view that ACh-evoked Na^+ and Cl^- influx are mediated by the $Na^+-K^+-2Cl^-$ cotransporter. These and intracellular H^+ studies (Saito et al. 1988), however, provide several lines of evidence to suggest that the basolateral membrane also possesses a pair of antiporters, Na^+-H^+ and $Cl^--HCO_3^-$. Stimulation with ACh evoked a substantial Na^+ influx via activation of the Na^+-H^+ antiporter (Saito et al. 1987b, 1988). The results of our microelectrode studies on mouse lacrimal acini (Nishiyama et al. 1988b) are in agreement with the view that the ACh-evoked Na^+ influx is mediated by multiple types of Na^+ transporter ($Na^+-K^+-2Cl^-$ cotransporter, Na^+-H^+ antiporter and others).

The Adrenergic Mechanism

α-Adrenergic Mechanism

Since the effects of α-adrenergic stimulation on the membrane potential of salivary gland acinar cells are almost identical to those of cholinergic stimulation, it would seem that α-adrenoceptor stimulation may cause fluid secretion in an identical manner to that of cholinergic stimulation. There have been many reports to support the view that α-adrenoceptor stimulation activates secretion via an increase in intracellular Ca^{2+} concentration which acts on the K^+-conductive pathways and causes K^+ release, K^+ reuptake and Na^+ uptake (see Petersen 1973).

β-Adrenergic Mechanism

Our microelectrode and K^+ flux studies (Iwatsuki and Nishiyama 1982; Nishiyama et al. 1988a) on mouse and rat parotid and mandibular glands have shown several lines of evidence suggesting that β-adrenoceptor stimulation evokes fluid secretion in a manner similar to that in the tracheal epithelium (Welsh et al. 1982) and in the rectal gland tubules of the spiny dogfish (Greger and Schlatter 1984). Stimulation with β-agonists (Katoh et al. 1983) or electrical field stimulation (Katoh et al. 1986) evokes K^+ uptake without causing a preceding K^+ release in the mandibular gland acinar cells of rat and mouse. The K^+ uptake evoked by β-agonists was confirmed to be mediated via the $Na^+-K^+-2Cl^-$ cotransporter (Nishiyama et al. 1988a). These and microelectrode studies (Nishiyama et al. 1988, unpublished data) together can be explained by postulating that β-receptor stimulation activates the adenylate cyclase/cyclic AMP-coupled pathway, in which cyclic AMP serves as an intracellular second messenger, activating the $Na^+-K^+-2Cl^-$ cotransport system at the basolateral membrane and opening the Cl^--conductive pathway at the luminal membrane. Direct evidence for cyclic AMP-activated Cl^--channels at the luminal membrane has been demonstrated in tracheal epithelium (Welsh 1986) and in the rectal gland epithelium of dogfish (Greger et al. 1985).

Recently, Cook et al. (1988), using whole-cell, patch-clamp recording techniques on rat mandibular gland acinar cells, have reported that isoproterenol evokes both K^+ and Cl^- current responses that are indistinguishable from those elicited by ACh, except, of cource, that they can be blocked selectively by propranolol. They also showed that cytosolic-free Ca^{2+} was essential for activating the isoproterenol-evoked current responses, whereas cyclic AMP, forskolin and cholera toxin all had no effect on the current responses. They concluded that β-receptor stimulation evoked K^+ and Cl^- currents via an increase in intracellular Ca^{2+}, but not via an increase in cyclic AMP. Evidence for a slight increase in intracellular Ca^{2+} evoked by isoproterenol has been demonstrated in rat parotid acini (Nauntofte and Dissing 1987). Iwatsuki and Nishiyama (1982) also reported that isoproterenol slightly activated the K^+-conductive pathway. More electrophysiological studies of β-receptor stimulation in salivary acinar cells are required.

Acknowledgement. The authors wish to thank Professor J.A. Young for his helpful advice and kind suggestion in preparing the manuscript. The authors thank also Miss Y. Aizawa for typing the manuscript.

References

Bundgaard M, Moller M, Poulsen JH (1977) Localization of sodium pumps in cat salivary glands. J Physiol (Lond) 273: 339–353

Case RM, Hunter M, Novak I, Young JA (1984) The anionic basis of fluid secretion by the rabbit mandibular salivary gland. J Physiol (Lond) 349: 619–630

Cook DI, Day ML, Champion MP, Young JA (1988) Ca^{2+} not cyclic AMP mediates the fluid secretory response to isoproterenol in the rat mandibular salivary gland: whole-cell patch clamp studies. Pflügers Arch 413: 67–76

Emmelin N, Grampp W, Thesleff P (1980) Sympathetically evoked secretory potentials in the parotid gland of the cat. J Physiol (Lond) 302: 183–195

Exley PM, Fuller CM, Gallacher DV (1986) Potassium uptake in the mouse submandibular gland is dependent on chloride and sodium and abolished by piretanide. J Physiol (Lond) 378: 97–108

Findlay I (1984) A patch-clamp study of potassium channels and whole-cell currents in acinar cells of the mouse lacrimal gland. J Physiol (Lond) 350: 179–195

Findlay I, Petersen OH (1985) Acetylcholine stimulates a Ca^{2+}-dependent Cl^- conductance in mouse lacrimal acinar cells. Pflügers Arch 403: 328–330

Gallacher DV, Morris AP (1986) A patch-clamp study of potassium currents in resting and acetylcholine stimulated mouse submandibular acinar cells. J Physiol (Lond) 373: 379–395

Gallacher DV, Petersen OH (1980) Electrophysiology of mouse parotid acini: effects of electrical flieds stimulation and ionophoresis of neurotransmitters. J Physiol (Lond) 305: 43–57

Gallacher DV, Petersen OH (1983) Stimulus-secretion coupling in mammalian salivary glands. In: Young JA (ed) Gastrointestinal physiology, vol 4. University Park Press, Baltimore, pp 593–660 (International Review of Physiology, vol 42)

Greger R, Schlatter E (1984) Mechanism of NaCl secretion in the rectal gland of spiny dogfish (Squalus acanthias) 1. Experiments in isolated in vitro perfused rectal gland tubules. Pflügers Arch 402: 63–75

Greger R, Schlatter E, Goglein H (1985) Cl^--channels in the apical cell membrane of the rectal gland "induced" by cAMP. Pflügers Arch 403: 446–448

Hannafin J, Kinne-Saffran E, Friedmann D, Kinner R (1983) Presence of a sodium-potassium chloride cotransport system in the rectal gland of Squalus acanthias. J Membr Biol 75: 73–83

Imai Y (1965a) Studies on the secretory mechanism of submaxillary gland of dog (part 1). J Physiol Soc Jpn 27: 304–312 (in Japanese)

Imai Y (1965b) Studies on the secretory mechanism of submaxillary gland of dog (part 2). J Physiol Soc Jpn 27: 313–324 (in Japanese)

Iwatsuki N, Nishiyama A (1982) Parotid acinar cells: ionic dependence of isoprenaline-evoked membrane potential changes. Pflügers Arch 393: 123–129

Iwatsuki N, Maruyama Y, Matsumoto O, Nishiyama A (1985) Activation of Ca^{2+}-dependent Cl^- and K^+ conductances in rat and mouse parotid acinar cells. Jpn J Physiol 35: 933–944

Kagayama M, Nishiyama A (1974) Membrane potential and input resistance in acinar cells from cat and rabbit submaxillary glands in vivo: effect of autonomic nerve stimulation. J Physiol (Lond) 242: 157–172

Katoh K, Nakasato M, Nishiyama A, Sakai M (1983) Activation of potassium transport induced by secretagogues in superfused submaxillary gland segments of rat and mouse. J Physiol (Lond) 341: 371–385

Katoh K, Kaneko K, Nishiyama A (1986) Effects of adrenergic neurotransmitter on K transport in superfused segments of rat submaxillary gland. Pflügers Arch 406: 1–5

Lau KR, Case RL (1986) Chloride activity in mandibular salivary gland cells during secretion. Biomed Res 7 [Suppl 2]: 181–184

Lundberg A (1955) The electrophysiology of the submaxillary gland of the cat. Acta Physiol Scand 35: 1–25

Lundberg A (1957a) The secretory potentials in the sublingual gland of the cat. Acta Physiol Scand 40: 21–34

Lundberg A (1957b) The mechanism of establishment of secretory potentials in sublingual gland cells. Acta Physiol Scand 40: 35–58

Lundberg A (1957c) Anionic dependence of secretion and secretory potentials in the perfused sublingual gland. Acta Physiol Scand 40: 101–112

Lundberg A (1958) Electrophysiology of salivary glands. Physiol Rev 38: 21–40

Manganel M, Turner RJ (1988) Coupled $Na^+ - H^+$ exchange in rat parotid basolateral membrane vesicles. J Membr Biol 102: 247–254

Martinez JR, Cassity N (1985) ^{36}Cl-fluxes in dispersed rat submandibular acini: effects of acetylcholine and transport inhibitors. Pflügers Arch 403: 50–54

Maruyama Y, Gallacher DV, Petersen OH (1983) Voltage and Ca^{2+}-activated K^+ channel in basolateral acinar cell membranes of mammalian salivary glands. Nature 302: 827–829

Nauntofte B, Dissing S (1987) Stimulation-induced changes in cytosolic calcium in parotid acini. Am J Physiol 253: G290–G297

Nauntofte B, Poulsen JH (1986) Effects of Ca^{2+} and furosemide on Cl^- transport and O_2 uptake in rat parotid acini. Am J Physiol 251: C175–C185

Nishiyama A, Petersen OH (1974) Membrane potential and resistance measurement in acinar cells from salivary glands in vitro: effect of acetylcholine. J Physiol (Lond) 242: 173–188

Nishiyama A, Katoh K, Saito Y, Wakui M (1980) Effect of neural stimulation on acinar cell membrane potentials in isolated pancreas and salivary gland segment. Membr Biochem 3: 49–66

Nishiyama A, Iwatsuki N, Takahashi H, Hayashi H, Katoh K (1988a) Potassium uptake evoked by cholinergic and β-adrenergic stimulation in submaxillary gland acinar cells. In: Davison JS, Shaffer EA (eds) Gastrointestinal and hepatic secretion. University Calgary Press, Calgary, pp 189–192

Nishiyama A, Takahashi H, Hayashi H (1988b) Electrogenic Na pump activity evoked by sustained stimulation with acetylcholine in mouse salivary and lacrimal gland acinar cells. In: Wong PYD, Young JA (eds) Exocrine secretion. Hong Kong University Press, Hong Kong, pp 129–132

Novak I, Young JA (1986) Two independent anion transport systems in rabbit mandibular salivary glands. Pflügers Arch 407: 649–656

Ozawa T, Saito Y, Nishiyama A (1988a) Mechanism of uphill chloride transport of the mouse lacrimal acinar cells: studies with Cl^--sensitive microelectrode. Pflügers Arch 412: 509–515

Ozawa T, Saito Y, Nishiyama A (1988b) Evidence for an anion exchanger in the mouse lacrimal gland acinar cell membrane. J Membr Biol 105: 273–280

Palfrey HC, Rao MC (1983) Na/K/Cl co-transport and its regulation. J Exp Biol 106: 43–54

Pedersen GL, Petersen OH (1973) Membrane potential measurement in parotid acinar cells. J Physiol (Lond) 234: 217–227

Petersen OH (1970a) Some factors influencing stimulation-induced release of potassium from the cat submandibular gland to fluid perfused through the gland. J Physiol (Lond) 208: 431–447

Petersen OH (1970b) The dependence of the transmembrane salivary secretory potential on the external potassium and sodium concentration. J Physiol (Lond) 210: 205–215

Petersen OH (1971) Secretory transmembrane potentials in acinar cells from the cat submandibular gland during perfusion with a chloride-free sucrose solution. Pflügers Arch 323: 91–95

Petersen OH (1973) Membrane potential measurement in mouse salivary gland cells. Experientia 26: 160–161

Petersen OH (1980) The electrophysiology of gland cells. Academic, London

Petersen OH, Gallacher DV (1988) Electrophysiology of pancreatic and salivary acinar cells. Annu Rev Physiol 50: 65–80

Petersen OH, Pedersen GL (1974) Membrane effects mediated by alpha- and beta-adrenoceptors in mouse parotid acinar cells. J Membr Biol 16: 353–362

Petersen OH, Poulsen JH (1968) Secretory potential, potassium transport and secretion in the cat submandibular gland during perfusion with sulphate Locke's solution. Experientia 24: 919–920

Pirani D, Evans LAR, Cook DI, Young JA (1987) Intracellular pH in the rat mandibular salivary gland: the role of $Na-H$ and $Cl-HCO_3$ antiports in secretion. Pflügers Arch 408: 178–184

Poulsen JH, Kristensen LO (1982) Is stimulation-induced uptake of sodium in rat parotid acinar cells mediated by a sodium/chloride co-transport system? In: Case RM, Garner A, Turnberg LA, Young JA (eds) Electrolyte and water transport across gastrointestinal epithelia. Raven, New York, pp 199–208

Poulsen JH, Oakley B (1979) Intracellular potassium ion activity in resting and stimulated mouse pancreas and submandibular gland. Proc R Soc Lond [Biol] 204: 99–104

Roberts ML, Petersen OH (1978) Membrane potential and resistance changes in salivary gland acinar cells by microiontophoretic application of acetylcholine and adrenergic agonists. J Membr Biol 39: 297–312

Roberts ML, Iwatsuki N, Petersen OH (1978) Parotid acinar cells: ionic dependence of acetylcholine-evoked membrane potential changes. Pflügers Arch 376: 159–167

Saito Y, Ozawa T, Hayashi H, Nishiyama A (1987a) The effect of acetylcholine on chloride transport across the mouse lacrimal gland acinar cell membranes. Pflügers Arch 409: 280–288

Saito Y, Ozawa T, Nishiyama A (1987b) Acetylcholineinduced Na^+ influx in the mouse lacrimal gland acinar cells: demonstration of multiple Na^+ transport mechanisms by intracellular Na^+ activity measurements. J Membr Biol 98: 135–144

Saito Y, Ozawa T, Suzuki S, Nishiyama A (1988) Intracellular pH regulation in the mouse lacrimal gland acinar cells. J Membr Biol 101: 73–81

Schneyer LH, Schneyer CA (1960) Electrolyte and inulin spaces of rat salivary glands and pancreas. Am J Physiol 199: 649–652

Schneyer LH, Yoshida Y (1969) Secretory potentials in rat submaxillary gland. Proc Soc Exp Biol Med 130: 190–196

Simon JAW, Bank HL (1984) Freeze-fracture and lead ion tracer evidence for a paracellular fluid secretory pathway in rat parotid glands. Anat Rec 208: 69–80

Suzuki K, Petersen OH (1985) The effect of Na^+ and Cl^- removal and of loop diuretics on acetylcholine-evoked membrane potential changes in mouse lacrimal acinar cells. Q J Exp Physiol 70: 437–445

Trautmann A, Marty A (1984) Activation of Ca-dependent K channels by carbamoylcholine in rat lacrimal glands. Proc Natl Acad Sci USA 81: 611–615

Turner RJ, George JN (1988) $Cl^- - HCO_3^-$ exchange is present with $Na^+/K^+/Cl^-$ cotransport in rabbit parotid acinar basolateral membranes. Am J Physiol 254: C391–C396

Turner RJ, George JN, Baum BJ (1986) Evidence for a $Na^+/K^+/Cl^-$-cotransport system in basolateral membrane vesicles from the rabbit parotid. J Membr Biol 94: 143–152

Wakui M, Nishiyama A (1980a) ACh-evoked complex membrane potentila changes in mouse submaxillary gland acini: a study employing channel blockers and atropine. Pflügers Arch 386: 251–259

Wakui M, Nishiyama A (1980b) Ionic dependence of acetyl-choline equilibrium potential of acinar cells in mouse submaxillary gland. Pflügers Arch 386: 261–267

Welsh MJ (1986) An apical-membrane chloride channel in human tracheal epithelium. Science 232: 1648–1650

Welsh MJ, Smith PL, Frizzell RA (1982) Chloride secretion by canine tracheal epithelium: II. The cellular electrical potential profile. J Membr Biol 70: 227–238

Physiology of Salivary Gland Exocytosis*

D. O. Quissell

Introduction

Three anatomically distinct pairs of major salivary glands (parotid, mandibular, and sublingual) and several different minor salivary glands are responsible for the production of saliva. This review article will focus primarily on the rat mandibular and parotid glands since most of our current understanding of the actual cellular processes involved in exocytosis has come from studies on these two tissues.

The primary control of salivary gland secretion is regulated by the autonomic nervous system. In general, parasympathetic stimulation leads to production of saliva at a rather high flow rate (Schneyer et al. 1972), while sympathetic stimulation leads to a much slower rate of saliva production, but of a more viscous nature.

Neurotransmitters evoke salivary gland secretion by binding to the basolateral surface receptors and, through the generation of specific intracellular second messengers, the intracellular mechanisms involved in the production of the primary secretory fluid and exocytosis are activated. The emphasis of this review will be on those more distal intracellular events that may be directly involved in the initiation and modulation of exocytosis.

Exocytosis is a cellular process by which cells are able to release synthesized material to the external environment. In the mammalian exocrine cell, the secretory material is first stored in the secretory granule, and following an appropriate cellular signal, the individual secretory granules migrate to the luminal plasma membrane, fuse with the membrane, and the secretory substances are discharged. Although fairly well defined morphologically (Hand 1987), the actual molecular basis of exocytosis and its regulation (stimulus-exocytosis coupling mechanism) still constitutes a poorly understood area of cell biology. In the rat mandibular gland, β-adrenergic receptor stimulation is an absolute requirement for mucin secretion (Quissell and Barzen 1980; Quissell et al. 1981; McPherson and Dormer 1984). Pure cholinergic or α-adrenergic receptor stimulation will not elicit significant mucin secretion. In the parotid gland of the rat and mouse,

---

* This work was supported by NIH Grants DE-07689 and DE-07201.

a pure cholinergic or α-adrenergic receptor-mediated response will elicit amylase release (Butcher and Putney 1980), albeit the rate of amylase secretion is significantly less than that observed following a pure β-adrenergic receptor-mediated response. In both the rat parotid and mandibular glands, adenosine $3',5'$-cyclic monophosphate (cyclic AMP) and calcium appear to play a major role in the stimulus-exocytosis coupling mechanism (Butcher and Putney 1980; Quissell et al. 1981). Cholinergic and α-adrenergic-mediated responses require extracellular calcium, whereas the β-adrenergic-mediated responses include changes in intracellular cyclic AMP levels (Butcher and Putney 1980; Quissell and Barzen 1980). Early studies had suggested that calcium may be the actual final mediator for exocytosis (Putney et al. 1977), and a unifying hypothesis was set forth which indicated that the final effector of parotid secretion was calcium. This simple view of rat salivary gland exocytosis and its control is no longer satisfactory, for cyclic AMP appears to be able to mediate rat parotid amylase release without the elevation of cytosolic calcium (Takuma and Ichida 1986a), and activation of the cyclic AMP pathway in rat mandibular gland is a prerequisite for mucin secretion.

Cyclic AMP Pathway

The predominate receptor involved in the direct stimulation of rat parotid and mandibular gland secretion is the β-adrenergic receptor. The activation of this receptor system results in a dramatic increase in cyclic AMP (Butcher and Putney 1980; Quissell et al. 1981). The mechanism by which β-adrenergic receptor stimulation leads to exocytosis via the increase in intracellular cyclic AMP is not well understood. Cyclic AMP is thought to mediate most, if not all, of its effects by the activation of a cyclic AMP-dependent protein kinase (A kinase or protein kinase A). Concomitant with an increase in intracellular cyclic AMP levels following β-adrenergic receptor stimulation, rat parotid and mandibular A kinase activity also increases, with the activation of A kinase remaining elevated throughout the entire secretory period (Baum et al. 1981a; Spearman and Butcher 1982; Quissell et al. 1983a). The extent of A kinase activation also correlates quite closely with the rate of exocytosis in both tissues (Baum et al. 1981b; Quissell et al. 1983a).

Two isoenzymes of A kinase have been identified and characterized in rat salivary glands. Both types are activated by the binding of cyclic AMP to the regulatory subunits which results in the dissociation of the holoenzyme to a regulatory subunit-cyclic AMP complex and an active catalytic subunit. The free catalytic subunit is then able to phosphorylate various protein substrates. Subcellular distribution studies indicated that the rat parotid and mandibular cells contain a cytosolic form of type I and type II and also contain a membrane-bound form of type-I A kinase (Baum et al. 1981a;

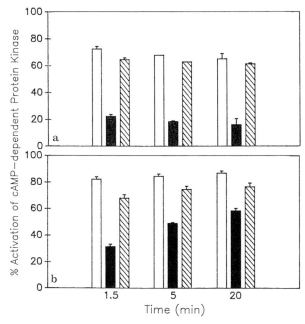

Time (min)

Fig. 1a, b. Cellular distribution and extent of activation of type-I and type-II kinase A in rat **a** parotid and **b** mandibular acinar cells following β-adrenergic receptor stimulation. Results are expressed as a percentage of activation in the stimulated cells compared to unstimulated cells (Quissell et al. 1988). Each value represents the mean value of at least four separate experiments and *vertical bars* represent ± SEM. *Open bars*, cytosol type I; *solid bars*, cytosol type II; *hatched bars*, microsomes type I

Quissell et al. 1988). Despite the fact that the type-II form comprises at least 65% of the total activity of both glands, recent studies indicate that following β-adrenergic receptor stimulation, both the cytosolic and microsomal form of type-I were activated to a far greater extent than the type-II form, supporting an important physiological role for the type-I form of the kinase (Fig. 1).

Since a cyclic AMP-dependent metabolic pathway has been implicated as the major pathway in the stimulus-exocytosis coupling mechanism for both the rat parotid and mandibular glands, protein phosphorylation and/or dephosphorylation may be one of the actual molecular mechanisms by which exocytosis is regulated. Recent studies support such a possible mechanism, but the problem that remains is to identify the phosphoprotein(s) that may be directly involved in the exocytotic pathway. Stimulation of β-adrenergic receptors in rat parotid and mandibular gland leads to the phosphorylation and dephosphorylation of several proteins (Jahn et al. 1980; Jahn and Söling 1981; Baum et al. 1981b; Freedman and Jamieson 1982a; Quissell et al. 1983b; Spearman et al. 1984). Of these, three proteins have been identified most consistantly in the rat parotid and mandibular acinar cells; 36-34 kDa (protein I), 26-24 kDa (protein II), and 22 kDa (protein III) phosphoproteins. Protein I has been identified as ribosomal protein S6 (Freedman and Jamieson 1982b; Jahn and Söling 1983; D. O. Quissell, unpublished data), whereas the function of the other two proteins is still quite obscure.

Protein III from the rat parotid has recently been purified and characterized (Thiel et al. 1988). Subcellular fractionation studies suggest that protein III is located in the endoplasmic reticulum. Because of its location (Thiel et al. 1988) and its slow rate of phosphorylation (Quissell et al. 1985) and dephosphorylation, this particular protein may not play a direct role in the stimulus-exocytosis coupling mechanism. However, it may still play an important physiological role in the regulation of calcium sequestration by the endoplasmic reticulum during β-adrenergic receptor stimulation (Plewe et al. 1984). Only one phosphorylation site has been identified (phosphoserine) per peptide and in vitro studies indicated that this particular site could be phosphorylated by cyclic AMP-dependent protein kinase. In vitro studies indicated that this particular sequence could be phosphorylated by the catalytic subunit of cyclic AMP-dependent protein kinase.

Of these phosphoproteins, only the 26-kDa phosphoprotein (protein II) appears to display the appropriate rate of phosphate turnover which would be compatible with a direct role in regulating rat parotid and mandibular exocytosis (Quissell et al. 1985, 1987). Phosphate turnover studies indicate that the in situ dephosphorylation rate for 26 kDa was quite rapid (apparent $t_{1/2} = 5\text{-}6$ min), whereas dephosphorylation rates for 21 kDa and 36 kDa were much slower ($t_{1/2} > 20$ min). The extent of phosphorylation of 26 kDa also correlated with the dose-response relation for β-adrenergic receptor-mediated secretion and with A kinase activation (Quissell et al. 1983a, 1985).

The 26-kDa phosphoprotein has recently been purified (D. O. Quissell, unpublished data) and as yet, it is unclear what its precise role may be in the exocytotic pathway. The protein appears to be an intrinsic membrane protein (Quissell et al. 1985), and the acceptor amino acid for endogenous

Table 1. Amino acid composition of the 26-kDa phosphoprotein

Amino acid	No. in peptide	Amino acid	No. in peptide
Aspartic acid	17	Tyrosine	3
Glutamic acid	28	Valine	12
Serine	26	Methionine	1
Glycine	43	Cysteine	—
Histidine	3	Isoleucine	8
Arginine	9	Leucine	18
Threonine	11	Phenylalanine	8
Alanine	14	Lysine	9
Proline	8		

phosphorylation is serine (Quissell et al. 1987). In vitro phosphorylation studies indicate that the 26-kDa phosphoprotein is an excellent substrate for A kinase. The amino acid composition of the 26 kDa phosphoprotein is given in Table 1.

In various biological systems, it is as important to terminate a biological response as it is to initiate it. Unfortunately, very little information is currently available regarding the actual identification and characterization of the protein phosphatases present in salivary gland tissues. In the guinea-pig parotid gland, protein phosphatases of the type 1 and 2A and 2B have been identified in the cytosolic fraction with most of type 1 and 2A in the inactive state. A microsomal-associated protein phosphatase has also been identified (Mieskes and Söling 1987).

Calcium Pathway

The importance of calcium in the exocytotic process of the salivary glands was first indicated by the studies of Douglas and Poisner (1963). However, the precise role for calcium in the regulation of secretion is not known nor is its role in exocytosis fully understood. Rat parotid and mandibular acinar cells pretreated with ethylene glycol-tetraacetic acid (EGTA), to deplete their intracellular stores of calcium, were greatly inhibited in their ability to secrete amylase (Butcher and Putney 1980) or mucins following adrenergic receptor stimulation (Quissell and Barzen 1980).

Cholinergic, α-adrenergic, and substance P receptor stimulation activates a number of calcium-dependent, intracellular responses that can lead to fluid or macromolecular secretion. In general, the evidence for these calcium-dependent processes comes from several different types of experimental approaches. Removal of extracellular calcium or the depletion of intra-cellular calcium stores greatly diminish or prevents fluid secretion or exocytosis. In the absence of receptor stimulation, the calcium ionophore, A23187, mimics the receptor-mediated response, and this mimic response is calcium dependent. Increases in intracellular free calcium levels following receptor stimulation also correlate with the secretory response.

In recent years, a considerable amount of information has been developed relating to the agonist-activated hydrolysis of inositol phospholipids and their subsequent role in regulating intracellular free calcium (Putney 1987). The focus of this discussion will be on those areas in which calcium may act as a direct effector of salivary gland exocytosis. Although the mechanism of calcium entry into the salivary gland and the release of calcium from intracellular stores is actively being determined (Hughes et al. 1988), these same inositol phospholipids may have other functions in the overall sequence of events during exocytosis.

The regulation of intracellular free calcium concentrations by the parotid and mandibular acinar cells before, during, and after stimulation has not been fully characterized. Several subcellular organelles have demonstrated an ability to bind or concentrate calcium (Nyjar and Pritchard 1971; Perec and Alonso 1971; Selinger et al. 1970). The microsomal fractions isolated from these tissue can accumulate calcium in an ATP-dependent manner (Terman and Gunter 1983; Watson and Siegel 1978; Kanagasuntheram and Randle 1976; Kanagasuntheram and Teo 1982a; Immelmann and Söling 1983; Hurley and Martinez 1985, 1986). Chlorpromazine, trifluoperazine and 4,4'-diisothiocyanostilbene-2,2'-disulfonate all inhibit calcium accumulation, but the mitochondrial transport inhibitors ruthenium red and carbonyl cyanide m-chlorophenylhydrazone had no effect on calcium transport. Marker enzyme analysis suggested that a specialized region of the endoplasmic reticulum may be involved.

The actual steady-state level of free intracellular calcium levels is modulated by the release or uptake of calcium from various intracellular stores such as the endoplasmic reticulum and mitochondria, the influx of calcium from the external milieu through various plasma membrane

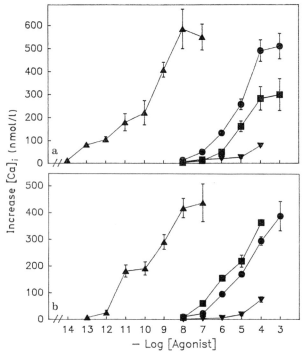

Fig. 2a, b. Calculated $[Ca^{2+}]_i$ of fura-2 loaded rat **a** parotid and **b** mandibular acinar cells. Intracellular free-calcium levels were calculated from the ratio of fluorescence (> 470 nm emissions) at two excitation wavelengths, 340 nm and 380 nm, after correction for autofluorescence, light scatter and fura-2 leakage. Values represent mean peak values obtained after stimulation of at least four separate experiments and *vertical bars* represent ± SEM. *Circles*, carbachol; *squares*, norepinephrine; *downward arrows*, isoproterenol; *upward arrows*, substance P

channels, and the removal of calcium via the plasma membrane Ca^{2+}-ATPase (Merrit and Rink 1987). Cholinergic, α-adrenergic, and substance P receptors stimulation lead to an increase in intracellular free calcium (Fig. 2). The increase in free calcium is due to the release of calcium from the endoplasmic reticulum and from calcium uptake (Merrit and Rink 1987). In recent years, a significant amount of data has developed that indicates that this particular stimulus-response coupling pathway involves inositol-1,4,5-trisphosphate (Hughes et al. 1988; Bonis et al. 1986; Henne et al 1987). Although it has not been demonstrated in all salivary gland tissues, this particular pathway would appear to be a ubiquitous second messenger.

β-Adrenergic receptor stimulation does not appear to increase intracellular free calcium concentration at physiological levels of stimulation (Takemura 1985; Takuma and Ichida 1986a; Dreux et al. 1986) nor does β-adrenergic receptor stimulation facilitate calcium efflux or influx. Calcium efflux is observed only after prolonged stimulation (McPherson and Dormer 1984; Butcher 1980; Dreux et al. 1986).

Unlike the cyclic AMP pathway, the major problem in determining the exact role of calcium in mediating cellular exocytosis is due to the complexity of the various intracellular calcium-dependent mechanisms. Calcium can mediate its effects through a vast number of different cellular events with some or all having a potential direct role in exocytosis. Calcium can directly bind to a large number of regulatory proteins such as calmodulin and calcimedins. It can act through a series of calcium-dependent protein kinases such as the calmodulin-dependent protein kinase and protein kinase C. It can activate or inhibit other important enzyme systems such as adenylate cyclase, phospholinses, etc. which can then lead to production of other intracellular messengers. It can also stimulate phosphodiesterases that, in turn, can modulate cellular cyclic AMP levels. All of these possibilities need to be further explored before a more complete understanding of the calcium-mediated events can be obtained.

Calmodulin is widely distributed in nature. It has been shown to be present in several different mammalian secretory tissues, including rat parotid and submandibular cells (Kanagasuntheram and Teo 1982b; Spearman and Butcher 1983; Arkle et al. 1986; Piascik et al 1986; Tojyo et al. 1987; Singh et al. 1986). Recent studies have implicated a role for calmodulin and calmodulin binding proteins in rat salivary gland exocytosis (Singh et al. 1986). Calmodulin clearly plays an important role in salivary gland calcium homeostatsis, and a plasma membrane calmodulin-dependent ATPase has been demonstrated. However, its precise direct role in cellular exocytosis is not understood, for it is unclear from the various studies using calmodulin antagonists if the effects observed on exocytosis are directly due to inhibition of the calmodulin-dependent secretory events or are secondary due to changes in intracellular calcium metabolism and/or nonspecific effects of these highly hydrophobic agents.

Just as protein phosphorylation may play an important role in mediating cellular exocytosis of the cyclic AMP dependent pathway, recent studies indicate that phosphorylation may play an important role during the calcium-dependent, phospholipid-dependent protein kinase (protein kinase C) activation that occurs during receptor stimulation due to a simultaneous increase in intracellular calcium and diacylglycerol. Phorbol esters, potent activators of protein kinase C, have been shown to induce rat parotid amylase and mandibular mucin secretion (Putney et al. 1984; Takuma and Ichida 1986b; Fleming et al. 1986). The stimulation is not calcium dependent, but when cellular calcium levels are increased via calcium ionophore, A23187, the secretory rate is augmented. Stimulation of guinea-pig parotid cells leads to translocation of protein kinase C from the cytosolic to the membrane fraction (Domenech and Söling 1987). Phosphorylation of the ribosomal protein S6 during receptor-mediated exocytosis has been shown to be catalyzed by protein kinase C (Padel and Söling 1985). Protein kinase C activity has been associated with rat parotid secretory granules, and two protein substrates have been identified (Baldys-Waglegorska et al. 1987). These data suggest that cytosolic protein kinase C may phosphorylate specific granule membrane proteins, but it remains to be seen whether these phosphorylation events directly contribute to the regulation of rat parotid exocytosis. A role for protein kinase C in the exocytotic process has not been demonstrated under all experimental conditions, however. Using dispersed rat mandibular acinar-intercalated duct cells, we were unable to demonstrate a role for protein kinase C during exocytosis. Phorbol esters were unable to elicit a secretory response, nor were they able to augment a response using the appropriate agonists. Endogenous protein phosphorylation was unaffected by the phorbol esters, and we were unable to observe any ribosomal S6 phosphorylation (Quissell et al., 1989). Thus, the role of this particular kinase in the exocytotic pathway may be very system dependent.

Speculation

The current hypothesis (Fig. 3), based on the above mentioned studies, suggests that there may exist within the rat parotid and mandibular acinar cell membrane fraction a "stimulus-coupled regulatory complex for exocytosis" in which the 26-kDa phosphoprotein is a subunit. The physiological function of the 26-kDa phosphoprotein is to transfer to the enzyme complex the cyclic AMP-mediated signal, and thus the 26-kDa protein is the actual regulatory site for cyclic AMP mediated exocytosis, with the extent of phosphorylation of the 26-kDa protein determining the actual rate of exocytosis (Quissell et al. 1985, 1987). In the rat parotid, since changes in intracellular calcium levels can also mediate an exocytotic process, there may be an additional protein present in the secretory complex, the role of which is to transfer to the enzyme complex the calcium-mediated signal. This protein could be calmodulin, another calcium-binding protein, or phosphoprotein.

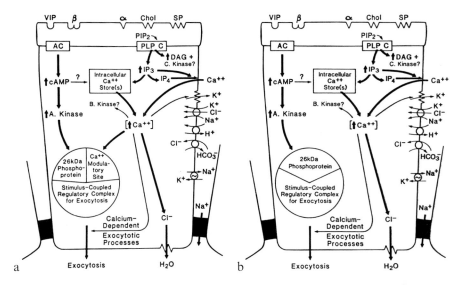

Fig. 3a, b. Current hypothesis summarizing the intracellular molecular events that appear to be directly involved during rat **a** parotid and **b** submandibular secretion. *VIP*, vasoactive intestinal peptide receptor; β, beta-adrenergic receptor; α, alpha-adrenergic receptor; *Chol*, cholinergic receptor; *SP*, substance P receptor; *AC*, adenylate cyclase; *PIP*, phosphatidylinositol 4-phosphate; *PLPC*, phospholipase C; *DAG*, diacylglycerol; IP_3, inositol 1,4,5-triphosphate; IP_4, inositol 1,3,4,5-tetrakisphosphate

References

Arkle S, Pickford PD, Schofield PS, Ward C, Argent BE (1986) Mechanism of the inhibitory effect of trifluoperazine on isoprenaline-evoked amylase secretion from isolated rat parotid glands. Biochem Pharmacol 35: 4121–4124

Baldys-Waglegorska A, Pour A, Moriarty CM, Dowd F (1987) The effect of calcium and cyclic AMP on amylase release in digitonin-permeabilized parotid gland cells. Biochim Biophys Acta 929: 190–196

Baum BJ, Colpo FT, Filburn CR (1981a) Characterization and relationship to exocrine secretion of rat parotid gland cyclic AMP-dependent protein kinase. Arch Oral Biol 26: 333–357

Baum BJ, Frieberg JM, Ito H, Roth GS, Filburn CR (1981b) Beta-adrenergic regulation of protein phosphorylation and its relationship to exocrine secretion in dispersed rat parotid gland acinar cell. J Biol Chem 256: 9731–9736

Bonis D, Giraird F, Rossignol B (1986) Inositol trisphosphate-induced Ca^{2+} release from rat parotid subcellular fractions. Biol Cell 57: 271–274

Butcher FR (1980) Regulation of calcium efflux from isolated rat parotid cells. Biochim Biophys Acta 630: 254–260

Butcher FR, Putney JW (1980) Regulation of parotid gland function by cyclic nucleotides and calcium. Adv Cyclic Nucleotide Res 13: 215–249

Domenech EM, Söling H-D (1987) Effects of stimulation of muscarinic and of beta-catecholamine receptors on the intracellular distribution of protein kinase C in guinea pig exocrine glands. Biochem J 242: 749–754

Douglas WW, Poisner AM (1963) The influence of calcium on the secretory response of the submaxillary gland to acetylcholine or to noradrenaline. J Physiol (Lond) 165: 528–541

Dowd F, Cheung P, Warren J, Faerber T, Traub D (1985) Comparison of cyclic AMP-dependent protein kinases from salivary glands of four species. J Dent Res 64: 1199–1203

Dowd F, Watson EL, Lau Y-S, Justin J, Pasienuik J, Jacobson KL (1987) Calcium-dependent protein kinase reactions associated with parotid gland secretory granule membranes. J Dent Res 66: 557–563

Dreux C, Imhoff V, Huleux C, Busson S, Rossignol B (1986) Forskolin, a tool for rat parotid secretion studies: ^{45}Ca efflux is not related to cAMP. Am J Physiol 251: C754–C762

Fleming N, Bilan PT, Sliwinski-Lis E (1986) Effects of a phorbol ester and diacylglycerols on secretion of mucin and arginine esterase by rat submandibular gland cells. Pflügers Arch 406: 6–11

Freedman SD, Jamieson JD (1982a) Hormone-induced protein phosphorylation. I. Relationship between secretagogue action and endogenous protein phosphorylation in intact cells from the exocrine pancreas and parotid. J Cell Biol 95: 903–908

Freedman SD, Jamieson JD (1982b) Hormone-induced protein phosphorylation. II. Localization to the ribosomal fraction from rat exocrine pancreas and parotid of a 29,000-dalton protein phosphorylated in situ in response to secretagogues. J Cell Biol 95: 909–917

Hand AR (1987) Functional ultrastructure of the salivary glands. In: Sreebny LM (ed) The salivary system. CRC, Boca Raton, pp 43–67

Henne V, Piiper A, Söling H-D (1987) Inositol 1,4,5-trisphosphate and 5'-GTP induce calcium release from different intracellular pools. FEBS Lett 218: 153–158

Hughes AR, Takemura H, Putney JW (1988) Kinetics of inositol 1,4,5-trisphosphate and inositol cyclic 1:2,4,5-trisphosphate metabolism in intact rat parotid acinar cells. J Biol Chem 263: 10314–10319

Hurley TW, Martinez JR (1985) Characterization of the kinetic and regulatory properties of high-affinity Ca^{2+}-ATPase activity in acinar preparation of rat submandibular salivary glands. Arch Oral Biol 30: 587–594

Hurley TW, Martinez JR (1986) Characterization and localization of two forms of active Ca^{2+} transport in vesicles derived from rat submandibular glands. Cell Calcium 7: 49–59

Immelmann A, Söling H-D (1983) ATP-dependent calcium sequestration and calcium/ATP stoichiometry in isolated microsomes from guinea pig parotid glands. FEBS Lett 162: 406–410

Jahn R, Söling H-D (1981) Phosphorylation of the same specific protein during amylase release evoked by beta-adrenergic or cholinergic agonists in rat and mouse parotid glands. Proc Natl Acad Sci USA 78: 6903–6906

Jahn R, Söling H-D (1983) Phosphorylation of the ribosomal protein S6 in response to secretagogues in the guinea pig exocrine pancreas, parotid and lacrimal gland. FEBS Lett 153: 71–76

Jahn R, Unger C, Söling H-D (1980) Specific protein phosphorylation during stimulation of amylase secretion by beta-agonists or dibutyryl adenosine 3',5'-monophosphate in the rat parotid gland. Eur J Biochem 112: 345–352

Kanagasuntheram P, Randle PJ (1976) Calcium metabolism and amylase release in rat parotid acinar cells. Biochem J 160: 547–564

Kanagasuntheram P, Teo TS (1982a) Parotid microsomal Ca^{2+} transport. Subcellular localization and characterization. Biochem J 298: 789–794

Kanagasuntheram P, Teo TS (1982b) Calmodulin-sensitive ATP-dependent calcium transport by the rat parotid endoplasmic reticulum. FEBS Lett 141: 233–236

McPherson MA, Dormer RL (1984) Mucin release and calcium fluxes in isolated rat submandibular acini. Biochem J 224: 473–481

Merrit JE, Rink TJ (1987) Regulation of cytosolic free calcium in fura-2 loaded rat parotid acinar cells. J Biol Chem 262: 17362–17369

Mieskes G, Söling H-D (1987) Protein phosphatases of the guinea-pig parotid gland. Eur J Biochem 167: 377–382

Nyjar MA, Pritchard ET (1971) Calcium binding by a plasma membrane fraction isolated from rat submandibular gland. Biochim Biophys Acta 323: 391–395

Padel U, Söling H-D (1985) Phosphorylation of the ribosomal protein S6 during agonist-induced exocytosis in exocrine glands is catalyzed by calcium-phospholipid-dependent protein kinase (protein kinase C). Eur J Biochem 151: 1–10

Perec CJ, Alonso GJ (1971) The effect of denervation on ATP dependent calcium uptake by microsomes of the submaxillary gland of rats. Experientia 27: 897–898

Piascik MT, Babich M, Jacobson KL, Watson EL (1986) Calmodulin activation and calcium regulation of parotid gland adlenylate cyclase. Am J Physiol 250: C642–C645

Plewe G, Jahn R, Immelmann A, Bode C, Söling H-D (1984) Specific phosphorylation of a protein in calcium accumulating endoplasmic reticulum from rat parotid glands following stimulation by agonists involving cAMP as second messenger. FEBS Lett 166: 96–103

Putney JW, Weiss SJ, Leslie BA, Marier SH (1977) Is calcium the final mediator of exocytosis in the rat parotid gland? J pharmacol Exp Ther 203: 144–155

Putney JW, McKinney JS, Aub DL, Leslie BA (1984) Phorbol ester-induced protein secretion in parotid gland. Relationship to the role of inositol lipid breakdown and protein kinase C activation in stimulus-secretion coupling. Mol Pharmacol 26: 261–266

Quissell DO, Barzen KA (1980) Secretory response of dispersed rat submandibular cells. II. Mucin secretion. Am J Physiol 238: C99–C106

Quissell DO, Barzen KA, Lafferty JL (1981) Role of calcium and cAMP in the regulation of rat submandibular mucin secretion. Am J Physiol 241: C76–C85

Quissell DO, Barzen KA, Deisher LM (1983a) Role of cyclic AMP-dependent protein kinase activation in regulating rat submandibular mucin secretion. Biochim Biophys Acta 762: 215–220

Quissell DO, Deisher LM, Barzen KA (1983b) Role of protein phosphorylation in regulating rat submandibular mucin secretion. Am J Physiol 245: G44–G53

Quissell DO, Deisher LM, Barzen KA (1985) The rate-determining step in cAMP-mediated exocytosis in the rat parotid and submandibular glands appear to involve analogous 26-kDa integral membrane phosphoproteins. Proc Natl Acad Sci USA 82: 3237–3241

Quissell DO, Deisher LM, Barzen KA (1987) Role of protein phosphorylation in rat salivary gland exocytosis. J Dent Res 66: 596–598

Quissell DO, Deisher LM, Barzen KA (1988) Subcellular distribution and activation of rat submandibular cAMP-dependent protein kinase following beta-adrenergic receptor stimulation. Biochim Biophys Acta 969: 28–32

Quissel DO, Barzen KA, Deisher LM (1989) Evidence against a direct role for protein kinase C in rat submandibular mucin secretion. Arch Oral Biol 34: 695–699

Selinger F, Naim E, Lassar M (1970) ATP-dependent calcium uptake by microsomal preparations from rat parotid and submaxillary glands. Biochim Biophys Acta 203: 326–334

Schneyer LH, Young JA, Schneyer CA (1972) Salivary secretions of electrolytes. Physiol Rev 52: 720–777

Singh J, Brady RC, Dedman JR, Quissell DO (1986) Subcellular distribution of calmodulin and its binding proteins within the rat submandibular gland. Am J Physiol 251: C403–C410

Spearman TN, Butcher FR (1982) Rat parotid gland protein kinase activation. Relationship to enzyme secretion. Mol Pharmacol 21: 121–127

Spearman TN, Butcher FR (1983) The effect of calmodulin antagonists on amylase release from the rat parotid gland in vitro. Pflügers Arch 397: 220–224

Spearman NT, Hurley KP, Olivas R, Ulrich RG, Butcher FR (1984) Subcellular location of stimulus-affected endogenous phosphoproteins in the rat parotid gland. J Cell Biol 99: 1354–1363

Takemura H (1985) Changes in cytosolic free calcium concentration in isolated rat parotid cells by cholinergic and beta-adrenergic agonists. Biochem Biophys Res Commun 131: 1048–1055

Takuma T, Ichida T (1986a) Does cyclic AMP mobilize Ca^{2+} for amylase secretion from rat parotid cells? Biochim Biophys Acta 887: 113–117

Takuma T, Ichida T (1986b) Phorbol ester stimulates amylase secretion from rat parotid cells. FEBS Lett 199: 53–56

Takuma T, Ichida T (1988) Amylase secretion from saponin-permeabilized parotid cells evoked by cyclic AMP. J Biochem 103: 95–98

Terman BI, Gunter TE (1983) Characterization of the submandibular gland microsomal calcium transport system. Biochim Biophys Acta 730: 151–160

Thiel G, Schmidt WE, Meyer HE, Söling H-D (1988) Purification and characterization of a 22-kDa microsomal protein from rat parotid gland which is phosphorylated following stimulation by agonists involving cAMP as second messenger. Eur J Biochem 170: 643–651

Tojyo Y, Uchida M, Matsumoto Y (1987) Inhibitory effects of calmodulin antagonists on isoproterenol- and dibutyryl cyclic AMP-stimulated amylase release from rat parotid acinar cells. Jpn J Pharmacol 45: 487–491

Watson EL, Siegel IA (1978) Factors affecting calcium accumulation and release in canine submandibular salivary microsomes. Arch Oral Biol 23: 323–328

Non-Adrenergic, Non-Cholinergic Control of Salivary Gland Function

D. A. Titchen and A. M. Reid

Introduction

It has been recognised for some time that the parasympathetic and sympathetic divisions of the autonomic nervous system may contribute to the regulation of salivary gland function (Babkin 1950; Burgen and Emmelin 1961; Young and Van Lennep 1979; Garrett 1982). Muscarinic cholinergic agonists and antagonists have been used to assess the role of the parasympathetic innervation. Effects of the muscarinic cholinergic innervation include vasodilation and profuse secretion of fluid of relatively low protein concentration. Similarly, the role of the sympathetic innervation has been judged from effects mediated by either α or β adrenoceptors and their block by the appropriate antagonists. Stimulation of α adrenoceptors may produce vasoconstriction, contraction of the myoepithelial cells and in some species, secretion. Stimulation of β adrenoceptors may result in vasodilation and has been shown in a number of species to lead to production of low volumes of fluid with high protein (or enzyme) concentration.

In addition to the generalisations referred to above, evidence has accumulated that mechanisms mediated by other than cholinergic or adrenergic receptors may be involved in control of salivary gland function. Heidenhain (1872) reported that vasodilation evoked by electrical stimulation of the parasympathetic innervation to the mandibular gland was not abolished by atropine (see Bloom and Edwards 1980). More recently there have been demonstrations of atropine-resistant parasympathetic control over both fluid and protein secretion from salivary glands. In this chapter such non-adrenergic, non-cholinergic (NANC) mechanisms and the transmitter substances that may mediate them are discussed. Consideration is also given to the importance of the mechanisms in the overall control of salivary gland function.

NANC Responses in Salivary Glands

Secretion of fluid and protein persisting after atropinisation has been reported following direct electrical stimulation of the parasympathetic

Young · Wong, Epithelial Secretion of Water and Electrolytes
© Springer-Verlag Berlin · Heidelberg 1990

innervation of salivary glands of the rat (Thulin 1976; Ekström et al. 1983 b), ferret (Ekström et al. 1988 b) and sheep (Reid and Titchen 1988 a, b). In each instance in which they have been studied, the parasympathetically mediated secretory responses of fluid obtained after atropine have been of a much lower level than those before. Ekström et al. (1988 b) reported that the atropine-resistant responses of the parotid and mandibular glands of the ferret obtained with parasympathetic nerve stimulation were 5% and 27%, respectively, of those obtained before administration of the antagonist. The total flow of saliva from the parotid gland of atropinized rats over an 80-min period of stimulation was only 15% of that in non-atropinised animals (Ekström et al. 1988 a). Similarly, parasympathetic reflex responses of the ovine parotid gland evoked by oesophageal distension were, after atropine, less than 10% of responses to similar stimulation before muscarinic blockade (Reid and Titchen 1988 a).

The much smaller overall fluid secretory response to parasympathetic stimulation after atropine is due not only to the lesser maximal rates of fluid secretion observed after atropine, but also because the response has a greater latency and in, addition, fades very quickly. Typical of this was the form of the reflex response of the ovine parotid gland before and after atropine (Reid and Titchen 1988 a). Before atropine, secretion of fluid was stimulated within seconds of application of the stimulus (oesophageal distension), and the response remained strong for the duration (15 min) of the stimulus. However after atropine there was a period of ca. 30 s before the response commenced, following which secretion was enhanced for only 3 to 4 min before fading. Similar latencies have also been observed with electrical stimulation of the parasympathetic innervation after atropine. Secretion of fluid from the ovine mandibular gland does not begin until ca. 60 s after commencement of stimulation after atropine (Reid and Titchen 1988 b). The latency between the start of stimulation and onset of secretion rose with both the mandibular and parotid glands of ferrets from ca. 1 to over 20 s (Ekström et al. 1988 b). The different temporal characteristics of the atropine-resistant responses can be explained as arising from the rapid release and action of acetylcholine which contributed to the secretory responses before, and slower release and action of other transmitters after atropine was given.

Demonstrations of fluid and protein secretion in response to parasympathetic nerve simulation after atropine have also involved relatively high frequencies of nerve stimulation. Ekström et al. (1988 b) noted that after atropine the threshold frequencies at which secretory responses were obtained rose from 0.2–0.5 Hz to 10–20 Hz for the parotid and from 2 to 10 Hz for the mandibular gland of the ferret. Higher frequencies of stimulation are more effective whether they are of preganglionic nerve fibres (such as to the mandibular gland of the sheep; Reid and Titchen 1988 b) or postganglionic fibres (such as to the parotid of the sheep; Reid and Titchen 1988 a, b). In demonstrating both vasodilation within, and secretion from the ovine mandibular gland in response to parasympathetic stimulation after atropine, Reid and Titchen (1988 b) employed a stimulus frequency of 40 Hz. At this frequency it was found that unlike the secretory response, the vasomotor response did not fatigue readily and also lasted for up to 15 min following periods of stimulation as short as 2 min.

Observation of reductions in vascular resistance in the mandibular gland of the cat by Andersson et al. (1982b) provided unequivocal evidence of the efficacy, after atropine, of higher frequencies of parasympathetic (preganglionic) nerve stimulation delivered intermittently; the same number of pulses delivered continuously at lower frequencies was less powerful. Similar results were obtained in a study of the effects of stimulation of postganglionic parasympathetic fibres on vascular responses in the ovine parotid gland (Andersson et al. 1982a). These and more recent observations of non-adrenergic sympathetic control over the vasculature of the cat mandibular gland (Bloom et al. 1987) illustrate the importance of both frequency and pattern of firing of autonomic nerves in control of salivary gland function. However, few investigations have been made of the frequency and form of efferent fibre discharges to salivary glands. Carr (1977) reported that in sheep anaesthetised with chloralose there was a background traffic of efferent impulses at 0.5–4 Hz in non-myelinated postganglionic fibres distributed to the ovine parotid. With reflex stimulation to parotid secretion discharge frequencies in excess of 20 Hz regularly occurred and the unitary activity changed from evenly distributed single action potentials to a patterned discharge of spikes in pairs and occasionally triplets. The interspike interval of the grouped spikes was between 8.6 and 14.4 ms resulting in instantaneous frequencies of ca. 100 Hz.

Even though the secretion of fluid with parasympathetic stimulation has been markedly reduced after atropine in all species, this has been less the case for secretion of protein. In their study of the rat parotid gland, Ekström et al. (1988a) found that total secretion of amylase with parasympathetic stimulation was as great after atropine as before. The lesser quantity of fluid secreted after atropine had an inversely higher concentration of amylase. This may be explained by the possibility that even before atropine the non-cholinergic transmitter(s) released from the parasympathetic innervation contributes most significantly to the initiation and maintenance of secretion of protein seen with parasympathetic stimulation.

Neuropeptides as NANC Transmitters

Amongst the criteria that must be satisfied in order to establish a substance as the mediator of a response in a tissue are: the substance must be synthesised and stored within nerves supplying the tissue; the substance must be released on stimulation of those nerves; and responses to exogenous application of the substance should mimic those to nerve stimulation. Consideration is given below to reports that using these criteria implicate the involvement of various neuropeptides in altering blood flow, secretion of fluid and secretion of protein from salivary glands.

Distribution of Neuropeptides in Salivary Glands

Of the species in which evidence has been obtained of involvement of NANC mechanisms in initiation of fluid secretion from salivary glands, details of the peptidergic innervation have been studied in both the rat and the sheep. Peptides that have been localised in nerve fibres close to secretory elements of salivary glands in the rat include substance P (SP), substance K (SK), vasoactive intestinal polypeptide (VIP) and calcitonin gene-related peptide (CGRP; Ekström 1987). Those that have been localised in ovine salivary glands (Table 1) include VIP, SP, CGRP as well as neuropeptide Y (NPY) and enkephalin (ENK) (Reid et al. 1988). The most notable difference in the innervation of the mandibular gland to that of the parotid in the sheep was the very high density of VIP immunoreactivity around the secretory endpieces (Reid et al. 1988). VIP immunoreactivity in nerve fibres to salivary glands has also been studied in a number of species in which, to date, there have been no direct demonstrations of NANC mechanisms involved in initiation of salivary secretion. In each of these species, including the cat (Lundberg 1981), pig (Kwun SY, Heywood LH, Reid AM, unpublished observations 1988) and man (Lundberg et al. 1984a), there are fibres staining for VIP surrounding both secretory and vascular tissue.

An interesting feature of neuropeptides is that they most commonly coexist with other neuropeptides and/or a classical neurotransmitter. Colocalisation studies have shown that in a number of tissues, sympathetic nerve terminals contain NPY in addition to noradrenalin (Sundler et al. 1986). This has been shown to be the case in the ovine salivary glands (Reid et al. 1988). Double staining techniques used in the study of ovine salivary glands showed that NPY was also present in VIP containing fibres around secretory elements of both parotid and mandibular glands. In the rat parotid gland, Al-Hadithi et al. (1988) found that VIP immunoreactive fibres

Table 1. The relative density and distribution of peptide immunoreactive nerve fibres around vascular, glandular and duct tissue in ovine parotid glands (after Reid et al. 1988)

	VIP	NPY	CGRP	SP	ENK
Secretory endpieces	*	***	*	*	*
Artery	**	***	**	**	*
Arterioles	***	***	**	**	–
Vein	***	***	*	*	**
Duct	*	*	*	*	–

VIP, vasoactive intestinal peptide; NPY, neuropeptide Y; CGRP, calcitonin gene-related peptide; SP, substance P; ENK, enkephalin; –, not identified; *, sparse; **, moderate; and ***, dense immunoreactivity to the peptides

contained SP. Around acinar secretory cells they identified both these peptides in large (90–120 nm) dense-cored vesicles of nerve terminals that also contained smaller agranular vesicles measuring 40–60 nm in diameter. They postulated that the smaller granules contained acetylcholine on the basis of the ultrastructural similarities of the nerve terminals they studied to those of cat exocrine glands studied by Lundberg (1981) in which both VIP and acetylcholine esterase (a marker for acetylcholine) were found. Although SP is not found in VIP-containing nerve fibres in the ovine salivary glands, it is located in the same fibres as CGRP. Coexistence of SP and CGRP has been noted in other tissues and a sensory role has been proposed for such fibres (Skofitsch and Jacobowitz 1985).

Release of Neuropeptides from Salivary Glands

Release of a neuropeptide may be inferred by demonstration of a significant increase in concentration of that peptide in the venous effluent from a tissue with stimulation of the nerves to that tissue. The first such demonstrations in studies of salivary glands were of increases in the concentration of VIP in the venous plasma from the cat mandibular gland by Bloom and Edwards (1980) and Lundberg et al. (1980). In atropinised cats Bloom and Edwards (1980) found the concentration of VIP rose from 48 ± 10 pmol/l before stimulation to 227 ± 56 pmol/l during stimulation of the parasympathetic innervation at 20 Hz. Following cessation of the 10-min stimulus, the level of VIP decreased abruptly. There was a close temporal association between the change in concentration of VIP and the change in blood flow through the gland during and after nerve stimulation, an important feature in implicating VIP as the mediator of the response. An increase in the concentration of VIP in the venous effluent from the mandibular gland with stimulation of its parasympathetic innervation has also been observed in the sheep (Reid AM, Shulkes A, Titchen DA, unpublished observations 1988), in which the release of VIP was more closely associated with secretory responses than with vascular changes within the gland.

In addition to VIP, peptide HI (PHI; peptide with N-terminal histidine and C-terminal isoleucine) is released from the cat mandibular gland during parasympathetic stimulation (Lundberg et al. 1984b). The two peptides appear in the venous effluent from the gland in near equimolar concentrations as may be expected, given that one sequence for each peptide is located on a common precursor gene (Itoh et al. 1983). It has recently been shown that stimulation of the sympathetic innervation to the cat mandibular gland results in release of NPY (Bloom et al. 1987), leading to the postulate that this peptide mediates the residual vasoconstrictor response to sympathetic stimulation following α and β adrenoceptor blockade.

Demonstration of release of peptides from the rat parotid gland has involved assay of the peptides in the gland before and after nerve stimulation. In this way it was shown that parasympathetic nerve stimulation for 20 and 60 min reduced the parotid gland content of VIP and SP by approximately 40% and 75%, respectively (Ekström et al. 1985). The reduction in content of these peptides corresponded with the rapid reduction in the NANC secretory response of the gland.

Effects of Exogenous Neuropeptides on Salivary Glands

Earlier literature on actions of SP and other tachykinins on salivary glands of the dog, hen and rat has been reviewed by Bertaccini (1976). Since then, a number of peptides has been shown to affect salivary gland fluid and/or protein secretion and/or blood flow. The examples cited below are not meant to be comprehensive, but indicative of the value of such studies in establishing that peptides may play an important role in regulating salivary gland function.

Some peptides on their own are stimulants to both secretion and increased blood flow, others exert one or more effects only in the presence of another transmitter. Effects differ among species. This is very evident with VIP, actions of which have been investigated in salivary glands of the cat, dog, ferret, human, pig, rabbit, rat and sheep. Of these species, VIP has been shown only to initiate secretion of fluid from salivary glands of the rat (Ekström et al. 1983a) and sheep (Reid and Heywood 1988; Reid and Titchen 1988a, c). Characteristically, effects of VIP on secretion of fluid are slow to appear and relatively prolonged, similar to effects of nerve stimulation after atropine. Ekström et al. (1983a) refer to a latency of 60–100 s between a bolus IV injection of VIP and the start of secretion which persisted for 240–360 s. In the rat, SP and SK stimulate secretion within 10 s and the secretion persists for 120–180 s. In both the rat and sheep, the secretion stimulated by VIP is of a high protein content. In sheep, VIP evoked mandibular secretion with concentrations of protein of ca. 4–6 mg/ml compared with ca. 1 mg/ml in saliva evoked by acetylcholine (Reid and Heywood 1988).

Although VIP does not stimulate fluid secretion in some species, it is responsible for augmentation of that initiated by other stimuli and for increases in secretion of protein. Lundberg (1981) showed that whilst VIP was not a secretomotor agonist of its own accord, it potentiated secretory responses to acetylcholine from the cat mandibular gland. This may be explained by the report that, in vitro, VIP increases the affinity of the glands' muscarinic receptors for acetylcholine by a factor of 10^5 (Lundberg et al. 1981, 1982). In the pig, Reid and Heywood (1986, 1988) demonstrated that VIP augmented both flow and protein concentration of secretion of the parotid and mandibular glands maintained by infusion of bethanecol. VIP was also reported by Larsson et al. (1986) to increase cyclic AMP in human mandibular gland tissue, as did a peptide with N-terminal histidine and C-terminal methionine (PHM) but not SP. However, neither VIP, PHM nor SP induced changes in K^+ secretion; it was concluded that none of the peptides causes secretion of fluid from the human gland, but that VIP and PHM modulate secretion of protein.

PHM is the human equivalent of PHI, and both peptides evoke vasodilation within salivary glands. However, PHI in the cat (Lundberg and Tatemoto 1982) is, in contrast to PHM in humans (Larsson et al. 1986), much less potent than VIP as a vasodilator. This led Larsson et al. (1986) to comment on the importance of using "species related peptides" in studies of exogenous peptides. Another potent vasodilator peptide is CGRP which in the rat is not of its own accord a secretomotor agonist (Ekman et al. 1986). This contrasts with the sheep, in which Edwards et al. (1988) found that CGRP stimulated mandibular secretion of very high protein concentration and caused a persisting reduction in the vascular resistance in the gland. Although these effects still occurred after administration of atropine, they were slower to appear and were significantly reduced, indicative of an interaction between CGRP and acetylcholine. A synergistic interaction between CGRP and SP has also been demonstrated on fluid secretion from the mandibular gland of the sheep (A.M. Reid and D.A. Titchen 1988, unpublished observations). Similarly, there is evidence of synergy between these two peptides in the rat (Ekman et al. 1986). These observations are of particular interest in that CGRP is generally associated with sensory nerves. How this peptide is normally involved, if at all, in the control of salivary section remains obscure.

Significance of NANC Mechanisms in Salivary Gland Function

The sole demonstration of reflex activation of NANC stimulation of salivary secretion has been, to date, the demonstration by Reid and Titchen (1988a) of stimulation of parotid secretion with oesophageal distension. This NANC response may operate during ingestion of freshly provided food, the scabrous nature and volume of which could be expected to provide considerable oesophageal stimulation. It is likely that NANC mechanisms are involved in a number of reflexes in prandial stimulation of parotid secretion in sheep. Such secretion is initially of a large volume with high concentration of protein (Patterson et al. 1982). Some of the high protein results from adrenergic stimulation, perhaps due to both the sympathetic innervation and circulating catecholamines, although β-adrenergic blockade (Patterson et al. 1982) or cervical sympathectomy (Carr et al. 1984) only reduces and does not abolish prandial increases in parotid export of protein. Since muscarinic cholinergic agonists provide intense stimulation of fluid, but not of protein secretion from the gland, it is suggested that NANC mechanisms may contribute significantly to the initial prandial secretory response. A feature of the initial prandial secretion of protein by the parotid is that the secretory response wanes relatively rapidly, declining to levels even less than those before provision of food. This could arise in part from exhaustion of NANC transmitter, which, as discussed above, is a feature of these responses when evoked experimentally.

The NANC mechanisms referred to above have been shown to make a strong contribution to neurally evoked changes in vascular resistance and protein secretion of salivary glands, but only a minor, if any, contribution to increases in fluid secretion. Their importance appears even more significant if account is taken of the considerable synergistic effects between different neuropeptides and between neuropeptides and cholinergic and/or adrenergic transmitters. Demonstrations that the NANC responses may be overlooked due to experimental use of unfavourable frequencies and modes of nerve stimulation and due to observation of effects at a time when the transmitter involved may already be exhausted by previous periods of nerve stimulation are also significant points to consider. These considerations lead us to suggest that the NANC responses may be more important in contributing to salivary gland responses during ingestion of food than has hitherto been recognised.

References

Al-Hadithi BAK, Stauber V, Mitchell J (1988) The co-localisation of substance P and VIP in cholinergic-type terminals of the rat parotid. J Anat 159: 83–92

Andersson PO, Bloom SR, Edwards AV (1982a) Parotid responses to stimulation of the parasympathetic innervation in bursts in weaned lambs. J Physiol (Lond) 330: 163–174

Andersson PO, Bloom SR, Edwards AV, Järhult J (1982b) Effects of stimulation of the chorda tympani in bursts on submaxillary responses in the cat. J Physiol (Lond) 322: 469–483

Babkin BP (1950) Secretory mechanisms of the digestive glands. Hoeber, New York

Bertaccini G (1976) Active polypeptides of non-mammalian origin. Pharmacol Rev 28: 127–177

Bloom SR, Edwards AV (1980) Vasoactive intestinal peptide in relation to atropine resistant vasodilation in the submaxillary gland of the cat. J Physiol (Lond) 300: 41–53

Bloom SR, Edwards AV, Garrett JR (1987) Effects of stimulating the sympathetic innervation in bursts on submandibular vascular and secretory function in cats. J Physiol (Lond) 393: 91–106

Burgen ASV, Emmelin NG (1961) Physiology of the salivary glands. Edward Arnold, London

Carr DH (1977) Reflex-induced electrical activity in single units of secretory nerves to parotid gland in nerves to the gut. In: Brooks FP, Evers PW (eds) Nerves and the gut. Slack, New Jersey, pp 79–85

Carr DH, Davey M, Titchen DA (1984) Sympathetic and adrenergic effects on protein secretion from the parotid of the sheep. In: Case RM, Lingard JM, Young JA (eds) Secretion: mechanisms and control. Manchester University Press, Manchester, pp 220–222

Edwards AV, Reid AM, Titchen DA (1988) Actions of exogenous calcitonin gene related peptide on the ovine submaxillary gland. Proc Aust Physiol Pharmacol Soc 19: 203P

Ekman R, Ekström J, Håkanson R, Sjögren S, Sundler F (1986) Calcitonin gene related peptide in rat salivary glands. J Physiol (Lond) 381: 36P

Ekström J (1987) Neuropeptides and secretion. J Dent Res 66(2): 524–530

Ekström J, Månsson B, Tobin G (1983a) Vasoactive intestinal peptide evoked secretion of fluid and protein from rat salivary glands and the development of supersensitivity. Acta Physiol Scand 119: 169–175

Ekström J, Månsson B, Tobin G, Garrett JR, Thulin A (1983b) Atropine-resistant secretion of parotid saliva on stimulation of the auriculo temporal nerve. Acta Physiol Scand 119: 445–449

Ekström J, Brodin E, Ekman R, Håkanson R, Månsson B, Tobin G (1985) Depletion of neuropeptides in rat parotid glands and declining atropine-resistant salivary secretion upon continuous parasympathetic nerve stimulation. Regul Pept 11: 353–359

Ekström J, Garrett JR, Månsson B, Tobin G (1988a) The effects of atropine and chronic sympathectomy on maximal parasympathetic stimulation of parotid saliva in rats. J Physiol (Lond) 403: 105–116

Ekström J, Månsson B, Olgart L, Tobin G (1988b) Non-adrenergic, non-cholinergic salivary secretion in the ferret. Q J Exp Physiol 73: 163–173

Garrett JR (1982) Adventures with autonomic nerves. Perspectives in salivary glandular innervations. Proc R Micr Soc 17: 242–253

Heidenhain R (1972) Über die Wirkung einiger Gifte auf die Nerven der Glandula submaxillaris. Pflügers Arch 5: 309–318

Itoh N, Obata K, Yanaihara N, Okamoto H (1983) Human preprovasoactive intestinal polypeptide contains a novel PHI-27-like peptide, PHM-27. Nature 304: 547–549

Larsson O, Dunér-Engström M, Lundberg JM, Fredholm BB, Änggård A (1986) Effects of VIP, PHM and substance P on blood vessels and secretory elements of the human submandibular gland. Regul Pept 13: 319–326

Lundberg JM (1981) Evidence for coexistence of vasoactive intestinal polypeptide (VIP) and acetylcholine in neurones of cat exocrine glands. Acta Physiol Scand [Suppl] 496: 1–57

Lundberg JM, Tatemoto K (1982) Vascular effects of the peptides PYY and PHI: comparison with APP and VIP. Eur J Pharmacol 83: 143–146

Lundberg JM, Änggård A, Fahrenkrug J, Hökfelt T, Mutt V (1980) Vasoactive intestinal polypeptide in cholinergic neurones of exocrine glands: functional significance of coexisting transmitters for vasodilation and secretion. Proc Natl Acad Sci USA 77: 1651–1655

Lundberg JM, Hedlund B, Bartfai T (1982) Vasoactive intestinal polypeptide enhances muscarinic binding in cat submandibular salivary gland. Nature 295: 147–149

Lundberg JM, Fahrenkrug J, Hökfelt T, Martling CR, Larsson O, Tatemoto K, Änggård A (1984a) Co-existence of peptide HI (PHI) and VIP in nerves regulating blood flow and bronchial smooth muscle tone in various mammals including man. Peptides 5: 593–606

Lundberg JM, Fahrenkrug J, Larsson O, Änggård A (1984b) Corelease of vasoactive intestinal polypeptide and peptide histidine isoleucine in relation to atropine-resistant vasodilation in cat submandibular salivary gland. Neurosci Lett. 52: 37–42

Patterson J, Brightling P, Titchen DA 1982) β-Adrenergic effects on composition of parotid salivary secretion of sheep on feeding. Q J Exp Physiol 67: 57–67

Reid AM, Heywood LH (1986) The effects of exogenous vasoactive intestinal polypeptide on secretion from the parotid salivary gland of the pig. Proc Aust Physiol Pharmacol Soc 17: 83P

Reid AM, Heywood LH (1988) A comparison of the effects of vasoactive intestinal polypeptide on secretion from the submaxillary gland of the sheep and pig. Regul Pept 20: 211–221

Reid AM, Titchen DA (1988a) Atropine-resistant secretory responses of the ovine parotid gland to reflex and direct parasympathetic stimulation. Q J Exp Physiol 73: 413–424

Reid AM, Titchen DA (1988b) Atropine-resistant parasympathetic responses of the ovine parotid and submaxillary glands. J Physiol (Lond) 396: 118P

Reid AM, Titchen DA (1988c) Effects of chronic denervation on the response of the ovine parotid to vasoactive intestinal polypeptide alone and with bethanechol. In: Davison JS, Shaffer EA (eds) Gastrointestinal and hepatic secretions: mechanism and control. University of Calgary Press, Calgary, pp 206–209

Reid AM, Furness JB, Titchen DA (1988) Neural peptides in the ovine salivary glands. In: Young JA, Wong PYD (eds) Exocrine secretion. Hong Kong University Press, Hong Kong, pp 157–160

Skofitsch G, Jacobowitz DM (1985) Calcitonin gene related peptide coexists with substance P in capsaicin sensitive neurons and sensory ganglia of the rat. Peptides 6: 747–754

Sundler F, Håkanson R, Ekblad E, Uddman R, Wahlestedt C (1986) Neuropeptide Y in the peripheral adrenergic and enteric nervous system. Int Rev Cytol 102: 243–269

Thulin A (1976) Motor and secretory effects of nerves on the parotid gland of the rat. Acta Physiol Scand 96: 506–511

Young JA, van Lennep EW (1979) Transport in salivary glands. In: Giebisch G, Tosteson DC, Ussing HH (eds) Membrane transport in biology IVB. Springer, Berlin Heidelberg New York, pp 563–674

2 Lacrimal Glands

Electrolyte Secretion by the Lacrimal Glands

Y. Saito, T. Ozawa, and A. Nishiyama

Introduction

Tear fluid contains electrolytes in plasma like concentrations together with some proteins (Botelho 1964; Kikkawa 1970; Alexander et al. 1972), and secretion is induced both by muscarinic and by α-adrenergic stimulation. The mechanisms responsible for NaCl entry into the acinar cells and into the acinar lumen have not been elucidated, however (Putney 1979; Petersen 1980), although during the last decade, substantial progress has been made in our understanding of the cellular mechanisms of lacrimal electrolyte secretion as a result of the introduction of several new investigative techniques. (1) Patch-clamp methods have demonstrated three types of ion channel activated by Ca^{2+}. (2) Ion-selective microelectrode studies have demonstrated the involvement of electroneutral ion transport mechanisms such as $Na^+ - H^+$ and $Cl^- - HCO_3^-$ exchange and $Na^+ - K^+ - 2Cl^-$ cotransport in agonist-induced turnover of NaCl. (3) Fluorescent probes have helped to visualize calcium release from intracellular stores and influx from the extracellular fluid. (4) Membrane fractionation techniques have opened up the way for analytical and biochemical studies of the plasma membranes and intracellular organelles. Furthermore, studies on the roles of inositol polyphosphate metabolism, cyclic AMP and Ca^{2+} in receptor-mediated signal transduction have provided clues about the regulatory mechanisms of exocrine secretion. In this review we shall focus on recent progress resulting from use of the above mentioned techniques as they relate to the lacrimal gland and propose a model of electrolyte secretion as shown in Fig. 1. Discussion on the role of β-adrenergic stimulation and agonist-induced protein phosphorylation (e.g. Jahn and Söling 1981, 1983; Mauduit et al. 1983; Dartt et al. 1984, 1988; Llano et al. 1987) in the secretory process has been omitted.

Young · Wong, Epithelial Secretion of Water and Electrolytes
© Springer-Verlag Berlin · Heidelberg 1990

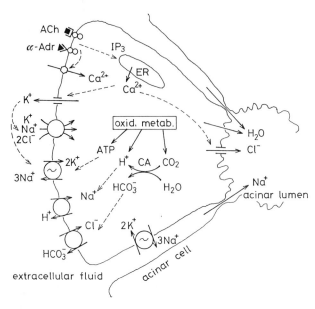

Fig. 1. Ion transport processes in the lacrimal acinar cell

Ion Channels

The application of cholinergic and α-adrenergic agonists to lacrimal acinar cells elicits biphasic changes in the membrane potential. An initial rapid hyperpolarization is followed by a transient small depolarization and subsequent sustained hyperpolarization with a concomitant decrease in the membrane resistances (Iwatsuki and Petersen 1978a, 1978b), and patch-clamp techniques have directly demonstrated the contribution of K^+, Cl^-, and nonselective monovalent cation channels to those agonist-induced changes in the membrane potentials (Findlay 1984; Marty et al. 1984; Trautmann and Marty 1984; Findlay and Petersen 1985; Evans and Marty 1986a, 1986b; Evans et al. 1986).

The K^+ channel, the so called "big K" channel, which has a very low selectivity for Na^+ and Cl^-, is activated by an increase in intracellular Ca^{2+} in the range of 10–100 nmol/l and by depolarization of the membrane potential (Findlay 1984; Trautmann and Marty 1984). Its location in the basolateral membrane is obvious, but whether it is also present in the luminal membrane is not known. It has been suggested that its role in secretion is to activate the Na^+-, K^+-ATPase and the $Na^+-K^+-2Cl^-$ cotransporter in the basolateral membrane by increasing the extracellular K^+ concentration (Petersen and Maruyama 1984) and to facilitate Cl^- exit into the acinar lumen by increasing the intracellular negativity (Saito et al. 1985, 1987a).

The Cl^- channel is activated by intracellular Ca^{2+} concentrations (Marty et al. 1984; Findlay and Petersen 1985) of 100–1000 nmol/l and membrane depolarization. The unit conductance is very small (1–2 pS) and the channel density is 5000–20000 per cell which is about 100 times greater than that of the K^+ channels (Marty et al. 1984). The Ca^{2+}-activated Cl^- conductance is partially blocked by furosemide and bumetanide in high concentrations (Evans et al. 1986). The localization of the Cl^- channel is still controversial (e.g., see Saito et al. 1987a) since the agonist-induced Cl^- current has been recorded only in whole-cell configurations of dispersed cells, although circumstantial evidence suggests its localization in the luminal membrane. A DIDS-inhibitable Cl^- conductance in the basolateral membrane that does not seem to be activated by ACh has also been demonstrated (Saito et al. 1987a). Further exploration is still necessary for the characterization of the various anion channels that seem to be present.

A calcium-activated, nonselective, monovalent cation channel with a unit conductance of 25 pS has been demonstrated in lacrimal cells (Marty et al. 1984). Its role in secretion is not clear, however, although Marty et al. (1984) have suggested that Na^+ influx is mediated by this channel in sustained secretion, because the intracellular Ca^{2+} concentration required to activate it is higher than 1000 nmol/l. On the other hand, the intracellular Ca^{2+} concentrations so far reported have rarely exceeded 1000 nmol/l during sustained agonist application (Ozawa et al. 1988c).

Na^+—K^+—$2Cl^-$ Cotransport

Coupled NaCl transport in the lacrimal gland was first suggested by Dartt et al. (1981), based on the finding that ACh-induced lacrimal secretion is inhibited by furosemide and by removal of Cl^- from the perfusate (Botelho et al. 1978). Suzuki and Petersen (1985) showed that the ACh null potential was shifted more negative by use of Cl^--free, NO_3^--containing solutions, Na^+-free solutions, or loop diuretics, and suggested that prevention of Cl^- accumulation into the acinar cells (by inhibiting $Na^+ - K^+ - 2Cl^-$ cotransport) decreased the contribution of the Cl^- conductance to the null potential and made the K^+ equilibrium potential dominant. On the other hand, Evans et al. (1986) suggested that the shift of ACh null potential by diuretics could be explained solely by direct blockade of the Ca^{2+}-activated Cl^- conductance. Direct evidence of uphill Cl^- accumulation into the acinar cells was provided by the measurement of intracellular Cl^- activity (A_i^{Cl}; Saito et al. 1985, 1987a). The A_i^{Cl} in the unstimulated condition was 30–35 mmol/l which is 1.4 times the equilibrium activity calculated from the membrane potential of about -40 mV. The addition of ACh (1 μmol/l) decreased A_i^{Cl} to about 20 mmol/l although the A_i^{Cl} was still 1.7 times the equilibrium activity because of the ACh-induced membrane hyperpolarization. Uphill Cl^- accumulation was significantly impaired in the absence of external Na^+ or

K^+ or in the presence of furosemide, and readmission of Na^+ or K^+ immediately increased Cl^- uptake (Ozawa et al. 1988a). ACh-induced Na^+ influx was inhibited by use of Cl^--free, NO_3^--containing solutions or in the presence of loop diuretics (Saito et al. 1987b). All of these findings are consistent with the presence of an $Na^+-K^+-2Cl^-$ cotransporter (Geck and Heinz 1986) although the stoichiometry is not known. Cl^- influx after cessation of ACh stimulation was only partially inhibited by either furosemide or DIDS alone, although, in combination, these drugs almost completely abolished the Cl^- influx. Thus, it was concluded that a parallel array of the $Na^+-K^+-2Cl^-$ cotransporter and $Cl^--HCO_3^-$ exchangers drives uphill Cl^- accumulation particularly when oxidative metabolism has been enhanced by a secretory stimulus (Ozawa et al. 1988a, 1988b).

Na^+-H^+ Exchanger

Amiloride inhibits Na^+ influx into the agonist-treated lacrimal glands (Parod and Putney 1980), and the inhibitory action has been attributed to blockade of a Na^+ conductance. Studies on the effects of amiloride on intracellular Na^+ activity (A_i^{Na}) and pH (pH_i), however, clearly demonstrate that a Na^+-H^+ exchanger plays the major role in ACh-induced Na^+ influx (Saito et al. 1988a, 1988b). The A_i^{Na} was 6 mmol/l in the unstimulated steady state and stimulation with ACh increased it to about 15 mmol/l. This ACh-induced increase in A_i^{Na} (Na^+ influx) was markedly reduced by amiloride without appreciable changes in the membrane potential or the input resistance. Acid loading the cell with CO_2/HCO_3^- buffered solution or by addition and withdrawal of NH_4^+ also caused a Na^+ influx that was susceptible to amiloride blockade. Similar findings have been obtained in a basolateral membrane vesicle preparation of rat lacrimal tissue (Mircheff et al. 1987).

The pH_i was 7.25 in intact unstimulated cells. The addition of ACh increased pH_i by about 0.1 unit, while the pH of the surrounding medium at the tissue surface was decreased. In the presence of amiloride or in a Na^+-free solution, ACh decreased pH_i monotonically (Saito et al. 1988a). The above findings indicate that stimulation with ACh enhances metabolic acid production. The ACh-induced increase in pH_i, therefore, may be the result of acid extrusion at a rate greater than the rate of acid production, probably due to *activation* of the Na^+-H^+ exchanger (see below).

The rate of acid extrusion from acid-loaded cells increased in a saturable manner as pH_i was reduced below 7.2, but, it was negligibly small (*inactivation*) when pH_i was about 7.2–7.3 (Saito et al. 1988b) even though a substantial driving force for Na^+-H^+ exchange (Aronson 1984) still existed. This kind of inactivation by higher pH_i and activation by agonist stimulation has been recognized in many other tissues although the mechanism of its regulation is not known. In other tissues regulatory roles for intracellular H^+ ion concentration, Ca^{2+}, protein kinase C, and tyrosine kinase have been suggested (see Grinstein and Rothstein 1986). In the inactive condition, the Na^+-H^+ exchanger is not reactivated by changes in extracellular pH or Na^+ concentration (Y. Saito et al., unpublished observations).

The rate of acid extrusion from acid-loaded cells is also a function of the extracellular Na^+ concentration, conforming to Michaelis-Menten kinetics, yielding an apparent K_m for Na^+ of 65 mmol/l and a V_{max} of 0.5 pH unit/min (Saito et al. 1988 b; unpublished observations). The apparent K_m value is similar to that reported for the exocrine pancreas (Dufresne et al. 1985; Hellmessen et al. 1985), but is one order higher than that reported for mostly inside-out oriented (Lambert et al. 1988) basolateral membrane vesicles from rat lacrimal gland (Mircheff et al. 1987). In addition, our study on the acid extrusion rate from the Na^+-depleted cell suggested that the apparent K_m value for intracellular Na^+ was lower than the normal activity of 6 mmol/l. These results indicate that activation and inactivation of the Na^+-H^+ exchanger and its transport rate are finely regulated at physiological ranges of pH_i and A_i^{Na} (Y. Saito et al., unpublished observations). The calculated net proton flux induced by ACh is comparable to the net Na^+ influx induced, suggesting that the major part ($>70\%$) of the ACh-induced Na^+ influx is mediated by the electroneutral Na^+-H^+ exchanger (Saito et al. 1988 a). This is consistent with the finding in the vesicle preparation that Na^+ fluxes driven by the proton gradient are significant (Mircheff et al. 1987), whereas a Cl^--dependent Na^+ flux was not detected (Lambert et al. 1988).

$Cl^--HCO_3^-$ Exchange

Evidence for the presence of a $Cl^--HCO_3^-$ exchanger in the lacrimal gland includes: (1) A_i^{Cl} is decreased (increased) by a sudden increase (decrease) in the extracellular HCO_3^- concentration; (2) pH_i is increased by Cl^- removal from the bicarbonate buffer solution; (3) the changes referred to in (1) and (2) above are inhibited by DIDS (Ozawa et al. 1988 b); (4) the presence of DIDS augments the ACh-induced increase of pH_i; and (5) the pH of the extracellular fluid after ACh stimulation becomes more acidic in the presence of DIDS than in its absence (Saito et al. 1988 a). The kinetic analysis of the $Cl^--HCO_3^-$ exchanger showed that the apparent K_m for the external Cl^- was about 50 mmol/l and the V_{max} was about 0.2 pH units/min. An interesting feature of this anion exchanger is that Na^+ appears to be required for its function since recovery of pH_i from the alkali load was enhanced only when both Cl^- and Na^+ ions were present in the bath solution (Y. Saito et al., unpublished data). It does not seem that the Na^+-H^+ exchanger is tightly coupled to the anion exchanger, however, since amiloride and DIDS had opposite effects on the ph_i of the ACh-treated cells (Saito et al. 1988a). Accordingly, the possibility of $Na^+ - (HCO_3^-)_n/Cl^-$ exchange can be suggested.

Studies on isolated membrane vesicles from rat lacrimal gland (Lambert et al. 1988) showed that the anion exchanger was electroneutral, was inhibited by SITS and furosemide, and had a $K_{0.5}$ for Cl^- of 6–10 mmol/l and an anion selectivity sequence of $SCN^- > NO_3^- > Cl^- > HCO_3^- > SO_4^{2-}$. Roughly 80% of the transporters were associated with the membranes of intracellular organelles, suggesting the presence of cytoplasmic pools of functional antiporters. The physiological role of the anion exchanger may be (1) pH recovery from the alkali load, and (2) Cl^- accumulation into the acinar cells against the electrochemical potential gradient.

Cellular Mechanisms of Lacrimal Secretion: A Model

Direct information on the ion transport processes in the luminal membrane is still very limited. From the above findings, however, we can postulate a mechanism for ion transport from the blood side to the acinar lumen (Fig. 1). The model differs from earlier ones (Marty et al. 1984; Petersen and Maruyama 1984) in that it includes several electroneutral ion transport mechanisms in the basolateral membrane. In particular, in the mouse and rat lacrimal glands, Na^+ influx mediated by $Na^+ - H^+$ exchange seems to be dominant, whereas in the mandibular salivary glands the $Na^+ - K^+ - 2Cl^-$ cotransporter dominates over the exchangers (Pirani et al. 1987).

The major steps of stimulus-secretion coupling can be described as follows. Binding of cholinergic and adrenergic agonists to the receptor sites activates phosphodiesterase followed by hydrolysis of phosphatidylinositol-4,5-bisphosphate to produce inositol-1,4,5-trisphosphate (IP_3) and diacylglycerol (Jones et al. 1979; Berridge 1984; Llano et al. 1987). IP_3 causes Ca^{2+} release from the endoplasmic reticulum (ER) (Streb et al. 1983, 1984; Putney 1986; Morris et al. 1987b). Agonist stimulation also increases Ca^{2+} influx from the extracellular fluid (ECF) (Keryer and Rossignol 1976; Parod and Putney 1978; Botelho and Dartt 1980; Parod et al. 1980) although the mechanism is unclear, via an unidentified, seemingly Na^+-dependent process (Ozawa et al. 1988c) similar to those reported for pancreas (Bayerdörffer et al. 1985) and salivary glands (Gallacher and Morris 1987; Morris et al. 1987). Increased cytosolic Ca^{2+} activates the basolateral K^+ channels allowing K^+ efflux into the basolateral extracellular space, and the Cl^- channels of the apical membrane, allowing Cl^- efflux into the acinar lumen. Stimulation of oxidative metabolism produces volatile and nonvolatile acids in the cytoplasm, and the CO_2 produced hydrates to yield H^+ and HCO_3^- ions (at a rate accelerated by carbonic anhydrease (CA) (Henniger et al. 1983)) and stimulates $Na^+ - H^+$ and $Cl^- - HCO_3^-$ exchangers at the basolateral border. The antiporters, together with the $Na^+ - K^+ - 2Cl^-$ cotransporter allow NaCl influx across the membrane. Increased intracellular Na^+ and extracellular K^+ concentrations activate the $Na^+ - K^+$ pump and cause Na^+ accumulation in the lateral intercellular space. A negative potential in the acinar lumen produced by activation of the apical Cl^- conductance and Na^+ accumulation in the lateral intercellular space causes Na^+ influx into the lumen down its electrochemical potential gradient through the leaky tight junction. Recent analytical and immunohistochemical studies have shown the presence of $Na^+ - K^+$ ATPase in the luminal membrane (Mircheff and Lu 1984; Wood and Mircheff 1986), so it is possible that a part of the intracellular Na^+ enters directly into the acinar lumen mediated by the luminal Na^+-, K^+-ATPase. Increased osmolality in the acinar lumen would cause water influx into the lumen via the paracellular and transcellular routes to produce an isotonic primary lacrimal fluid.

References

Alexander JH, Van Lennep EW, Young JA (1972) Water and electrolyte secretion by the exorbital lacrimal gland of the rat studied by micropuncture and catheterization techniques. Pflügers Arch 337: 229–309

Aronson PS (1984) Electrochemical driving force for secondary active transport: Energetics and kinetics of $Na^+ - H^+$ exchange and Na^+-glucose cotransport. In: Blaustein MP, Lieberman M (eds) Electrogenic transport: fundamental principles and physiological implications. Raven, New York, pp 49–70

Bayerdörffer E, Eckhardt L, Haase W, Schulz I (1985) Electrogenic calcium transport in plasma membrane of rat pancreatic acinar cells. J Membr Biol 84: 45–60

Berridge MJ (1984) Inositol trisphosphate and diacylglycerol as second messengers. Biochem J 220: 345–360

Botelho SY (1964) Tears and the lacrimal gland. Sci Am 211(6): 78–86

Botelho SY, Dartt DA (1980) Effect of calcium antagonism or chelation on rabbit lacrimal gland secretion and membrane potentials. J Physiol (Lond) 304: 397–403

Botelho SY, Fuenmayor N, Hisada M (1978) Flow and potentials during perfusion of lacrimal gland with electrolyte solutions. Am J Physiol 235: C8–C12

Dartt DA, Möller M, Poulsen JH (1981) Lacrimal gland electrolyte and water secretion in the rabbit: localization and role of $(Na^+ + K^+)$-activated ATPase. J Physiol (Lond) 321: 557–569

Dartt DA, Donowitz M, Joshi VJ, Mathiu RS, Sharp WG (1984) Cyclic nucleotide-dependent enzyme secretion in the rat lacrimal gland. J Physiol (Lond) 352: 375–384

Dartt DA, Mircheff AK, Donowitz M, Sharp WG (1988) Ca^{2+}- and cAMP-induced protein phosphorylation in lacrimal gland basolateral membranes. Am J Physiol 254: G541–G551

Dufresne M, Bastie MJ, Vaysse N, Creach Y, Hollande E, Ribet A (1985) The amiloride sensitive Na^+/H^+ antiport in guinea pig pancreatic acini: characterization and stimulation by caerulein. FEBS Lett 187: 126–130

Evans G, Marty A (1986a) Calcium-dependent chloride current in isolated cells from rat lacrimal glands. J Physiol (Lond) 378: 437–460

Evans G, Marty A (1986b) Potentiation of muscarinic and adrenergic responses by an analogue of guanosine 5'triphosphate. Proc Natl Acad Sci USA 83: 4099–4103

Evans G, Marty A, Tan YP, Trautmann A (1986) Blockage of Ca-activated Cl conductance by furosemide in rat lacrimal glands. Pflügers Arch 406: 65–68

Findlay I (1984) A patch-clamp study of potassium channels and whole-cell currents in acinar cells of the mouse lacrimal gland. J Physiol (Lond) 350: 179–195

Findlay I, Petersen OH (1985) Acetylcholine stimulates a Ca^{2+}-dependent Cl^- conductance in mouse lacrimal acinar cells. Pflügers Arch 403: 328–330

Gallacher DV, Morris AP (1987) The receptor-regulated calcium influx in mouse submandibular acinar cells is sodium dependent. J Physiol (Lond) 384: 119–130

Geck P, Heinz E (1986) The $Na^+ - K^+ - 2Cl^-$ cotransport system. J Membr Biol 91: 97–105

Grinstein S, Rothstein A (1986) Mechanism of regulation of the Na^+/H^+ exchanger. J Membr Biol 90: 1–12

Hellmessen W, Christian AL, Fasold H, Schulz I (1985) Coupled $Na^+ - H^+$ exchange in isolated acinar cells from rat exocrine pancreas. Am J Physiol 249: G125–G136

Henniger RA, Schulte BA, Spicer SS (1983) Immunolocalization of carbonic anhydrase isozymes in rat and mouse salivary and exorbital lacrimal glands. Anat Rec 207: 605–614

Iwatsuki N, Petersen OH (1978a) Membrane potential, resistance, and intracellular communication in the lacrimal gland: effects of acetylcholine and adrenaline. J Physiol (Lond) 275: 507–520

Iwatsuki N, Petersen OH (1978b) Intracellular Ca^{2+} injection causes membrane hyperpolarization and conductance increase in lacrimal acinar cells. Pflügers Arch 377: 185–187

Jahn R, Söling HD (1981) Protein phosphorylation during secretion in the rat lacrimal gland. A general role of EC-protein in stimulus-secretion coupling in exocrine organs? FEBS Lett 131: 28–30

Jahn R, Söling HD (1983) Phosphorylation of the ribosomal protein S6 in response to secretagogues in the guinea pig exocrine pancreas, parotid and lacrimal gland. FEBS Lett 153: 71–76

Jones LM, Cockcroft S, Michell RH (1979) Stimulation of phosphatidylinositol turnover in various tissues by cholinergic and adrenergic agonists, by histamine and by caerulein. Biochem J 182: 669–676

Keryer G, Rossignol B (1976) Effect of carbachol on ^{45}Ca uptake and protein secretion in rat lacrimal glands. Am J Physiol 230: 99–104

Kikkawa T (1970) Secretory potentials in the lacrimal gland of the rabbit. Jpn J Ophthalmol 14: 247–262

Lambert RW, Bradley ME, Mircheff AK (1988) $Cl^- - HCO_3^-$ antiport in rat lacrimal gland. Am J Physiol 255: G367–G373

Llano I, Marty A, Tanguy J (1987) Dependence of intracellular effects of GTPγS and inositoltrisphosphate on cell membrane potential and on external Ca ions. Pflügers Arch 409: 499–506

Marty A, Tan YP, Trautmann A (1984) Three types of calcium-dependent channel in rat lacrimal glands. J Physiol (Lond) 357: 293–325

Mauduit P, Herman G, Rossignol B (1983) Effect of trifluoperazine on ^3H-labeled protein secretion induced by pentoxifylline, cholinergic or adrenergic agonists in rat lacrimal gland. A possible role of calmodulin? FEBS Lett 152: 207–211

Mircheff AK, Lu CC (1984) A map of membrane population isolated from rat exorbital gland. Am J Physiol 247: G651–G661

Mircheff AK, Ingham CE, Lambert RW, Hales KL, Hensley CB, Yiu SC (1987) Na^+/H^+ antiporter in lacrimal acinar cell basal-lateral membranes. Invest Ophthalmol Vis Sci 28: 1726–1729

Morris AP, Fuller CM, Gallacher DV (1987a) Cholinergic receptor regulates a voltage insensitive but Na^+-dependent calcium influx pathway in salivary acinar cells. FEBS Lett 211: 195–199

Morris AP, Gallacher DV, Irvine RF, Petersen OH (1987b) Synergism of ins(1,4,5)P$_3$ with ins(1,3,4,5)P$_4$ in activating Ca^{2+}-dependent K^+ channels. Nature 330: 653–655

Ozawa T, Saito Y, Nishiyama A (1988a) Mechanism of uphill chloride transport of the mouse lacrimal acinar cells: studies with Cl^- sensitive microelectrode. Pflügers Arch 412: 509–515

Ozawa T, Saito Y, Nishiyama A (1988b) Evidence for an anion exchanger in the mouse lacrimal gland acinar cell membrane. J Membr Biol 105: 273–280

Ozawa T, Takahashi H, Saito Y, Nishiyama A (1988c) Effect of cholinergic stimulation on intracellular Ca^{2+} concentration of the lacrimal gland acinar cells. In: Wong PYD, Young JA (eds) Exocrine secretion. Hong Kong University Press, Hong Kong, pp 137–139

Parod RJ, Putney JW (1978) The role of calcium in the receptor mediated control of potassium permeability in the rat lacrimal gland. J Physiol (Lond) 281: 371–381

Parod RJ, Putney JW (1980) Stimulus-permeability coupling in rat lacrimal gland. Am J Physiol 239: G106–G113

Parod RJ, Leslie BA, Putney JW (1980) Muscarinic and α-adrenergic stimulation of Na and Ca uptake by dispersed lacrimal cells. Am J Physiol 239: G99–G105

Petersen OH (1980) The electrophysiology of gland cells. Academic, London

Petersen OH, Maruyama Y (1984) Calcium-activated potassium channels and their role in secretion. Nature 307: 693–696

Pirani D, Evans LAR, Cook DI, Young JA (1987) Intracellular pH in the rat mandibular salivary gland: the role of $Na - H$ and $Cl - HCO_3$ antiports in secretion. Pflügers Arch 408: 178–184

Putney JW (1979) Stimulus-permeability coupling: role of calcium in the receptor regulation of membrane permeability. Pharmacol Rev 30: 209–245

Putney JW (1986) A model for receptor-regulated calcium entry. Cell Calcium 7: 1–12

Saito Y, Ozawa T, Hayashi H, Nishiyama A (1985) Acetylcholine-induced change in intracellular Cl^- activity of the mouse lacrimal acinar cells. Pflügers Arch 405: 108–111

Saito Y, Ozawa T, Hayashi H, Nishiyama A (1987a) The effect of acetylcholine on chloride transport across the mouse lacrimal gland acinar cell membrane. Pflügers Arch 409: 280–288

Saito Y, Ozawa T, Nishiyama A (1987b) Acetylcholine-induced Na^+ influx in the mouse lacrimal gland acinar cells. Demonstration of multiple Na^+ transport mechanisms by intracellular Na^+ activity measurements. J Membr Biol 98: 135–144

Saito Y, Ozawa T, Suzuki S, Nishiyama A (1988a) Intracellular pH regulation in the mouse lacrimal gland acinar cells. J Membr Biol 101: 73–81

Saito Y, Ozawa T, Nishiyama A (1988b) $Na^+ - H^+$ and $Cl^- - HCO_3^-$ antiporters in the mouse lacrimal gland acinar cells. In: Wong PYD, Young JA (eds) Exocrine secretion, Hong Kong University Press, Hong Kong, pp 161–163

Streb H, Irvine RF, Berridge MJ, Schulz I (1983) Release of Ca^{2+} from a nonmitochondrial intracellular store in pancreatic acinar cells by inositol-1,4,5-trisphosphate. Nature 306: 67–69

Streb H, Bayerdörffer E, Haase W, Irvine RF, Schulz I (1984) Effect of inositol-1,4,5-trisphosphate on isolated subcellular fractions of rat pancreas. J Membr Biol 81: 241–253

Suzuki K, Petersen OH (1985) The effect of Na^+ and Cl^- removal and of loop diuretics on acetylcholine-evoked membrane potential changes in mouse lacrimal acinar cells. Q J Exp Physiol 70: 437–445

Trautmann A, Marty A (1984) Activation of Ca-dependent K channels by carbamylcholine in rat lacrimal glands. Proc Natl Acad Sci USA 81: 611–615

Wood RL, Mircheff AK (1986) Apical and basal-lateral Na/K-ATPase in rat lacrimal gland acinar cells. Invest Ophthalmol Vis Sci 27: 1293–1296

3 Exocrine Pancreas

Electrolyte Transport in Pancreatic Ducts*

I. Novak

Exocrine secretion in the pancreas is regulated by two hormones, secretin and cholecystokinin-pancreozymin (CCK). CCK stimulates release of pancreatic enzymes and a fluid that is quite similar to plasma in its ionic composition. Secretin, on the other hand, stimulates secretion of fluid that is isotonic with plasma, but quite different in ionic composition. The most striking difference is in the bicarbonate and chloride concentrations, which also change with the secretory rate (Fig. 1). At low secretory rates, HCO_3^- and Cl^- concentrations are plasma-like, but at high secretory rates the HCO_3^- concentration rises to approach a plateau of 120-140 mmol/l (in cat, dog and human) and 80 mmol/l (in rat). Simultaneously, the Cl^- concentration falls to 20-50 mmol/l, depending on the species. The concentrations of Na^+ and K^+ do not change with secretory rate and remain plasma-like in most species (see Novak 1988).

Various theories have been put forward to account for the origin of pancreatic secretion, in particular its anionic composition. Dreiling and Janowitz (1959) postulated in their "exchange theory" that the primary secretion is rich in HCO_3^-, and that subsequently, as the fluid passes through the ductal system, it is modified by exchange of HCO_3^- for Cl^-. In the "unicellular theory", Rothman and Brooks (1965) proposed that Cl^- and HCO_3^- secretion occur in the same cell since they observed interdependence between Cl^- and HCO_3^- outputs. In the "admixture theory", originally proposed by Lim et al. (1936) and elaborated by others (see Novak 1988), it is postulated that pancreatic juice is a mixture of two components – one high in enzymes and Cl^-, originating in acini, the other high in HCO_3^-, originating in ducts. Evidence from micropuncture and other studies on intact glands supports the admixture theory and points to the small interlobular ducts as the site of HCO_3^- secretion (see Novak 1988).

---

* Parts of the author's work quoted in this review were supported by Alexander von Humboldt Foundation and the Medical Foundation, University of Sydney.

Young · Wong, Epithelial Secretion of Water and Electrolytes
© Springer-Verlag Berlin · Heidelberg 1990

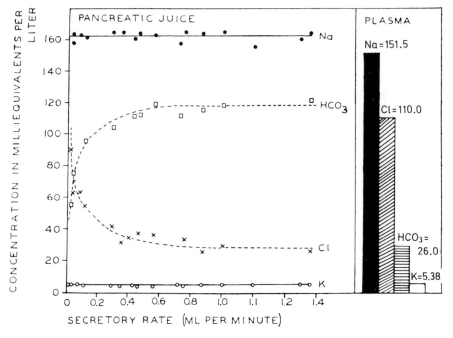

Fig. 1. Relation between the rate of secretin-stimulated secretion and the concentration of Na^+, K^+, Cl^- and HCO_3^- in the pancreatic juice of the dog (from Bro-Rasmussen et al. 1956)

Until recently, the main source of information about electrolyte transport in pancreatic ducts was derived from in vivo and in vitro studies of intact glands, which are composed of acini (80%), ducts ($< 5\%$) and endocrine cells (2%) (Bolender 1974). Several transport models have been derived from these studies (De Pont et al. 1982; Kuijpers et al. 1984; Swanson and Solomon 1975; Schulz 1971), but in order to test the models it is essential to have direct access to the basolateral and luminal membranes of the epithelium and to know the electrochemical gradients across the epithelium and cell membranes. Only a handful of electrophysiological studies on intact glands has been published (see Novak 1988). The transepithelial potential of free-flowing inter- and intralobular ducts has been reported to lie between -2 and $-9\,mV$ (lumen negative), although most measurements reported have not been corrected for liquid junction and diffusion potentials (Schulz et al. 1969; Swanson and Solomon 1975; see Novak 1988). Secretin has been shown to increase the luminal negativity, but only in the main duct (Way and Diamond 1970), which is not involved in secretion (Swanson and Solomon 1973). In microelectrode studies a relatively low cell potential of -20 to $-40\,mV$ has been recorded (Swanson and Solomon 1975; Greenwell 1975) which hyperpolarized on stimulation (Greenwell 1975). Contrary to

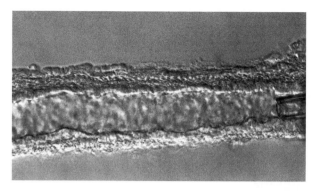

Fig. 2. An interlobular duct isolated from the rat pancreas and perfused in vitro. Part of the perfusion pipette is seen at the *right* side of the picture. The inside diameter of the duct is about 30 μm

this finding, the cell potential measured with a potential-sensitive dye depolarized from -80 to -70 mV on stimulation (Schulz 1980).

Recently, new efforts have been made to isolate pancreatic duct epithelium by tissue culture (Harris and Coleman 1987), separation of ducts from tissue digests of whole pancreas (Stuenkel et al. 1988) and separation of ductal tissue from pancreases in which acinar atrophy had been induced with a copper-deficient diet (Argent et al. 1986). Our method for isolation of intra- and interlobular pancreatic ducts is to dissect them from fresh, untreated rat pancreas and to microperfuse them in vitro (Fig. 2; Novak and Greger 1988a). With direct access to both sides of the epithelium and application of electrophysiological techniques, we were able to define the conductive and nonconductive properties of the basolateral and luminal membranes. From data obtained in such studies a new model for ductal electrolyte transport has been proposed (Fig. 5; Novak and Greger 1988b). Evidence for the model is summarized below, and is related to what is known about electrolyte secretion in intact glands.

Cellular Mechanism of Electrolyte Transport in Small Pancreatic Ducts

Basic Electrophysiological Properties

The epithelium of small inter- and intralobular pancreatic ducts, which are capable of iso-osmotic salt and water transport, can be classified as "leaky", i.e. the resistance of the paracellular route is far less than the combined resistances of the basolateral and luminal membranes (Novak and Greger 1988a, 1989). The specific transepithelial resistance (R_{te}) is between 80-90

$\Omega\,cm^2$. The epithelium is capable of developing a small transepithelial potential (PD_{te}) of about $-1\,mV$ (lumen negative) in the absence of exogenous agonists, when the transport systems are operating at a basal level. Upon stimulation, PD_{te} increases up to $-5\,mV$ (Novak and Greger 1988b, 1989). The resting cellmembrane potential measured across the basolateral membrane of duct cells (PD_{bl}) is $-63\,mV$, and it responds to various experimental manipulations in the bath or luminal perfusate (see below).

The Basolateral Membrane

Na^+-, K^+-ATPase

In most epithelia the prime driving force for salt and water transport is the Na^+-, K^+-ATPase. The requirement of Na^+ and K^+ for pancreatic secretion suggested that the Na^+-, K^+-ATPase also plays a role in HCO_3^- secretion (see Novak 1988). Indeed, histochemical studies in the cat and rat pancreas have shown that the small interlobular and intralobular ducts have the highest densities of the pump (Bundgaard et al. 1981; Madden and Sarras 1987). Correspondingly, ouabain was also found to be a potent inhibitor of secretin-stimulated secretion in the cat and rabbit pancreas (Case and Scratcherd 1974; Kuijpers et al. 1984; Swanson and Solomon 1975). In the rat pancreas, however, even high doses of the inhibitor had a slow and incomplete effect on secretin-evoked secretion, and consequently the role of the pump current in ductal transport has been questioned (Evans et al. 1986). Hence, we have reinvestigated whether the inhibitor had an effect in isolated perfused rat ducts. Ouabain (3 mmol/l) in a bath solution with a low K^+ concentration (in order to increase the pump sensitivity to the inhibitor) had a biphasic effect on PD_{bl} of duct cells (Novak and Greger 1988a). In the first phase PD_{bl} depolarized instantaneously by $5\,mV$, indicating that the pump current was inhibited. This event was followed by a slower depolarization due to a running down of ion gradients after the Na^+-, K^+-ATPase inhibition.

K^+ Channels

Basolateral K^+ channels have been well described in many secretory epithelia. In salivary glands the opening of K^+ channels on stimulation explains the long-standing observation of K^+ transients, i.e. increase in K^+ concentration in venous effluent shortly after stimulation (Petersen and Maruyama 1984). In pancreas no such transients have been observed, and the K^+ concentration in pancreatic juice is plasma-like in most species, except for the rat (Sewell and Young 1975). Perhaps this was the reason why no K^+ channels were postulated in any of the models for pancreatic duct

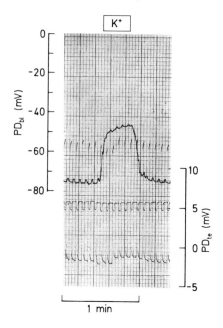

Fig. 3. The effect of an increase in bath K^+ concentration (from 5 to 20 mmol/l) on the basolateral membrane potential (PD_{bl}) of a pancreatic duct cell. PD_{te}, transepithelial potential of pancreatic duct

secretion. In fact, the intact rat pancreas stimulated with secretin was found to be insensitive to K^+ channel blockers (Evans et al. 1986). Yet clearly secretion is dependent on extracellular K^+ (Case and Scratcherd 1974), and since the ducts have the Na^+-, K^+-ATPase, it is clear that accumulated K^+ must leave the cell by some mechanism.

In the isolated perfused duct, a K^+ conductance on the basolateral membrane of duct cells has been clearly demonstrated (Fig. 3). It is inhibited by Ba^{2+} (1 mmol/l), but not by tetraethylammonium (TEA^+; 50 mmol/l) (Novak and Greger 1988a), and there is an indication that this conductance is sensitive to intracellular pH (Novak and Greger 1988a, 1989). The exact nature of this K^+ channel will need to be determined by patch-clamp studies on these ducts.

In tissue-cultured ducts obtained from copper-deficient rats, Argent and coworkers (1987a) applied the patch-clamp technique to study ion channels. They reported a large-conductance K^+ channel in inside-out patches (236 pS in 150 mM KCl). High Ca^{2+} concentrations on the internal surface increased the frequency of opening of this channel, but in the micromolar Ca^{2+} concentration range the channel remained largely closed and its open probability was increased by membrane depolarization. In these ducts the channel is rarely observed in the cell-attached configuration.

Na^+—H^+ Antiport

The Na^+-, K^+-ATPase creates a Na^+ gradient across the cell membrane that drives the Na^+-dependent transport of another ion or substrate. In pancreatic ducts, one simple solution to achieve HCO_3^- transport would be to couple the entry of Na^+ to the entry of HCO_3^- ion directly in a process that would be somewhat analogous to the SITS-sensitive $Na^+ - 2(3)HCO_3^-$ carrier that was first described in renal proximal tubules of amphibia (Boron and Boulpaep 1983). In rat pancreatic ducts, however, there is no evidence for such a transport system. PD_{bl} depolarized only upon addition of HCO_3^-/CO_2 or CO_2, but not when HCO_3^- alone was added to the bath as one would predict, for example, for a $2Na^+ - HCO_3^-$ carrier. This deloparization was not acutely dependent on bath Na^+, nor was it inhibited by addition of SITS to the bath (Novak and Greger 1988a).

Another way to achieve HCO_3^- transport would be to couple Na^+ influx to H^+ efflux. Such a $Na^+ - H^+$ antiport, located on the basolateral membrane, was included in many models (Swanson and Solomon 1975; De Pont et al. 1982; Scratcherd et al. 1981). Evidence for the antiport was based on the observation that lipid-soluble weak acids (substituted for HCO_3^-) were able to support up to 40% of pancreatic secretion. The use of amiloride as a $Na^+ - H^+$ exchange inhibitor, however, was not very successful. Amiloride had no effect on secretion of the in vitro rabbit pancreas (Kuijpers et al. 1984), or on the in vivo pig pancreas (Grotmol et al. 1986b). In the cat pancreas, 2-4 mmol/l amiloride inhibited up to 45% secretion, but since it also inhibited 25% of the Na^+-, K^+-ATPase activity in isolated membranes, it was concluded that the action of the blocker was nonspecific (Wizemann and Schulz 1973).

Some investigators have proposed other transport systems as alternative explanations for HCO_3^- transport. Grotmol and coworkers (1986a) postulated a basolateral proton pump on the basis of observations made on the in vivo pig pancreas that pancreatic HCO_3^- secretion was inhibited by decreased plasma pH and a nonspecific pump inhibitor, NN'-dicyclohexylcarboiimidine (DCCD). Kuijpers and coworkers (1984) proposed another transport system for the rabbit pancreas, a complex Na^+-H^+-Cl^--HCO_3^- carrier, which would bring Na^+ and HCO_3^- into the cell, and Cl^- and H^+ into interstitium. Such a carrier was described as furosemide and SITS sensitive, but not amiloride sensitive. Studies of perfused rat pancreatic ducts indicate that the presence of such a carrier is unlikely in this tissue. First, ducts were not affected by furosemide or SITS added to the bath (Novak and Greger 1988a). Second, there was no change in PD_{bl} when HCO_3^- (without CO_2) was added to the bath. With addition of HCO_3^-, for example, one would expect hyperpolarization of PD_{bl} if such a complex carrier were present on the basolateral membrane of pancreatic duct cells (Novak and Greger 1988a). Influx of HCO_3^- would increase the cell pH, which in turn would increase the K^+ conductance, and thus hyperpolarize the cell membrane. At the same time, operation of the carrier would lead to depletion of cell Cl^-, resulting in a decrease of Cl^- conductance, which duct cells do show (see below), and this would also hyperpolarize the cell membrane.

Reexamining the proposal of the basolateral Na^+-H^+ antiport, we tested the rat pancreatic ducts for sensitivity to amiloride (1 mmol/l) and the amiloride derivative EIPA (5-ethyl-isopropyl-6-bromoamiloride; 0.1 mmol/l). Both inhibitors had a clear effect on duct cell PD_{bl}, which depolarized by 5 and 10 mV, respectively (Novak and Greger 1988a and c, 1989). The most plausible explanation for the effect of these inhibitors is that they cause a fall in intracellular pH, which in turn reduces the basolateral K^+ conductance and thus depolarizes the cell. Further evidence for the antiport has been provided by recent findings of Stuenkel et al. (1988) who measured intracellular pH using 2',7'-bis(carboxyethyl)-5(6)-carboxyfluorescein (BCCF) in a suspension of duct fragments. Removal of extracellular Na^+ acidified duct cells (from pH 7.4 to 6.4), and amiloride (1 mmol/l, prevented the Na^+-dependent pH recovery.

The Luminal Membrane

Ductal HCO_3^- transport depends on provision of CO_2, which is mainly derived from plasma or bath perfusate CO_2, although some may also be provided endogenously by cell metabolism. Within the cell, CO_2 is hydrated by carbonic anhydrase, which is abundant in pancreatic ducts (see Schulz 1987), to liberate H^+ and HCO_3^-. H^+ leaves the cell via the basolateral $Na^+ - H^+$ antiport, and HCO_3^- is secreted into the lumen. In the past, the transport step of HCO_3^- across the luminal membrane represented perhaps the most speculative part of the cellular mechanism of pancreatic HCO_3^- secretion. In several previous models arising from studies on intact glands it has been suggested that HCO_3^- moves across the luminal membrane via a HCO_3^- channel (De Pont et al. 1982; Kuijpers et al. 1984; Scratcherd et al. 1981), a Cl^--HCO_3^- antiport (Scratcherd et al. 1981), or as CO_2 which is then hydrated in the lumen to form HCO_3^- and H^+, after which the proton is pumped into the cell by a proton pump (Schulz 1971; Swanson and Solomon 1975).

Cl^- Channels

In recent years Cl^- channel blockers have been used to characterize conductive properties of Cl^- transporting as well as HCO_3^- transporting epithelia. Two of these blockers, originally developed for the thick ascending limb of Henle's loop (Wangemann et al. 1986), 5-nitro-2-(3-phenylpropylamino)-benzoate (NPPB) and 3',5'-dichlorodiphenylamine-2-carboxylate (DCl-DPC) were tested on isolated perfused ducts. Luminal infusion of the inhibitors (10^{-5} mol/l) produced 8-10 mV hyperpolarization of PD_{bl} (Fig. 4) and about a 60% increase in the fractional resistance of the luminal membrane (Novak and Greger 1988b). Both changes in the membrane potential and resistance are consistent with inhibition of a luminal Cl^- conductance. In order to verify that there is a Cl^- conductance in the luminal membrane, the electromotive force (EMF) for Cl^- was

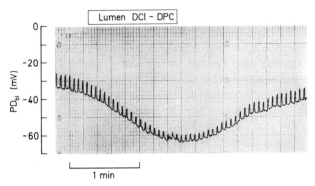

Fig. 4. The effect of a luminally applied Cl^- channel blocker, DCl-DPC (10^{-5} mol/l), on the basolateral membrane potential (PD_{bl}) of a pancreatic duct cell. A change in the height of the current-induced voltage deflections indicates an increase in the fractional resistance of the luminal membrane

increased by lowering the luminal concentration of Cl^- from 150 to 30 mmol/l. Such a maneouvre depolarized PD_{bl} by about 10 mV, indicating that indeed there is a Cl^- conductance on the luminal membrane (Novak and Greger 1988c, 1989).

Our conclusion is strengthened by a report of Argent and coworkers (Argent et al. 1987b, Gray et al. 1988) who demonstrated anion channels in rat pancreatic ducts in patch-clamp studies. They describe large-conductance anion channels (415 pS in 150 mmol/l Cl^-) in inside-out patches derived both from luminal and basolateral membranes, but the function of these is unclear (Argent et al. 1987b). Such an anion conductance was not detected in the basolateral membrane of perfused rat pancreatic ducts, where a change in bath Cl^- concentration or addition of Cl^- channels blockers had no effect (Novak and Greger 1988b). The small-conductance anion channels (4.5 pS in 150 mmol/l Cl^- solution) detected in cell-attached patches appear more relevant, as the addition of 10 nmol/l secretin to the bath increased their open state probability (Gray et al. 1988).

Considering that the pancreatic duct cells have luminal Cl^- channels, and the pancreatic ducts secrete HCO_3^-, the obvious question is how HCO_3^- enters the lumen. One solution would be if the Cl^- channel was also permeable to HCO_3^-. Although no selectivity sequence for pancreatic duct cells is known yet, in epithelial Cl^- channels studied so far, P_{Cl^-} (permeability for Cl^-) has been at least 2.5 times higher than $P_{HCO_3^-}$ (Reinhardt et al. 1987; Bormann et al. 1987). Hence, for HCO_3^- to take this route in the presence of Cl^-, intracellular HCO_3^- would have to be at least 2.5 times higher than Cl^-, so that the intracellular pH would be in the order of 7.7–8.0, and/or cellular Cl^- would have to be kept below equilibrium by an active extrusion mechanism. Neither of these solutions appears likely, and our finding that the initial event of cyclic AMP-mediated secretion is HCO_3^- independent, but involves Cl^- channels (Novak and Greger 1988b), speaks in favour of an important role of Cl^- channels in pancreatic ductal secretion.

$Cl^-–HCO_3^-$ Antiport

One of the simplest ways to achieve HCO_3^- secretion that we have proposed is to incorporate a $Cl^-–HCO_3^-$ antiport in the luminal membrane in parallel with the Cl^- channels (Novak and Greger 1987, 1988b). This hypothesis has been tested in perfused ducts by using SITS as an antiport inhibitor. Luminally applied SITS (0.1 mmol/l) hyperpolarized PD_{bl} by 8 mV (Novak and Greger 1988b). It is postulated that blocking of the exchange would cause a fall in intracellular Cl^- and a consequential decrease in the Cl^- conductance. Simultaneously, there would also be a rise in cell pH, which could increase the basolateral K^+ conductance. Either or both of these changes would lead to membrane hyperpolarization, as we indeed observed.

Our proposal for the luminal $Cl^-–HCO_3^-$ antiport has recently been supported by the findings of Stuenkel et al. (1988). Removal of extracellular Cl^- from a duct suspension in a HCO_3^--containing medium increased the cell pH, and this was reversed by restitution of Cl^-. DIDS prevented both the Cl^--free induced increase in cell pH and also pH recovery after addition of Cl^-. Although Stuenkel et al. (1988) cannot conclude in which membrane the exchanger lies, our results on perfused ducts show that SITS acts only from the luminal, not the basolateral side (Novak and Greger 1988a, b). Hence, the location of the exchanger must be luminal.

Effect of Stimulation

Although there is good evidence that secretin acts via cyclic AMP to evoke pancreatic HCO_3^- secretion (Argent et al. 1986; Schulz 1980), the cellular mechanism of cyclic AMP action has been rather speculative (see Schulz 1987). We have tested both dibutyryl cyclic AMP (db-cAMP) and secretin on isolated perfused ducts and found them to have very similar effects, except for the time course of their actions, i.e. secretin activated faster than db-cAMP, but it took longer for the duct to come to a resting level after secretin removal (Novak and Greger 1988b, 1989). Upon stimulation, PD_{te} increased from the resting level of -1 mV (lumen negative with respect to bath) to a stimulated level of up to -5 mV. The most dramatic effect was observed on the cell potential: PD_{bl} depolarized by 26 mV (i.e. from -62 to -36 mV). Simultaneously, R_{te} decreased by about 10%, and the fractional resistance of the luminal membrane decreased dramatically. Clearly, the primary event on stimulation was opening of an anion conductance on the luminal membrane. This is most likely to have been the Cl^- channel since there is a pronounced Cl^- conductance during stimulation (Novak and Greger 1989), since the Cl^- channels blockers are effective in duct cells (Novak and Greger 1988b), and since the onset of membrane depolarization is independent of extracellular HCO_3^-/CO_2 (Novak and Greger 1988b). In several epithelia, e.g. shark rectal gland, trachea, nasal epithelium (cf. Greger and Kunzelmann 1989), the primary step in cyclic AMP-mediated secretion is also the opening of Cl^- channels. Yet there are other epithelia, e.g. salivary and lacrimal glands, in which secretion is mediated via a Ca^{2+} transduction pathway and involves regulation of K^+ channels (Petersen and Maruyama 1984) or both K^+ and Cl^- channels (Cook et al. 1988). In pancreatic ducts opening of K^+ channels cannot be the initiating step in cyclic AMP-induced secretion since we would have observed hyperpolarization, not depolarization of PD_{bl}. Nevertheless, opening of basolateral K^+ channels is important in transporting pancreatic ducts, e.g. inhibition of K^+ exit with Ba^{2+} abolishes secretin or db-cAMP induced increases in PD_{te} and it increases R_{te} (Novak and Greger 1989). In fact, during stimulation the increase in the luminal Cl^- conductance and ensuing depolarization would increase the driving force for K^+ exit across the basolateral membrane. It seems, however, that the depolarization alone cannot keep the K^+ channel opened and some other regulatory mechanism is involved (Novak and Greger 1988b, 1989).

The results of our studies have led us to propose a new model for pancreatic HCO_3^- secretion (Fig. 5; Novak and Greger 1988b). Our data verify that the basolateral membrane contains the Na^+-, K^+-ATPase and provide more solid evidence for the basolateral Na^+-H^+ exchanger. In this respect the new working model agrees with earlier proposed models obtained on intact glands (De Pont et al. 1982; Kuijpers et al. 1984; Swanson

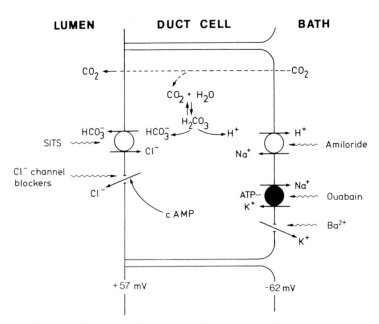

Fig. 5. The cellular model of electrolyte transport in the small pancreatic ducts as established from electrophysiological studies of isolated perfused rat pancreatic ducts (from Novak and Greger 1988b)

and Solomon 1975). Results from the perfused duct preparation, however, demonstrate that the basolateral membrane contains a K^+ conductance and that the luminal membrane contains a Cl^- conductance and a $Cl^- - HCO_3^-$ antiport. The key event during stimulation is the opening of Cl^- channels via a cyclic AMP-activated pathway, which leads to Cl^- efflux from the cell into the duct lumen down an electrochemical gradient. Subsequently Cl^- reenters the cell in exchange for HCO_3^-, as determined by chemical gradients. Thus Cl^- is recirculated across the luminal membrane, and there is a resulting net secretion of HCO_3^- into the duct lumen. Protons left in the cell are extruded by the $Na^+ - H^+$ exchanger, for which the Na^+-, K^+-ATPase provides the Na^+ gradient, and the basolateral K^+ channels allow recirculation of K^+. The transcellular current from lumen to interstitium is thus carried by a net rheogenic exit step for HCO_3^- on the luminal membrane, by K^+ ions crossing the basolateral K^+ channels, and by the excess number of Na^+ ions pumped by the electrogenic Na^+-, K^+-ATPase. Increase in the lumen negativity creates a favourable gradient for passive entry of cations, but as yet it is not known how cations reach the lumen of secreting ducts. The only published studies of transepithelial ductal diffusion potentials have been carried out on the main duct, which shows negligible selectivity for cations ($P_{Li^+} : P_{Na^+} : P_{K^+} : P_{Rb^+} : P_{Cs^+} = 1.08 : 1.00 : 1.10 : 1.09 : 1.12$) in contrast to definite selectivity for anions ($P_{F^-} : P_{Br^-} : P_{Cl^-} : P_{I^-} : P_{HCO_3^-}$ $= 0.44 : 1.38 : 1.08 : 2.05 : 0.60$) (Greenwell 1977). Since rat pancreatic juice has K^+ concentrations higher than in plasma, it is tempting to postulate that some K^+ can be secreted transcellularly. However, no K^+ conductance was found on the luminal membrane (Novak and Greger 1988c, 1989). It thus seems most likely that following an increase in PD_{te} (lumen negative), K^+, and more importantly, Na^+ reach the lumen paracellularly, with water following iso-osmotically.

In order to verify the model, measurements of intracellular Cl^- and pH in resting and stimulated ducts are required. Furthermore, it will be important to establish whether and how K^+ channels, and possibly $Na^+ - H^+$ and $Cl^- - HCO_3^-$ antiports, are regulated. Nevertheless, we can make several predictions. For the model to work, Cl^- should be above equilibrium. Since there is no $Na^+ - K^+ - 2Cl^-$ symport to bring Cl^- into the cell (Novak and Greger 1988a), one way to do so would be via the $Cl^- - HCO_3^-$ antiport. Consequently, for ductal HCO_3^- secretion to take place, there needs to be a steady supply of luminal Cl^-, and of course of intracellular HCO_3^-. In the case of Cl^-, this would be no problem in the experimental situation in perfused ducts since the lumen is perfused with Cl^--rich solutions. It may also be no problem in vivo since the Cl^--rich fluid required for ductal transport could be provided by the acini. Secretin, apart from stimulating ducts, may also act on acini, which have secretin receptors, and we know that at least enzyme secretion is induced by the hormone (Kimura et al. 1987; Schulz 1980; Trimble et al. 1987). It is quite possible that secretin also stimulates Cl^- secretion in acini. In the case of intracellular HCO_3^-, provision of extracellular HCO_3^-/CO_2 is needed to keep the transport running (Novak and Greger 1988b), and we expect the intracellular HCO_3^- to be above equilibrium across the luminal membrane. Whether the Na^+-H^+ antiport or the $Cl^--HCO_3^-$ antiport is stimulated via a cyclic AMP-dependent pathway remains to be established.

Although there are still many questions unanswered, the model explains the long-standing observations that pancreatic HCO_3^- secretion is dependent on the presence of Cl^-, and is sensitive to Cl^- transport inhibitors such as SITS and furosemide (in high doses), which probably act luminally (see Novak 1988). Involvement of Cl^- in HCO_3^- secretion, and the idea that some Cl^- might come from acini to be exchanged with HCO_3^- by ducts leads us to reassess the unicellular theory of pancreatic juice formation (see above). Nevertheless, small pancreatic ducts are responsible for the production of a HCO_3^--rich, Cl^--poor fluid which is then modified in the large ducts by exchange of luminal HCO_3^- for plasma Cl^-, a process which is most apparent at low secretory rates (Fig. 1). It remains to be clarified what the cellular mechanism of Cl^- and HCO_3^- transport in larger ducts is, and how this differs from the smaller secreting ducts.

References

Argent BE, Arkle S, Cullen MJ, Green R (1986) Morphological, biochemical and secretory studies on rat pancreatic ducts maintained in tissue culture. Q J Exp Physiol 71: 633–648

Argent BE, Arkle S, Gray MA, Greenwell JR (1987a) Two types of calcium-sensitive cation channels in isolated rat pancreatic duct cells. J Physiol (Lond) 386: 82 P

Argent BE, Gray MA, Greenwell JR (1987b) Characteristics of a large conductance anion channel in membrane patches excised from rat pancreatic duct cells in vitro. J Physiol (Lond) 394: 146 P

Bolender RP (1974) Stereological analysis of the guinea pig pancreas. Analytical model and quantitative description on nonstimulated pancreatic cells. J Cell Biol 61: 269–287

Bormann J, Hamill OP, Sakmann B (1987) Mechanism of anion permeation through channels gated by glycine and γ-aminobutyric acid in mouse cultured spinal neurones. J Physiol (Lond) 385: 243–286

Boron WF, Boulpaep EL (1983) Intracellular pH regulation in the renal proximal tubule of the salamander. Basolateral HCO_3^- transport. J Gen Physiol 81: 53–94

Bro-Rasmussen F, Killmann SA, Thaysen JH (1956) The composition of pancreatic juice as compared to sweat, parotid saliva and tears. Acta Physiol Scand 37: 97–113

Bundgaard M, Møller M, Poulsen JH (1981) Localization of sodium pumps in cat pancreas. J Physiol (Lond) 313: 405–414

Case RM, Scratcherd T (1974) The secretion of alkali metal ions by the perfused cat pancreas as influenced by the composition and osmolality of the external environment and by inhibitors of metabolism and Na^+,K^+-ATPase activity. J Physiol (Lond) 242: 415–428

Cook DI, Day ML, Champion MP, Young JA (1988) Ca^{2+} not cyclic AMP mediates the fluid secretory response to isoproterenol in the rat mandibular salivary gland: whole-cell patch-clamp studies. Pflügers Arch 413: 67–76

De Pont JJHHM, Jansen JWCM, Kuijpers GAJ, Bonting SL (1982) A model for pancreatic fluid secretion. In: Case RM, Garner A, Turnberg LA, Young JA (eds) Electrolyte and water transport across gastrointestinal epithelia. Raven, New York, pp 11–20

Dreiling DA, Janowitz D (1959) The secretion of electrolytes by the human pancreas. Am J Dig Dis 4: 137–144

Evans LAR, Pirani D, Cook DI, Young JA (1986) Intraepithelial current flow in rat pancreatic secretory epithelia. Pflügers Arch 407: S107–S111

Gray MA, Greenwell JR, Argent BE (1988) Secretin-regulated chloride channel on the apical plasma membrane of pancreatic duct cells. J Membr Biol 105: 131–142

Greenwell JR (1975) The effects of cholecystokinin-pancreozymin, acetylcholine and secretin on the membrane potentials of mouse pancreatic cells in vitro. Pflügers Arch 353: 159–170

Greenwell JR (1977) The selective permeability of the pancreatic duct of the cat to monovalent ions. Pflügers Arch 367: 265–27

Greger R, Kunzelmann K (1989) Epithelial chloride channels. In: Young JA, Wong P (eds) Epithelial secretion of water and electrolytes. Springer, Berlin Heidelberg New York, pp 3–13

Grotmol T, Buanes T, Raeder MG (1986a) NN'-dicyclohexylcarboiimidine (DCCD) reduces pancreatic $NaHCO_3$ secretion without changing pancreatic tissue ATP levels. Acta Physiol Scand 128: 547–554

Grotmol T, Buanes T, Brøs O, Raeder MG (1986b) Lack of effect of amiloride, furosemide, bumetanide and triamterene on pancreatic $NaHCO_3$ secretion in pigs. Acta Physiol Scand 126: 593–600

Harris A, Coleman L (1987) Establishment of tissue culture system for epithelial cells derived from human pancreas. A model for the study of cystic fibrosis. J Cell Sci 87: 695–703

Kimura T, Imamura K, Eckhardt L, Schulz I (1987) Ca^{2+}-, phorbol ester-, and cAMP-stimulated enzyme secretion from permeabilized rat pancreatic acini. Am J Physiol 250: G698–G708

Kuijpers GAJ, Van Nooy IGP, De Pont JJHHM, Bonting SL (1984) The mechanism of fluid secretion in the rabbit pancreas studied by means of various inhibitors. Biochim Biophys Acta 778: 324–331

Lim RKS, Ling SM, Liu AC, Yuan IC (1936) Quantitative relationship between the basic and other components of the pancreatic secretion. Chin J Physiol 10: 475–492

Madden ME, Sarras MP (1987) Distribution of Na^+,K^+-ATPase in rat exocrine pancreas as monitored by K^+-NPPase cytochemistry and [^{3}H]-ouabain binding: a plasma membrane protein found primarily to be ductal cell associated. J Histochem Cytochem 35: 1365–1374

Novak I (1988) Pancreatic HCO_3^- secretion. In: Häussinger D (ed) pH Homeostasis – mechanism and control. Academic, London, pp 447–470

Novak I, Greger R (1987) Cellular mechanism of bicarbonate transport in isolated perfused pancreatic ducts. Acta Physiol Scand 129: 13A

Novak I, Greger R (1988a) Electrophysiological study of transport systems in isolated perfused pancreatic ducts. Properties of the basolateral membrane. Pflügers Arch 411: 58–68

Novak I, Greger R (1988b) Properties of the luminal membrane of isolated perfused rat pancreatic ducts. Effect of cyclic AMP and blockers of chloride transport. Pflügers Arch 411: 546–553

Novak I, Greger R(1988c) Ion transport systems of isolated perfused rat pancreatic ducts. Pflügers Arch 411: R74

Novak I, Greger R (1989) Effect of stimulation on isolated perfused rat pancreatic ducts. Role of Cl^- and K^+ channels. Pflügers Arch (in preparation)

Petersen OH, Maruyama Y (1984) Calcium-activated potassium channels and their role in secretion. Nature 307: 693–696

Reinhardt, Bridges RJ, Rummel W, Lindemann B (1987) Properties of anion-selective channel from rat colonic enterocyte plasma membrane reconstituted into planar phospholipid bilayers. J Membr Biol 95: 47–57

Rothman SS, Brooks FP (1965) Pancreatic secretion in vitro in "Cl^--free", "CO_2-free", and low-Na^+ environment. Am J Physiol 209: 790–796

Schulz I (1971) Influence of bicarbonate-CO_2- and glycodiazine buffer on the secretion of the isolated cat's pancreas. Pflügers Arch 329: 283–306

Schulz I (1980) Bicarbonate transport in the exocrine pancreas. Ann NY Acad Sci 341: 191–209

Schulz I (1987) Electrolyte and fluid secretion in the exocrine pancreas. In: Johnson LR (ed) Physiology of gastrointestinal tract, vol 1. Raven, New York, pp 1147–1171

Schulz I, Yamagata A, Weske M (1969) Micropuncture studies on the pancreas of the rabbit. Pflügers Arch 308: 277–290

Scratcherd T, Hutson D, Case RM (1981) Ionic transport mechanism underlying fluid secretion by the pancreas. Philos Trans R Soc Lond [Biol] 296: 167–178

Sewell WA, Young JA (1975) Secretion of electrolytes by the pancreas of the anaesthetized rat. J Physiol (Lond) 252: 379–396

Stuenkel EL, Machen TE, Williams JA (1988) pH regulatory mechanism in rat pancreatic ductal cells. Am J Physiol 254: G925–G930

Swanson CH, Solomon AK (1973) A micropuncture investigation of the whole tissue mechanism of electrolyte secretion by the in vitro rabbit pancreas. J Gen Physiol 62: 407–429

Swanson CH, Solomon AK (1975) Micropuncture analysis of the cellular mechanisms of electrolyte secretion by the in vitro rabbit pancreas. J Gen Physiol 65: 22–45

Trimble ER, Bruzzone R, Biden TJ, Meehan CJ, Andreu D, Merrifield RB (1987) Secretin stimulates cyclic AMP and inositol triphosphate production in rat pancreatic acinar tissue by two fully independent mechanisms. Proc Natl Acad Sci USA 84: 3146–3150

Wangemann P, Wittner M, Di Stefano A, Englert HC, Lang HJ, Schlatter E, Greger R (1986) Cl^--channel blockers in the thick ascending limb of the loop of Henle. Pflügers Arch 407: S128–S141

Way LW, Diamond JM (1970) The effect of secretin on electrical potential differences in the pancreatic duct. Biochim Biophys Acta 203: 298–307

Wizemann V, Schulz I (1973) Influence of amphotericin, amiloride, ionophores, and 2,4-dinitrophenol on the secretion of the isolated cats pancreas. Pflügers Arch 339: 317–338

The Role of Ion Channels in the Mechanism of Pancreatic Bicarbonate Secretion *

M. A. Gray, J. R. Greenwell and B. E. Argent

Ion Channels on Pancreatic Duct Cells

The current model for pancreatic duct cell bicarbonate secretion is shown in Fig. 1a. It is based on data derived from secretory studies on intact glands (see Case and Argent 1989), together with recent electrophysiological and intracellular pH measurements made on small pancreatic ducts (Gray et al. 1988b; Novak and Greger 1988a, 1988b; Stuenkel et al. 1988). The functions of this secretion are to flush digestive enzymes (secreted by acinar cells) along the ductal tree and into the duodenum and to provide an alkaline environment for the action of these enzymes on food in the gut.

Here we describe the regulated ion channels (Fig. 1a, b), the activity of which underlies the potassium and chloride conductances on the basolateral and apical membranes of the duct cell (Novak and Greger 1988a, 1988b) and which play a fundamental role in electrogenic bicarbonate secretion. However, in passing, it should be noted that patch-clamp studies have now identified a number of other channels in duct cells (Fig. 1b), although at the moment their functions remain unknown.

Basolateral Potassium Conductance

The role of the basolateral potassium conductance is to recycle K^+ accumulated by the Na^+-, K^+-ATPase and to provide a pathway for current flow across the basolateral membrane during secretion (Fig. 1a). The best candidate for the underlying channel (Fig. 1b) is a voltage-dependent, Ca^{2+}-activated, maxi-K^+ channel (Argent et al. 1987a), which has many properties in common with those described in other glandular epithelia (Petersen 1986). There are about 20 of these large conductance K^+ channels in the plasma membrane of each duct cell, and the channel density is about 1 per $19\ \mu m^2$ of plasma membrane.

---

* This work was supported by the Medical Research Council (UK).

Young · Wong, Epithelial Secretion of Water and Electrolytes
© Springer-Verlag Berlin · Heidelberg 1990

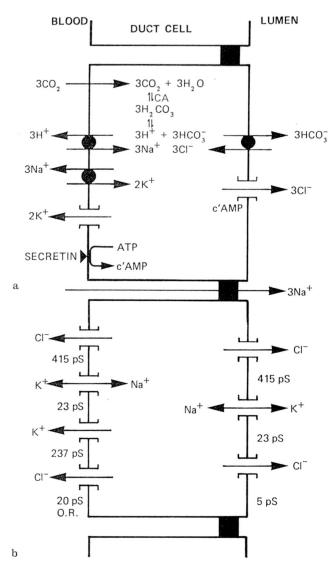

Fig. 1a. Cellular model for electrogenic bicarbonate secretion by pancreatic duct cells. *CA*, carbonic anhydrase. **b** Summary of conductance, distribution and selectivity of ion channels on rat and human pancreatic duct cells as determined using the patch-clamp technique. Conductance data are taken from experiments on excised patches. The channels are: 25 pS non-selective cation (Argent et al. 1987a); 237 pS maxi-K^+ (Argent et al. 1987a); 415 pS voltage-dependent anion (Argent et al. 1987b); 20 pS chloride, *OR*, outward rectifier, the slope conductance at a membrane potential of 0 mV is given (Gray et al. 1988a); 5 pS chloride (Gray et al. 1988b). The 5 pS chloride channel on the apical membrane, and the 237 pS maxi-K^+ channel on the basolateral membrane are involved in electrogenic bicarbonate secretion

What is the evidence that activity of this channel underlies the basolateral potassium conductance of the intact cell? From the pharmacological point of view it is not conclusive. Both the potassium conductance (Novak and Greger 1988a) and the maxi-K^+ channel are blocked by barium. However, tetraethylammonium (TEA), which also blocks the channel, has only a small depolarizing effect on the duct cell membrane potential (Novak and Greger 1988a). Moreover, we have recently found that whole-cell potassium currents can be completely blocked by barium, whereas in the presence of TEA, a small residual current persists. Taken together with the results of Evans et al. (1986), who showed that neither barium nor TEA has any effect on secretin-stimulated fluid secretion from the perfused rat pancreas, these data may indicate that other, as yet unidentified, potassium channels are present in the basolateral membrane.

However, strong evidence of a role for the maxi-K^+ channel in bicarbonate transport comes from the effect of secretory stimulants on channel activity. One can predict from the model shown in Fig. 1a that channel activity should increase following stimulation in order to balance the increased secretory current flowing across the apical membrane. This is in fact the case: the proportion of total time that maxi-K^+ channels on intact duct cells are open (their open-state probability) is markedly elevated by secretin, dibutyryl cyclic AMP and forskolin. As activity of this channel is voltage dependent (Argent et al. 1987), such an effect could result from the depolarization that occurs following exposure to these stimulants (Gray et al. 1988c; Novak and Greger 1988b). However, this is not the only explanation since whole-cell potassium currents can be markedly activated by intracellular cyclic AMP, and, in excised patches, the maxi-K^+ channel can be activated by exposing the cytoplasmic face of the membrane to a solution containing ATP and the catalytic subunit of A-kinase (M.A. Gray, J.R. Greenwell, B.E. Argent unpublished observations). Under these experimental conditions the membrane potential is clamped, so both results provide evidence for an additional activation pathway involving phosphorylation mediated by protein kinase A.

Apical Chloride Conductance

Three lines of evidence suggest that a small conductance (5 pS) chloride channel is responsible for the apical membrane chloride conductance. (1) The channel is located only on the apical membrane and is active in cell-attached patches (Gray et al. 1988b). (2) Both channel activity and a chloride conductance can be detected on unstimulated cells (Gray et al. 1988b; Novak and Greger 1988b). (3) Secretin, cyclic AMP and forskolin all increase channel activity (Gray et al. 1988b). This last effect causes the stimulant-induced depolarization of the duct cell (Gray et al. 1988c; Novak and Greger 1988b) and a decrease in the fractional resistance of the apical plasma membrane (Novak and Greger 1988 b). We originally identified this channel on rat duct cells (Gray et al. 1988 b), but it is also present in the human pancreas (Argent et al. 1988; Gray et al. 1988 a). It provides luminal chloride for the $Cl^- - HCO_3^-$ exchanger and is an important control point in the secretory mechanism.

Even under the most favourable experimental conditions, only 23% of all patches on the apical plasma membrane contained this small conductance channel. However, when present, it typically occurred in clusters that usually contained two or three, but occasionally up to nine, active channels (Figs. 2a, 3a, 4a, 6). The open-state probability is not markedly voltage dependent (Figs. 2a, 3a), indicating that the channel will be active at potentials (-50 to -60 mV) measured across the apical membrane in microperfused ducts (Novak and Greger 1988 b).

Proof that this channel selects for chloride is shown in Fig. 2. When equal chloride concentrations are present on both sides of excised patches the current/voltage (I/V) relation is linear, and the currents always reverse at a membrane potential of 0 mV, that is, when there is no chemical or electrical driving force for chloride diffusion across the patch (Fig. 2b). However, if a threefold chloride concentration gradient is created across the membrane, there is a marked leftward shift of the I/V plot, and the channel currents now reverse at a membrane potential of -26 mV (Fig. 2b). This is exactly the predicted shift for a channel that selects for chloride over sodium and potassium. Using a similar approach it is possible to estimate that the $Cl^- : HCO_3^-$ permeability ratio is about 5:1, making it appear very unlikely that significant amounts of bicarbonate enter the lumen directly via the channel.

Figure 3 shows the characteristics of this channel in intact cells. Provided there is no bicarbonate in the bath medium, the cell-attached I/V plot is linear and the single channel conductance about 5 pS, regardless of whether the recording pipette contains a Na^+-rich or a K^+-rich solution (Fig. 3b, c). Exposing the cells to a medium containing bicarbonate causes a slight outward rectification of the single channel currents, that is, outward currents are conducted slightly more easily than inward currents (Fig. 3d, e). We think it unlikely that this results from a direct action of bicarbonate on the channel since we did not observe a similar rectification with excised patches.

_____➤

Fig. 2a, b. Small chloride channel in excised patches. **a** Channel currents recorded from an inside-out patch excised from the apical surface of a rat pancreatic duct cell. Both extracellular (pipette) and intracellular (bath) faces of the membrane were bathed in a Na^+-rich solution containing Cl^- in a concentration of 150 mmol/l. Low pass filtered at 200 Hz. The membrane potential (Vm) is indicated adjacent to the records. An upward deflection from the closed state (*horizontal line*) represents outward current and a downward de-flection inward current. **b** Single-channel I/V plots. *, data from the experiment shown in **a**. o, same experiment after a threefold chloride concentration gradient had been created across the patch by replacing bath chloride with sulphate, keeping sodium and potassium con-centrations constant. (From Gray et al. 1988 b)

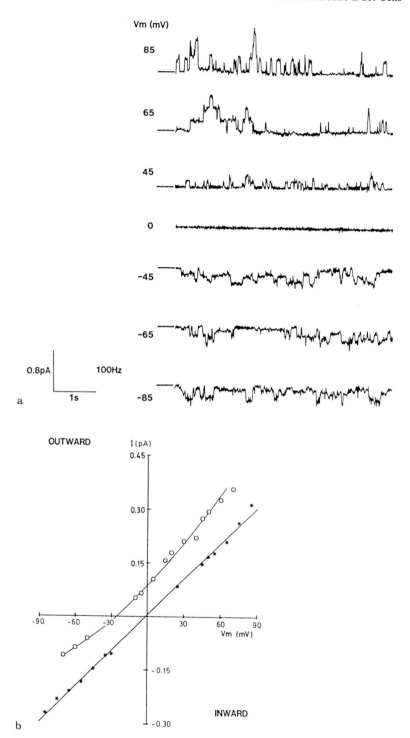

Under all conditions tested, currents flowing through the channel reversed at pipette potentials near to 0 mV, that is, close to the resting membrane potential of the cell (Fig. 3b–e). Initially, this observation caused us some concern since it indicates that intracellular chloride is in electrochemical equilibrium and that the model for electrogenic bicarbonate secretion shown in Fig. 1a would not work. However, all our patch-clamp experiments were performed at room temperature, under which conditions activity of the $Cl^- - HCO_3^-$ exchanger (Fig. 1a), the only transport element available to accumulate chloride, would be markedly inhibited (Hoffmann et al. 1979). Furthermore, the resting chloride conductance of the apical membrane (which we detect as channel activity in unstimulated cells) would ensure that any residual chloride gradient was rapidly dissipated.

Most important of all, the activity of this small conductance chloride channel can be increased by secretin, the physiological regulator of pancreatic bicarbonate transport, by forskolin, a drug which activates the catalytic subunit of adenylate cyclase, and by dibutyryl cyclic AMP. Since there is ample evidence that secretin uses cyclic AMP as an intracellular messenger (see Case and Argent 1989), physiological regulation of the channel is almost certainly achieved by phosphorylation catalyzed by protein kinase A.

As illustrated in Fig. 4, short-term exposure of duct cells to secretin causes a marked increase in total current flow across cell-attached patches. This effect is accompanied by an increase in the number of channels that are open simultaneously, as can be seen from the current records themselves (Fig. 4a) and from the associated current amplitude histograms (Fig. 4b). For reasons discussed below, we believe that this is caused by an increase in the open-state probability of individual ion channels (Fig. 4c), rather than an increase in the total number of channels in the patch. This change in open-state probability is achieved by a large reduction in the time that the channel spends in the closed state (Fig. 4e), coupled with a slight increase in the open time (Fig. 4d). Said another way, each channel opens more frequently and stays open for slightly longer. All these effects of secretin were fully reversed upon withdrawal of the hormone, but this usually took between 8 and 10 min (Fig. 4a–e).

Fig. 3a – e. Small chloride channel in cell-attached patches. **a** Channel currents recorded from a patch on the apical surface of a rat pancreatic duct cell. Low pass filtered at 300 Hz. Solutions: bath, Na^+ rich; pipette, K^+ rich. The pipette potential (V_p) is shown adjacent to each record. In cell-attached recordings the total voltage across the patch is equal to the cell membrane potential minus V_p. **b – e** Single channel I/V plots. **b** Bath, Na^+ rich; pipette, K^+ rich (11 patches). **c** Bath, Na^+ rich; pipette, Na^+ rich (14 patches). **d** Bath, Na^+ rich containing 25 mmol/l bicarbonate; pipette, K^+ rich (3 patches). **e** Bath, Na^+ rich containing 25 mmol/l bicarbonate; pipette, Na^+ rich (2 patches). Solutions contained 150 mmol/l Cl^- in absence of bicarbonate and 125 mmol/l Cl^- when bicarbonate was present. (From Gray et al. 1988b)

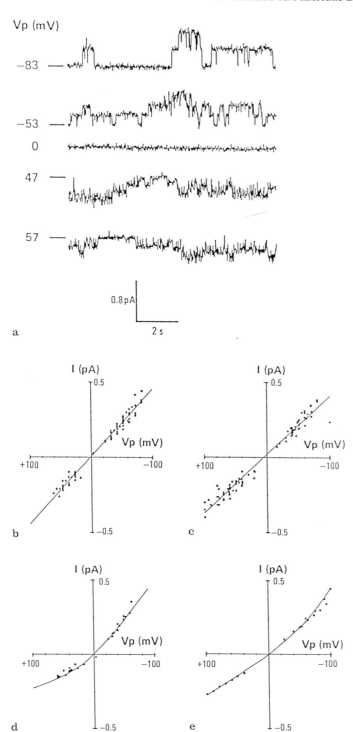

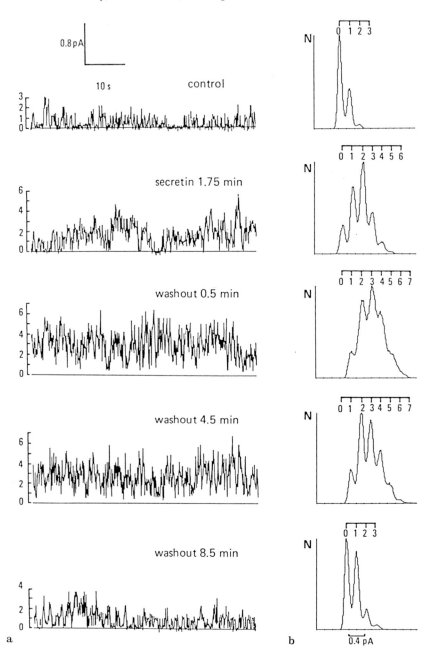

Fig. 4a, b.

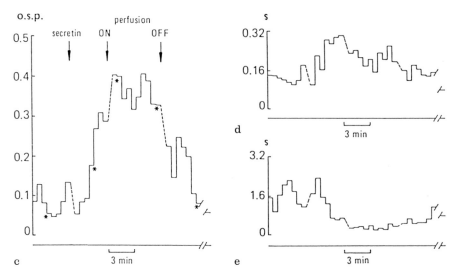

Fig. 4a – e. Regulation of chloride channel activity by secretin (10 nmol/l). **a** Channel currents in a cell-attached patch on an isolated rat pancreatic duct cell. The times indicate the period between either addition or washout of secretin from the bath and the start of each trace. Low pass filtered at 300 Hz. Solutions; bath, Na^+ rich; pipette, K^+ rich, both containing 150 mmol/l Cl^-. *Vertical scale* indicates the number of channels open simultaneously. Because outward currents flowing through the channel are easier to resolve this patch was voltage clamped at $V_p = -50$ mV. Thus, chloride ions will be moving from the recording pipette into the cell. **b** Current amplitude histograms derived by analysis of the corresponding tracings. Data sampled at 2.2 kHz. *Horizontal scale* indicates number of channels open simultaneously. **c – e** Effects of 10 nmol/l secretin on **c** the open-state probability; **d** mean open time and **e** mean closed time of the chloride channel. Same experiment as **a** and **b**. *Arrow 'secretin'* indicates when the hormone was added to the bath (volume 1.5 ml), and *arrows 'perfusion on'* and *'perfusion off'* when the perfusion flow (5 ml/min) was switched. *Dashed lines* indicate access to screened cage, and *stars* the mid-point of recordings shown in **a**. For illustrative purpose data collected over 4.5 min towards the end of the experiment have been omitted. Open-state probability, mean open and mean closed times were calculated from data sampled at 2.2 kHz into 33 s bins, and assuming a total of eight channels in the patch which was the maximum number observed to open simultaneously. Binomial analysis of the data also suggested that eight channels were present, and that this number did not change following stimulation. (From Gray et al. 1988 b)

Figure 5 shows the effects of forskolin and dibutyryl cyclic AMP on channel activity. In this experiment the open-state probability increased threefold after exposure of the duct cell to the stimulants. However, unlike the response to secretin, the effect of these stimulants on channel activity reversed within 2 min of their washout from the bath.

One other important, albeit negative, finding was that stimulants never caused the appearance of channel activity in quiescent patches from intact cells. This makes it very unlikely that short-term stimulation can increase the total number of active channels in a patch either by activating dormant channels or by causing the insertion of new channel proteins into the

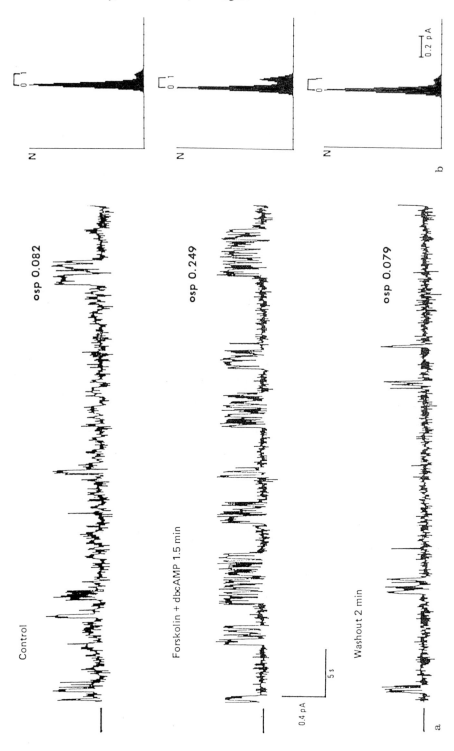

membrane. Under these conditions we believe that the major effect is on the open-state probability of channels that are already active. The experiment shown in Fig. 5 provides confirmation of this idea since multiple channel openings were not observed, making it likely that there was only one active channel present throughout the experiment.

For technical reasons it is not possible to examine the effects of prolonged exposure to stimulants during continuous cell-attached monitoring of channel activity. However, if duct cells were stimulated for periods up to 45 min and then patch clamped, we noticed (in addition to the increase in open-state probability) a marked increase, from 10% to 23%, in the proportion of patches that contained active chloride channels. Initially, we took this to indicate that prolonged stimulation had caused insertion of new channels into the apical membrane. However, an alternative explanation is the disaggregation of large channel clusters into smaller ones.

We tested for cluster disaggregation by comparing the number of channels (N) in patches derived from unstimulated cells with the number of channels in patches derived from stimulated cells (Fig. 6). The distribution profile for N in unstimulated cells suggested that there are two populations of patches: one with $N = 1-5$ and a second with $N = 6-9$. In contrast, N was never greater than 5 in patches obtained from stimulated cells. This supports the idea of cluster disaggregation following long-term stimulation, but does not exclude a simultaneous increase in channel numbers.

Thus, depending on the experimental conditions, stimulation appears to affect two aspects of channel function. Short-term stimulation causes an increase in the open-state probability of individual channels (Figs. 4, 5), and long-term exposure has an additional effect on either the total number, or the distribution, of channels in the apical membrane (Fig. 6).

Recently, the characteristics of Ca^{2+}- and cyclic AMP-activated chloride channels in the apical membranes of a number of chloride secreting epithelial cells have been described (for reviews see Frizzell 1987). Most of these channels have much larger conductances than the secretin-regulated channel we have identified on pancreatic duct cells. Two other, larger conductance chloride channels are present on the duct cell (Fig. 1 b; Argent et al. 1987 b; Gray et al. 1988 a), but neither appears to be hormonally regulated, and at the moment their functions are unknown. A small

---

Fig. 5a, b. Regulation of chloride channel activity by 1 mmol/l dibutyryl cyclic AMP and 1 μmol/l forskolin. **a** Single channel currents recorded at $V_p = -40$ mV from a cell-attached patch on the apical surface of a rat pancreatic duct cell. Bath and pipette contained a Na^+-rich solution with 150 mmol/l Cl^-. Low pass filtered at 300 Hz. *Top trace*, control; *middle trace*, starts 1.5 min after addition of stimulants to the bath; *bottom trace*, starts 2 min after bath washout. The open-state probability of the channel over the period of these recordings is shown to the *right* and *above* each trace. **b** Current amplitude histograms derived by analysis of the corresponding tracings. Data sampled at 2.2 kHz. (From Gray et al. 1988 b)

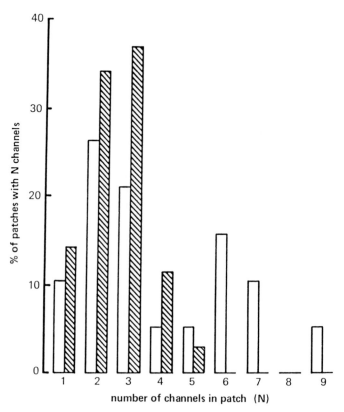

y-axis: % of patches with N channels
x-axis: number of channels in patch (N)

Fig. 6. Number of chloride channel in patches obtained from unstimulated and stimulated rat pancreatic duct cells. The number of channels (N) in a patch was taken as the maximum number of simultaneous single-channel current steps observed during the first 45 s of recording immediately after establishing a giga-seal. *Open columns*, 19 patches from unstimulated cells; *shaded columns*, 35 patches from cells stimulated with a mixture of secretin (10 nmol/l, dibutyryl cyclic AMP (0.1–1 nmol/l) and forskolin (1 µmol/l) for between 5 and 45 min (From Gray et al. 1988 b)

conductance (1–2 pS), Ca^{2+}-activated anion channel has been identified on the chloride-secreting lacrimal acinar cell by noise analysis of whole-cell currents (Marty et al. 1984). However, this channel has not been further characterized or localized to the apical membrane using single-channel recording techniques.

Finally, the identification of a cyclic AMP-regulated chloride channel on pancreatic duct cells may explain the reduced pancreatic bicarbonate secretion that occurs in the inherited disease cystic fibrosis (Kopelman et al. 1985). In airway epithelia, the underlying genetic defect is expressed as abnormal regulation of apical chloride channels by intracellular cyclic AMP (Schoumacher et al. 1987; Li et al. 1988). Since one of the functions of pancreatic ductal secretions is to flush enzymes out of the gland, stasis, followed by activation of these hydrolytic enzymes within the ductal tree, may well initiate the pathological changes that occur in the pancreases of cystic fibrosis patients.

References

Argent BE, Arkle S, Gray MA, Greenwell JR (1987a) Two types of calcium-sensitive cation channels in isolated rat pancreatic duct cells. J Physiol (Lond) 386: 82P

Argent BE, Gray MA, Greenwell JR (1987b) Characteristics of a large conductance anion channel in membrane patches excised from rat pancreatic duct cells in vitro. J Physiol (Lond) 394: 146P

Argent BE, Coleman L, Gray MA, Greenwell JR, Harris A (1988) Anion-selective channel on the apical plasma membrane of human pancreatic duct cells in vitro. J Physiol 403: 49P

Case RM, Argent BE (1989) Pancreatic secretion of electrolytes and water. In: Schultz SG (ed) Handbook of Physiology, Section 6, Vol. III, American Physiological Society, Bethesda, pp 383–417

Evans LAR, Pirani D, Cook DI, Young JA (1986) Intraepithelial current flow in rat pancreatic secretory epithelia. Pflügers Arch 407 [Suppl 2]: S107–S111

Frizzell RA (1987) Cystic fibrosis: a disease of ion channels. Trends Neurosci 10: 190–193

Gray MA, Coleman L, Harris A, Greenwell JR, Argent BE (1988a) Chloride channels on human pancreatic duct cells. In: Wong PYD, Young JA (eds) Exocrine secretion. Hong Kong University Press, Hong Kong, pp 73–75

Gray MA, Greenwell JR, Argent BE (1988b) Secretin-regulated chloride channel on the apical plasma membrane of pancreatic duct cells. J Membr Biol 105: 131–142

Gray MA, Greenwell JR, Argent BE (1988c) Ion channels in pancreatic duct cells: characterization and role in bicarbonate secretion. In: Mastella G, Quinton PM (eds) Cellular and molecular basis of cystic fibrosis. San Francisco Press, San Francisco, pp 205–216

Hoffman EK, Simonsen LO, Sjoholm C (1979) Membrane potential, chloride exchange, and chloride conductance in Ehrlich mouse ascites tumour cells. J Physiol (Lond) 296: 61–84

Kopelman H, Durie P, Gaskin K, Weizman Z, Forstner G (1985) Pancreatic fluid secretion and protein hyperconcentration in cyctic fibrosis. N Engl J Med 312: 329–334

Li M, McCann D, Liedtke CM, Nairn AC, Greengard P, Welsh MJ (1988) Cyclic AMP-dependent protein kinase opens chloride channels in normal but not cystic fibrosis airway epithelium. Nature 331: 358–360

Marty A, Tan YP, Trautmann A (1984) Three types of calcium-dependent channel in rat lacrimal glands. J Physiol (Lond) 357: 293–325

Novak I, Greger R (1988a) Electrophysiological study of transport systems in isolated perfused pancreatic ducts: properties of the basolateral membrane. Pflügers Arch 411: 58–68

Novak I, Greger R (1988b) Properties of the luminal membrane of isolated perfused rat pancreatic ducts. Effect of cyclic AMP and blockers of chloride transport. Pflügers Arch 411: 546–553

Petersen OH (1986) Calcium-activated potassium channels and fluid secretion by exocrine glands. Am J Physiol 251: G1–G13

Schoumacher RA, Shoemaker RL, Halm DR, Tallant EA, Wallace RW, Frizzell RA (1987) Phosphorylation fails to activate chloride channels from cystic fibrosis airway cells. Nature 330: 752–754

Stuenkel EL, Machen TE, Williams JA (1988) pH regulatory mechanisms in rat pancreatic ductal cells. Am J Physiol 254: G925–G930

The Metabolic Basis of Secretion by the Exocrine Pancreas*

T. Kanno

Energy Metabolism

The term metabolism is used to refer to all the chemical and energy transformations that occur in the body. This chapter sets the stage for consideration of the production and utilization of energy in the exocrine pancreas.

The pancreatic acinar cells comprise 89% of the pancreatic cell mass in the guinea pig and 77% in the rat (see Case 1978). The major energy consumer in the pancreas is thus likely to be the acinar cells. There is evidence from studies on fragments of rat pancreatic tissue that mitochondria supply more than 90% of the energy needed by the pancreas, that ATP pools are renewed at least every 23 s, and that protein biosynthesis depends on a common pool of ATP supplied by oxidative phosphorylation and glycolysis (Bauduin et al. 1969). As to the utilization of energy, ATP may be hydrolyzed in every step of secretion: uptake of raw materials from the extracellular space, biosynthesis of secretory substances, intracellular transport of secretory granules, exocytosis of secretory granules, concomitant secretion of electrolytes, formation of second and third messengers, and protein phosphorylation. The need for ATP in the synthesis of secretory and nonsecretory (e.g. membrane protein) elements occurring *pari passu* in the process of the transport and exocytosis of zymogen granules was denied by Jamieson and Palade (1971) who studied slices of guinea pig pancreas. They suggested that the energy requirements for zymogen discharge may be related to the fusion of the granule membrane with the apical plasmalemma. Vilmart-Seuwen et. al (1986) attempted to specify a widespread hypothesis on the requirement of ATP for exocytosis. They measured ATP pools in different strains of *Paramecium tetraurelia*, synchronously exocytosing trichocysts, and concluded that: (a) membrane fusion during exocytosis did not require the presence of ATP, (b) the occurrence of membrane fusion might involve the elimination of ATP from primed fusogenic sites, and (c)

---

* This investigation was supported by Ministry of Education, Science, and Culture of Japan Grants-in-Aid 61 440 025 for scientific research.

most of the ATP consumption measured in the course of exocytosis seemed to be related to other processes, probably to recovery phenomena.

ATP is also hydrolyzed by the Na^+-, K^+-ATPase to produce Na^+ and K^+ gradients across the membrane of the acinar cell. The activity of the Na^+-, K^+-ATPase may be responsible for secretion of electrolytes in the acinar cells. Thus, fluid secretion is also an important index of energy consumption in the acinar cells. ATP may mainly be supplied by a concomitant increase in ATP synthesis in the mitochondria of the pancreatic acinar cells.

The activities of mitochondria in the processes of secretion have been studied in our laboratory by monitoring the redox states of the electron transfer system. The redox state of cytochromes in mitochondria in the isolated perfused rat pancreas can easily be monitored with a scanning organ spectrophotometer (Kanno et al. 1981, 1983; Shibuya and Kanno 1985; Kanno and Matsumoto 1986; Matsumoto and Kanno 1988; Kanno 1988). This technique has the advantage of allowing simultaneous measurement of secretory responses (protein output and fluid secretion) and the redox state of cytochromes during continuous stimulation (Kanno 1987).

Redox Response Versus Secretory Response to Various CCK-8 Concentrations

The redox response was recorded with a scanning organ spectrophotometer when the isolated perfused rat pancreas (with the duodenum still attached) was continuously stimulated with the C-terminal octapeptide of cholecystokinin (CCK-8) at high (pharmacological) concentration (50–500 pmol/l). The preparation was first perfused with a Ca^{2+}-free solution for about 30 min to reach steady levels, after which the absorption spectrum of the cytochromes was measured. The tip of the light guide of the scanning organ spectrophotometer was placed on the surface of the preparation and the difference between the stored initial average of 16 scannings of absorption spectra and the subsequent average was continuously computed and displayed as the difference spectrum every 16 s throughout the experiments. The steady levels of the final set of measurements made after perfusion had been stopped were considered to represent the maximum reduction levels for the cytochromes. At the maximum reduction levels, the differences betweeen the optical density at 575 nm and that of cytochrome aa_3 (605 nm), at 575 nm and that of cytochrome b (562 nm), or at 540 nm and that of cytochrome $c+c_1$ (550 nm) were considered to represent 100% reduction of the respective cytochromes. The changes in redox states of the cytochromes were expressed as percentage reductions. Figure 1 shows an example of the time course of the redox states of the cytochromes and the difference spectra taken before, during, and after perfusion with solutions containing CCK-8 (200 pmol/l) and the maximum reduction state (Shibuya and Kanno 1985). Cytochrome reduction reached peak levels of about 30% of the respective maximum

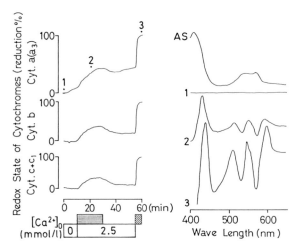

Fig. 1. Time course of the redox state of cytochromes (*Cyt*), aa_3, b, and $c+c_1$ (*left*) recorded before, during, and after perfusion with standard solutions containing CCK-8 (200 pmol/l); *number* and *dots* on the *top line* (cyt $a(a_3)$) correspond to time when difference spectra (*right*) were recorded. *Stippled bar* indicates the periods of perfusion with 200 pmol/l CCK-8 solution and *hatched bar* the period when perfusion was stopped. *AS*, absolute spectrum

levels about 10 min after the start of perfusion with the CCK-8 solutions. The redox state of these cytochromes returned to the resting levels when the CCK-8 solution was replaced with the standard solutions.

During the measurements of redox states of the cytochromes, perfusates were collected from the common duct and subjected to analysis for pancreatic digestive protein. Thus, dose–response relations were obtained for the redox and the secretory responses to various concentrations of CCK-8 (Fig. 2; Kanno and Matsumoto 1986). A previous study in our laboratory showed that the protein output and cytochrome reduction were enhanced when the concentration of CCK-8 was increased (Shibuya and Kanno 1985). The protein output and cytochrome reduction were further examined in the following experiments by changing the CCK-8 concentration over a much wider range. There is a distinct discrepancy between the dose-dependent redox response and the dose-dependent secretory response (Fig. 2; Kanno and Matsumoto 1986). A sigmoidal relation was obtained between the concentration of CCK-8 in the solutions perfusing the pancreas and the level of reduction of cytochromes recorded from the pancreas, whereas a bell-shaped relation was obtained between the concentration of CCK-8 and the protein output. Continuous stimulation of the pancreas with a physiological CCK-8 concentration, 10 pmol/l or lower, induced a small, but distinct increase in protein output and little, if any, change in the redox state of the cytochromes. Continous stimulation with CCK-8 (30 pmol/l) caused maximum protein output and only a small parallel reduction of cytochromes. Continuous stimulation with CCK-8 at an extremely high concentra-

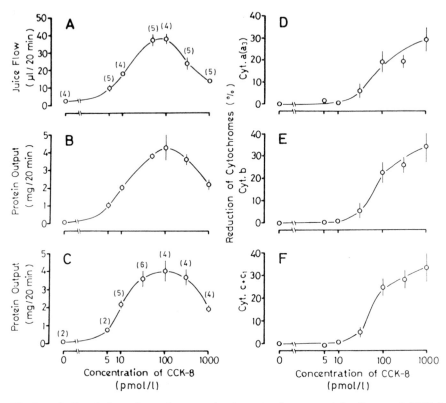

Fig. 2a – f. Correlation of cytochrome reduction, protein output, juice flow, and CCK-8 concentration. Juice flow (a) and protein output (b) were obtained from experiments on "draining preparations" (Kanno 1987). Protein output (c) and cytochrome reduction (d – f) were obtained from experiments on "flushing preparations" (Kanno 1987). Protein output and juice flow are total amount of protein and flow in a sample collected for 20 min of stimulation with CCK-8 in different concentrations. Reduction of cytochromes is the mean of 20-min measurements during the respective CCK-8 stimulations. Numbers in parentheses indicate the numbers of experiments. (From Kanno and Matsumoto 1986)

tion (1 nmol/l), which has been shown to produce the morphological changes of acute pancreatitis (see Kanno 1988), induced only a slight increase in protein output, but a large reduction of cytochromes. The pattern of the dose-response relation for CCK-8-induced protein output was identical to that for CCK-8-induced fluid secretion measured in the preparation when these two responses were measured simultaneously. Thus, the relation between the redox response and the protein output can be regarded as the relation between the redox response and fluid secretion.

Because it is known that fluid secretion in the pancreas requires a considerable expenditure of metabolic energy in the form of ATP hydrolysis by the Na^+-, K^+-ATPase in the plasma membrane of the acinar cells (Hootman et al. 1983), the dose-dependent cytochrome reduction might be a sign of relative hypoxia caused by excess increase in fluid secretion under conditions of limited supply of O_2 to the acinar cell. In fact, it is well documented that the parallel cytochrome reduction in isolated mitochondria may be a sign of the transition from the resting state (state 4) to the anoxic state (state 5; Chance and Williams 1956). This view may be an adequate explanation for the following experiments.

The influence of hypoxia on the redox state and protein output induced by continuous stimulation with CCK-8 (50 pmol/l) was examined in the isolated perfused rat pancreas with the duodenum still attached (Kanno 1988). The Po_2 of the perfusing solution equilibrated with 95% O_2 was about 430 mmHg, and the O_2 concentration of the perfusing solution was decreased by equilibration with gas mixtures containing 75, 50, and 25% O_2, respectively. The protein output was decreased when the O_2 concentration was lowered, whilst the resting level of the redox state was reduced and the CCK-8-induced cytochrome reduction was enhanced when Po_2 was lowered. In contrast, protein output and fluid secretion were increased, and the CCK-8-induced cytochrome reduction was nullified when the O_2 supply was increased (Matsumoto and Kanno 1988). In this experiment, we were able to increase perfusion flow rate without inducing oedema by first excising the duodenum from the isolated rat pancreas. The parallel reduction of the cytochromes was not detected even when the preparation was continuously stimulated with CCK-8 at higher concentrations (30 pmol/l, 100 pmol/l, and 1 nmol/l) at a perfusion rate of 3 ml/min, which was about three times higher than the maximum rate used in the isolated pancreas with the duodenum still attached.

If the activity of the Na^+-, K^+-ATPase is a prime determinant of the CCK-8-induced parallel cytochrome reduction, then inhibition of the activity with ouabain may result in the disappearance of the parallel reduction. Addition of ouabain (1 mmol/l) to the perfusing solution 25 min before continuous stimulation with CCK-8 (50 or 200 nmol/l) almost completely inhibited the secretory responses, but the parallel cytochrome reduction was still recorded in the isolated perfused rat pancreas with duodenum (H. Kuriyama and T. Kanno, unpublished data quoted by Kanno 1988). This result supports the view that the activity of the Na^+-, K^+-ATPase may not be the sole determinant of the parallel cytochrome reduction.

The rate of mitochondrial respiration is governed by the interplay of four factors, among which the cytoplasmic [ATP]/[ADT] [P_i] ratio serves as the primary signal for an altered need for energy production (Erecińska and Wilson 1982). However, we have shown that the cytoplasmic [ATP]/[ADP] [P_i] ratio remained almost constant during continuous stimulation with acetylcholine (ACh; Matsumoto et al. 1988). In these experiments, we used phosphorus nuclear magnetic reasonance (^{31}P NMR) at the organ level for non-invasive measurements of compounds such as ATP, ADP, inorganic phosphate (P_i), sugar phosphate, creatine phosphate, and tissue pH. Continuous stimulation with ACh (0.1 µmol/l) caused marked and sustained increases in secretory responses in the absence of detectable change in the tissue levels of phosphorus compounds, whilst the tissue pH was decreased slightly by 0.05 pH unit.

$[Ca^{2+}]_c$ As an Intracellular Signal for Accelerating the Electron Transfer System

The increase in cytosolic free calcium, $[Ca^{2+}]_c$ which is the intracellular signal for stimulus-secretion coupling, may also be a signal for accelerating the electron transfer system. The view that mitochondrial Ca^{2+} transport regulates the free-Ca^{2+} concentration of the mitochondrial matrix, $[Ca^{2+}]_m$, has recently been proposed (Hansford 1985; Denton and MacCormack 1985). Three key dehydrogeneses in mammalian mitochondria have been found to be activated by Ca^{2+} with a half-maximum effect at about 1 µmol/l. Hormones, neurotransmitters, and other extracellular signals, which stimulate ATP-requiring processes such as secretion or muscle contraction by increasing $[Ca^{2+}]_c$, could also increase intramitochondrial oxidative metabolism and, hence, promote the replenishment of ATP (Denton and McCormack 1985). In this manner, the formation of reducing power for oxidative phosphorylation can be accelerated under the very conditions under which ATP synthesis is likely to increase (Denton and McCormack 1985). This view is compatible with the following results.

Continuous stimulation of the isolated perfused pancreas with CCK-8 (20 pmol/l) caused a gradual, but large increase in protein output and a slight parallel reduction of cytochromes. When $CaCl_2$ was removed from the extracellular environment, the secretory response was strongly inhibited and the parallel cytochrome reduction disappeared. Both responses were regained immediately after the replacement of the Ca^{2+}-deficient solution (containing CCK-8) with a standard solution containing 2.5 $CaCl_2$ (2 mmol/l) and no CCK-8 (Shibuya and Kanno 1985). An almost linear relation was found between the magnitude of the protein output in response to CCK-8 (50 pmol/l) and extracellular Ca^{2+} concentration ($[Ca^{2+}]_o$) in the range of 0.5–2.5 mmol/l. Similar relations were also found between the levels of reduction of cytochromes and $[Ca^{2+}]_o$ (Fig. 3; Kanno and Matsumoto 1986).

Balance Between Consumption and Production of Energy During Stimulus-Secretion Coupling

Since it is known that oxidative phosphorylation supplies more than 90% of the energy for the pancreas (Bauduin et al. 1969), change in tissue O_2 tension (Po_2) may reflect an overall alteration of energy production. Pancreatic acinar Po_2 has recently been measured in anaesthetized rats using recessed-

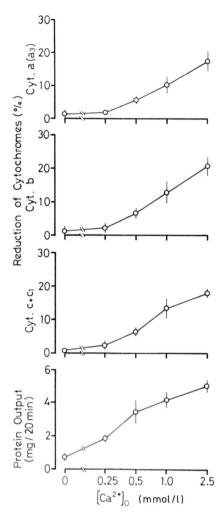

Fig. 3. Correlation of cytochrome reduction, protein output, and $[Ca^{2+}]_o$. Protein output is the total quantity of protein in a sample collected for 20 min of continuous stimulation with CCK-8 (50 pmol/l). Reduction of cytochromes is the mean of 20-min measurement during continuous stimulation with CCK-8. Values are means $\pm$ SEM of four experiments. (From Kanno and Matsumoto 1986)

tip microelectrodes (Harper et al. 1986). Bolus injection of CCK-8 (4 µg/kg body weight) induced a decrease in Po_2 from a resting level (average 3.3 kPa) to a minimum level of 1.8 kPa, while not directly affecting pancreatic blood flow. In such oxygen environments, substantial concentration gradients may occur from the extracellular space to the mitochondria. In fact, a significant oxygen gradient within about 1 µm of the mitochondria was estimated in single-cell suspensions of rat hepatocytes under conditions of mild hypoxia (of about 2 kPa Po_2; Jones and Kennedy 1982). Thus, even though the blood circulation was maintained in the anaesthetized rat, it seems highly likely that stimulation with CCK-8 at a pharmacological concentration may cause a $[Ca^{2+}]_c$-dependent acceleration of oxidative phosphorylation that in turn may cause parallel cytochrome reduction in the absence of discernible changes in the tissue levels of phosphorus compounds.

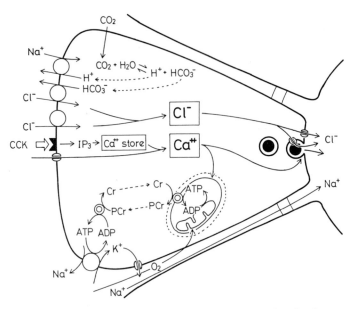

Fig. 4. Schematic representation of the cellular events in stimulus-secretion coupling in a pancreatic acinar cell. Continuous stimulation with CCK at a physiologically low concentration induces Ca^{2+} entry, which maintains a sustained secretory response in which production and consumption of energy are well balanced. Stimulation with CCK at a pharmacologically high concentration induces release of Ca^{2+} from store sites and Ca^{2+} entry, which are responsible for the dual phases of the secretory responses. The transient initial component of the response may be mediated by inositol 1,4,5-triphosphate (IP_3). CCK also activates the Na^+-, K^+-ATPase, the Na^+-H^+ and the $Cl^--HCO_3^-$ antiports and the unique Cl^- transport system. ATP for the Na^+-, K^+-ATPase may be supplied via the cytoplasmic creatine kinase (CPK) system from phosphocreatine (PCr). PCr is supplied by diffusion from the mitochondrial CPK system. The respiratory chain in a mitochondrion supplies ATP to the mitochondrial CPK system. O_2 is supplied to the respiratory chain. An increase in $[Ca^{2+}]_c$ induces a parallel reduction of cytochromes

In skeletal muscle, high-energy phosphates are transferred across the cytosol to the site of ATP consumption predominantly in the form of phosphocreatine because the degree of diffusibility of creatine is higher than that of ATP (see Murakami et al. 1988). The existence of this system has been confirmed in the rat mandibular gland (Murakami et al. 1988). If this system also exists in the rat exocrine pancreas, the main route for energy transfer from mitochondria to the Na^+-, K^+-ATPase in the exocrine pancreas of the rat can be proposed as a modification of that presented by Murakami et al. (1988) for the rat mandibular gland. In the modified model (Fig. 4), the cardinal role of $[Ca^{2+}]_c$ in the secretory and redox responses to CCK-8 is stressed as in the previous model (Kanno 1988).

References

Bauduin H, Colin M, Dumont GE (1969) Energy sources for protein synthesis and enzymatic secretion in rat pancreas in vitro. Biochim Biophys Acta 174: 722–733

Case RM (1978) Synthesis, intracellular transport and discharge of exportable proteins in the pancreatic acinar cell and other cells. Biol Rev 53: 211–354

Chance B, Williams GR (1956) The respiratory chain and oxidative phosphorylation. In: Nord FF (ed) Advances in enzymology and related subjects of biochemistry, vol 17. Interscience, New York, pp 65–134

Denton RM, McCormack JG (1985) Ca^{2+} transport by mammalian mitochondria and its role in hormone action. Am J Physiol 249: E543–E554

Erecińska M, Wilson DF (1982) Regulation of cellular energy metabolism. J Membr Biol 70: 1–40

Hansford RG (1985) Relation between mitochondrial calcium transport and control of energy metabolism. Rev Physiol Biochem Pharmacol 102: 1–72

Harper SL, Pitts VH, Granger DN, Kvietys PR (1986) Pancreatic tissue oxygenation during secretory stimulation. Am J Physiol 250: G316–G322

Hootman SR, Ernst SA, Williams JA (1983) Secretagogue regulation of Na^+-K^+ pump activity in pancreatic acinar cells. Am J Physiol 245: G339–G349

Jamieson JD, Palade GE (1971) Condensing vacuole conversion and zymogen granule discharge in pancreatic exocrine cells: metabolic studies. J Cell Biol 48: 503–552

Jones DP, Kennedy FG (1982) Intracellular oxygen supply during hypoxia. Am J Physiol 243: C247–C252

Kanno T (1987) The perfused pancreas for studying exocrine secretion. In: Poisner AM, Trifaró JM (eds) In vitro methods for studying secretion. Elsevier, Amsterdam, pp 45–61

Kanno T (1988) Roles of mitochondria in stimulus-secretion coupling in pancreatic acinar cells. In: Thorn NA, Treiman M, Petersen OH (eds) Molecular mechanisms in secretion. Munksgaard, Copenhagen, pp 315–323

Kanno T, Matsumoto T (1986) Influence of extracellular $[Ca^{2+}]$ on secretory and redox responses to CCK-8 in perfused rat pancreas. Am J Physiol 251: C10–C16

Kanno T, Ikei N, Nakase Y (1981) Simultaneous measurements of cholecystokinin-induced changes in absorption spectrum of cytochromes, NAD(P)H-fluorescence, and enzyme output in isolated perfused rat pancreas. Biomed Res 2: 281–389

Kanno T, Saito A, Ikei N (1983) Dose-dependent effects of acetylcholine stimulating respiratory chain and secretion of isolated perfused rat pancreas. Biomed Res 4: 175–186

Matsumoto T, Kanno T (1988) Optical absorbance changes induced by CCK-8 under limited O_2 supply in isolated perfused rat pancreas. Am J Physiol 254: C727–C734

Matsumoto T, Kanno T, Seo Y, Murakami M, Watari H (1988) Phosphorus nuclear magnetic resonance in isolated perfused rat pancreas. Am J Physiol 254: G575–G579

Murakami M, Seo Y, Watari H (1988) Dissociation of fluid secretion and energy supply in rat mandibular gland by high dose of ACh. Am J Physiol 254: G781–G787

Shibuya I, Kanno T (1985) Calcium-dependent secretory and redox response to CCK-8 in isolated perfused rat pancreas. Am J Physiol 248: C228–C234

Vilmart-Seuwen J, Kersken H, Stürzl R, Plattner H (1986) ATP keeps exocytosis sites in a primed state but is not required for membrane fusion: an analysis with *Paramecium* cells in vivo and in vitro. J Cell Biol 103: 1279–1288

4 Endocrine Pancreas

Ion Channels in Insulin-Secreting Cells: Their Role in Stimulus-Secretion Coupling

M. J. Dunne and O. H. Petersen

Introduction

The maintenance of homeostatic blood-glucose levels is a complex, regulated process mainly controlled by a single molecule – insulin. This polypeptide hormone, synthesised and stored in the pancreatic β cells of the islets of Langerhans, is released by the process of exocytosis in response to an elevated concentration of glucose in the plasma (Hedeskov 1980). The key intracellular regulator of insulin secretion is a rise in the cytosolic concentration of free calcium ions ($[Ca^{2+}]_i$), a rise that it totally dependent upon calcium outside the cell (Wollheim and Biden 1987).

In the 1960s our understanding of stimulus-secretion coupling in insulin-secreting cells took a major step forward when Dean and Matthews (1968) published the first intracellular recordings with glass microelectrodes from β cells. In this series of experiments, Dean and Matthews were able to show that the extracellular application of a number of substances known to elicit insulin secretion, including glucose and glyceraldehyde, resulted in both a depolarisation of the β cell membrane and a modification of the cell's electrical behaviour, including the generation of spike potentials. Later, Matthews and Sakamoto (1975) demonstrated that the voltage-gated spike potentials were due to the inward movement of Ca^{2+}.

There was now a discussion as to how glucose evoked its effects. Did glucose bind to a membrane receptor to provoke stimulation, or was glucose fuelling cellular metabolism to provoke the response? Fortunately, Matthews and Sakamoto (1975) were able to answer these questions by demonstrating that inhibitors of sugar transport and metabolism prevented both insulin secretion from the cells and carbohydrate-evoked electrical activity, thus making the fuel hypothesis generally accepted (Hedeskov 1980; Wollheim and Biden 1987).

The link between carbohydrate metabolism and membrane depolarisation was demonstrated in 1975 by Sehlin and Taljedal to be a decrease in the

Young · Wong, Epithelial Secretion of Water and Electrolytes
© Springer-Verlag Berlin · Heidelberg 1990

permeability of the cell membrane to potassium ions. However, it was not until some 10 years later that the identity of this potassium conductance pathway was identified through the use of the improved patch-clamp recording technique to study single-channel currents (Hamill et al. 1981).

Patch-clamp experiments of insulin-secreting cells have been carried out on a number of preparations, including human and rodent β cells (Ashcroft et al. 1984, 1987; Cook and Hales 1984; Findlay et al. 1985b; Rorsman and Trube 1985) as well as clonal insulin-secreting cells (Dunne et al. 1986; Sturgess et al. 1986). Fortunately, it turns out that the properties of the different channels so far described show very little species differentiation.

The effect of 10 mmol/l glucose on the membrane potential of a single pancreatic β cell is demonstrated in Fig. 1. The whole-cell voltage record is taken from an individual rat β-cell in the current-clamp mode. When the cell is directly challenged with the sugar, there is a lag time of approximately 1 min which is followed by a clear depolarisation of the membrane and the initiation of Ca^{2+} spike potentials. These action potential-like spikes are then maintained throughout the duration of the experiment.

Only one particular type of K^+ channel is operational in intact unstimulated insulin-secreting cells – a channel that is selectively closed when cells are challenged with either glucose or glyceraldehyde (Ashcroft et al. 1984; Dunne et al. 1986). Since this channel is exactly the same as the one shown to be inhibited by the intracellular application of ATP (Cook and Hales 1984; Rorsman and Trube 1985), closure of the ATP-sensitive K^+ channel in intact cells initiates the membrane depolarisation.

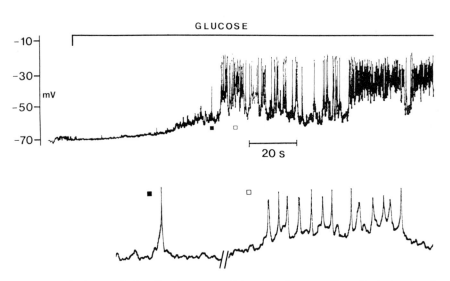

Fig. 1. Patch-clamp, whole-cell voltage record (current-clamp configuration) showing the effect of glucose (10 mmol/l) on the membrane potential of a cultured rat β cell. The record begins 300 s after the recording configuration was generated. *Expanded inserts* come from the periods indicated by the *solid* and *open squares*

Properties of ATP-Sensitive Potassium Channels

Two types of ATP-sensitive K^+ channel (K_{ATP} channel) exist in the membranes of insulin-secreting cells (Dunne et al. 1986). Both these channels, the large and the small K_{ATP} channel, appear to have the same biophysical characteristics (differing only in unit conductance) and are controlled in a similar manner by both external and internal molecules. Hence, we have restricted our discussion to the larger of the two channels.

The frequency of K_{ATP} channel openings in studies on the intact cell is extremely low and typified by very brief and infrequent openings from one to two channels. However, when either a detergent, such as saponin, is used to make holes in the plasma membrane (outside the isolated patch from where the recording is made) thereby equilibrating the cell interior with the bath solution ("open-cell"), or when a patch of membrane is excised from the cell, many more channel open events become apparent with much longer dwell times (Petersen and Dunne 1988). Experiments of this type, in which the internal solution is equilibrated with an ATP-free bath solution, indicate that in the intact cell, the ATP-sensitive K^+ channels are tonically inhibited by some endogenous molecule, which is probably ATP (Dunne et al. 1986; Petersen and Findlay 1987).

The density of K_{ATP} channels in intact cells has been investigated. Rorsman and Trube (1985) report that of the 500 or so K^+ channels present in the intact cell, less than 1% are active in the resting cell. In our studies the density of channels is considerably higher than the 500 or so predicted by Rorsman and Trube (1985). Assuming that the average open-tip area of a 5 MΩ pipette is around 2.5 μm^2 (Sakmann and Neher 1983) and that in the open-cell preparation there are on average 12 ± 1 active K_{ATP} channels per patch (Dunne et al. 1986), the mean number of channels per μm^2 will be about five. As the diameter of an intact cell is approximately 12.5 μm, the total number of channels per cell must be somewhere in the region of 2400. However, as some patches have upwards of 55 active K_{ATP} channels, giving an average cell density of more than 10000 channels, the possibility may exist that there are regions or "hot spots" where the density of K^+ channels is extraordinarily high.

K_{ATP} channels express a degree of inward current rectification by preferentially allowing K^+ ions to enter the cell whilst restricting their efflux (Ashcroft et al. 1984; Dunne et al. 1986). This rectification is probably due to the intracellular content of Na^+ and/or Mg^{2+} ions (Findlay 1987). The frequency of channel openings and closures is relatively unaffected by the potential of the membrane (Ashcroft 1988) and is not thought to be influenced by changes in the internal free Ca^{2+} concentration (Cook and Hales 1984). K_{ATP} channels are, however, regulated in a complex manner by a variety of internally applied nucleotides.

The principal effect of ATP on K^+ channels is to evoke closure. The ATP action is characterised by: (a) being mediated through the free ATP ionic complex ATP^{4-}, (b) the nucleotide acting specifically from the membrane inside, ATP will not close channels when it is added to the external membrane surface since ATP^{4-} is non-hydrophobic, (c) reducing both the mean open time of the channels and the number of channel-open events per burst, (d) having no effect on the single-channel conductance and (e) being independent of the membrane potential of the cell.

ATP also has a number of stimulatory influences on channels. First, internal ATP has been found effectively and dramatically to reverse the run down of K^+ channels. This effect is dose dependent, influenced by the length of exposure of the membrane to ATP and cannot be mimicked by either non-hydrolyzable analogues of ATP or by Mg^{2+}-free, ATP-containing solutions (Findlay and Dunne 1986; Trube et al. 1986; Ohno-Shosaku et al. 1987). This indicates that the process of maintaining channel integrity involves at least one ATP-fuelled protein phosphorylation step. Secondly, high concentrations of ATP (5 mmol/l) added to the inside of the membrane for extended periods of time result, after an initial period of complete channel inhibition, in a clear recovery of channel openings (Findlay and Dunne 1986). Finally, ATP will also evoke direct K^+ channel activation, at concentrations ranging from 10 to 50 µmol/l (Dunne et al. 1988 a).

The action of ADP is complicated. In general, low concentrations of ADP, less than 0.5 mmol/l, open channels, whereas higher concentrations close K^+ channels (Dunne and Petersen 1986a; Kakei et al. 1986). ADP-β-S, a non-hydrolyzable analogue of the nucleotide, consistently fails to open K^+ channels (Dunne and Petersen 1986a; Dunne et al. 1988b). These somewhat unpredictable and varied effects of ADP when added alone are not apparent when ADP is added to patches where K^+ channels are inhibited by ATP. Under these conditions ADP will invariably open, or reactivate channels in a dose-dependent manner, even when the concentration of ADP is very low in comparison with that of ATP (Dunne et al. 1988b). Interestingly, this effect of ADP can be mimicked by ADP-β-S, implying that competitive interactions between ATP and ADP in the intact cell may be important in determining the ability of K^+ channels to open. The reduced and non-reduced forms of the pyridine nucleotides also influence channel behaviour. High concentrations (> 500 µmol/l) inhibit channels, whereas low concentrations (< 500 µmol/l) of each nucleotide open channels (Dunne et al. 1988 a).

The actions of the guanosine nucoeotides have also been studied. GTP, GDP and their non-hydrolyzable analogues all open K_{ATP} channels, at concentrations ranging between 10 µmol/l and 2 mmol/l (Dunne and Petersen 1986b). Can the effects of the guanosine nucleotides be explained by the possible involvement of a transducer-type G protein? On the basis of the experiments carried out in the original study by Dunne and Petersen (1986b) apparently not, since the action of GDP should be the opposite to that of GTP, and the effects of GTP, GDP and their analogues should be distinguishable. However, recent experiments carried out in our laboratory have shown that the alumino-fluoride complex, AlF_4^-, which is known to have effects on a number of G protein regulated systems (Bigay et al. 1987), will also evoke a potent and dose-dependent (1 to 10 mmol/l) activation of K_{ATP} channels (Dunne et al. 1989). It is therefore possible to model the effects of the guanosine nucleotides and the activation of K^+ channels evoked by AlF_4^-, in terms of G proteins, if we assume there are a number of different control inputs to the K_{ATP} channel. The effects of GTP, GDP and GTP and GDP analogues could be explained by the nucleotides binding to an 'activating site' on the channel, or its control unit(s), a binding domain that is distinct from the putative transducing G protein site.

Due to the link between K^+ channel closure and the initiation of insulin secretion, it is not surprising that the pharmacology of these channels is of particular interest to the treatment of insulin-regulation disorders. The sulphonamide drug diazoxide, which has been used clinically to treat insulinomas, inhibits insulin secretion through the specific activation of K_{ATP} channels (Trube et al. 1986). This activation requires the presence of soluble cytosolic molecules since the effects of the drug are only ever consistently observed in the presence of internal ATP (Dunne et al. 1987). The structurally related sulphonylurea drugs tolbutamide, glibenclamide and glipizide have been used for many years in the treatment of non-insulin-dependent diabetes (type II), as each will provoke the stimulation of insulin secretion. Patch-clamp studies have shown that these drugs specifically close K_{ATP} channels, without influencing the gating of other K^+ channels both in intact cells as well as excised patches and open cells (Sturgess et al. 1985; Trube et al. 1986; Dunne et al. 1987; Zunkler et al. 1988a). Inhibition of channels by tolbutamide occurs independently of the availability of Mg^{2+} ions (Dunne et al. 1987) and is enhanced by ADP (Zunkler et al. 1988b), indicating that the differing effects of the sulphonylureas and diazoxide are mediated by the drugs binding to different sites on the channel, or control units, in the plasma membrane.

Since the potent sulphonylurea compound glibenclamide has an extremely high affinity for the K^+ channel ($K_D = 0.06$ nmol/l), and is therefore around 1000 times more effective at closing them than tolbutamide, the drug may ultimately be used in the purification and isolation of the channel (Petersen 1988b). As the availability of functional expression system is essential for successful cloning, it is interesting that Ashcroft and her collaborators (1988) have recently reported that membrane patches obtained from *Xenopus laevis* oocytes injected with poly(A^+) mRNA from the HIT-T15 insulin-secreting cells express both ATP- and Ca^{2+}-sensitive K^+ channels.

The intricate control of the K_{ATP} channel gating becomes even more complex when we consider that the channel is also influenced by a Ca^{2+}- and phospholipid-dependent protein kinase C input (Petersen 1988b). Wollheim et al. (1988) first demonstrated that potent activators of kinase C, such as phorbol esters (PMA) and cell-permeable diacylglycerols (DC_{10}), promote the release of insulin through the specific closure of ATP-sensitive K^+ channels in intact cells. The direct action of protein kinase C activators on K^+ channels inhibited by ATP and ADP has also been investigated in our laboratory, with interesting results (unpublished data). When applied in the open-cell recording configuration, PMA was able to close K^+ channels with a time course comparable to that seen in the intact cell, but later in the experiment the phorbol ester was also able to evoke a clear activation of channels, similar to that reported in intact cells by Ribalet et al. (1988). Novel biphasic effects of phorbol esters have also been reported in other regulated systems, such as the Ca^{2+} channels in cardiac cells (Lecarda et al. 1988).

Properties of Calcium- and Voltage-Sensitive Potassium Channels

The Ca^{2+}- and voltage-activated K^+ channel in insulin-secreting cells is very similar to the channels described in a number of exocrine, endocrine, muscle and nerve cells (Petersen and Maruyama 1984). With a high unit conductance of between 200 and 300 pS in symmetrical K^+-rich solutions, the channel is inoperative in intact resting cells (-70 mV membrane potential), but open during membrane depolarisations (Findlay et al. 1985a; Petersen and Findlay 1987). The relation between channel open-state probability and membrane potential is characterised by a saturating sigmoidal curve that is shifted to more negative potentials as $[Ca^{2+}]_i$ increases. The sensitivity of the channel to changes in the internal Ca^{2+} concentration is high, between 10^{-6} and 10^{-7} mol/l, with significant levels of channel openings being observed at negative potentials in the elevated Ca^{2+}-containing solutions (Findlay et al. 1985a). The Ca^{2+}- and voltage-activated K^+ channel is also influenced by changes in the internal pH of the cells (Cook et al. 1984).

Properties of Voltage-Sensitive Calcium Channels

The purpose of carbohydrate-induced K_{ATP} channel closure is to evoke a membrane depolarisation that is required for the opening of voltage-gated Ca^{2+} channels (Petersen and Findlay 1987). Whole-cell, inward Ca^{2+} currents have been described in neonatal rat β cells (Satin and Cook 1985, 1988), mouse β cells (Rorsman and Trube 1986; Plant 1988a) and clonal insulin-secreting cells (Findlay and Dunne 1985; Rorsman et al. 1986). However, only two studies have identified single Ca^{2+} channel currents, using Ba^{2+} ions as the current charge carrier. In the original investigation of Ca^{2+} channels, Velasco et al. (1988) described a 30-pS channel whose gating was promoted by depolarising the membrane potential from -70 to -20 mV. The channel showed little inactivation over a 200 ms period, indicative of the L-type Ca^{2+} channel described in heart cells (Reuter 1983).

The only other study of Ca^{2+} channels (Rorsman et al. 1988) largely confirmed the findings of Velasco et al. (1988) by describing a 24-pS, L-type, voltage-activated channel sensitive to the Ca^{2+}-channel agonist BAY K8644.

Significantly, in potassium-depolarised intact RINm5F insulin-secreting cells, Velasco et al. (1988) also found that the gating of the L-type Ca^{2+} channel was influenced by glyceraldehyde. D-glyceraldehyde enhanced the open probability of channels by increasing the mean channel open time and causing a corresponding decrease in the longer of the two mean closed times, as well as decreasing the threshold potential for voltage activation. This result may have important physiological implications. In RINm5F cells, D-glyceraldehyde depolarises the membrane by about 50 mV (Dunne et al. 1986). If the sugar only influenced the gating of the Ca^{2+}-channels via the depolarization, then the probability of opening would be very low (approximately 0.01, Velasco et al. 1988). However, because of its modulation of channel gating, a depolarization of 50 mV evokes a significant increase in the degree of channel gating (open probability $= 0.12$).

The mechanism by which glyceraldehyde modulates Ca^{2+} channels is unknown. There is evidence to suggest that cyclic AMP favours the opening of Ca^{2+} channels in insulin-secreting cells (Prentki and Matschinsky 1987), and cytosolic cyclic AMP has been shown to open Ca^{2+} channels in the heart (Cachelin et al. 1983). However, cyclic AMP levels have been shown to vary very little in response to 10 mmol/l D-glyceraldehyde in these cells (Wollheim et al. 1984). One interesting possibility is that during stimulation, Ca^{2+} channels could be modulated by a kinase C-mediated phosphorylation process in a similar manner to that seen for the ATP-sensitive K^+ channel (Petersen 1988 b).

Properties of Voltage-Sensitive Sodium Channels

The only study to date in which both voltage-gated Na^+ currents and single Na^+ channels have been presented is that of Plant (1988b). Using the whole-cell patch-clamp technique applied to primary cultured pancreatic β cells, tetrodotoxin-sensitive Na^+ currents were generated by the application of a depolarising voltage to the membrane from a holding potential or prepulse potential more negative than -80 mV. Similarly, single Na^+ channel currents, opening with an amplitude of 1 pA at -30 mV, were also recorded from outside-out patches. However, because the Na^+ currents were found to be inactive at potentials more positive than -80 mV, Plant (1988b) concludes that these channels are unlikeky to play a major role in stimulus-secretion coupling. Whether these voltage-inactivation characteristics are indeed an intrinsic property of the channels in insulin-secreting cells or simply artefacts of the particular recording configurations remains to be determined.

Properties of Non-specific Cation Channels

Non-specific cation channels (Ca^{2+}-NS) have currently only been described in the clonal insulin-secreting cell line CR1-G1 (Sturgess et al. 1986). These channels have a conductance of 25 pS, are activated by changes in the internal concentration of Ca^{2+} and inhibited by adenine nucleotides with a potency series of AMP > ADP > ATP > adenosine. One postulated role for these channels is to maintain the rhythmical pattern of electrical activity experienced by the cells in the presence of sustained exposure to carbohydrate (Fig. 1), thereby behaving in a similar manner to the non-selective cation channels described in heart cells (Partridge and Swandulla 1988). However, since in the CR1-G1 cells the levels of calcium required to open the channels is in the millimolar range, the physiological significance of these channels is doubtful.

Carbohydrate-Induced Insulin Secretion

The effect of glucose on the membrane potential of a single pancreatic β cell has been demonstrated in Fig. 1. In Fig. 2 we have summarised the current knowledge relating to the involvement of the various ion channels described in the regulation of insulin secretion.

The following sequence of events is proposed for carbohydrate-induced insulin secretion: in the resting cell the membrane potential, as in most cell types, is determined by a transmembrane K^+ gradient maintained by the $Na^+ - K^+$ pump and the presence of open ATP-sensitive K^+ channels. At concentrations high enough to elicit insulin release, the metabolism of either glucose or glyceraldehyde evokes a decrease in the potential difference across the plasma membrane (a membrane depolarisation), by a decrease in the open probability of the K_{ATP} channels. The link that couples carbohydrate metabolism to the closure of channels is unknown, but may involve changes in the concentration and/or activity of the adenosine or pyridine nucleotides, and/or the activation of a calcium- and phospholipid-dependent protein kinase C, via the metabolic generation of 1,2 diacylglycerol. Membrane depolarisation opens a voltage-dependent Ca^{2+} gate through which Ca^{2+} ions can enter the cell. At the point of opening of the Ca^{2+} channels the membrane potential will be around $-20\,mV$, and this depolarisation coupled with the ensuing rise in the cytosolic concentration of Ca^{2+} will cause the calcium- and voltage-dependent K^+ channel to open. The opening of the high-conductance channel will tend to depolarise the membrane, thereby closing the Ca^{2+} gate. Closure of Ca^{2+} channels will decrease $[Ca^{2+}]_i$ which, coupled with a return towards the high-resting negative membrane potential, will tend to close the large K^+ channel. As these channels close, a renewed depolarisation of the membrane is generated,

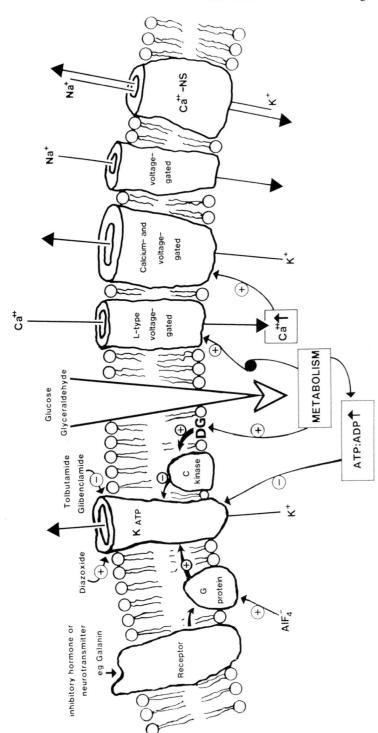

Fig. 2. Single-ion channels in the plasma membrane of insulin-secreting cells and their regulatory inputs. K_{ATP}, the ATP-sensitive potassium channel; $Ca^{++}-NS$, the non-selective cation channel

promoting opening of the voltage-dependent Ca^{2+} channels. A cycle of channel openings and closures has, therefore, been initiated, which leads to repetitive firing of Ca^{2+} action-potential spikes. The culmination of these changes in potential is the generation of finely controlled waves of Ca^{2+} influx, as recently demonstrated by Grapengiesser et al. (1988), which is the key intracellular signal for the secretion of insulin by exocytosis from the cell, granular fusion with the plasma membrane and release at the point of contact. As the extracellular glucose concentration drops below the normal resting level, reopening of the ATP-sensitive K^+ channel and closure of other channels results, establishing once again the normal resting conditions.

This proposed scheme of events does raise a number of issues. First, how are the ATP-sensitive K^+ channels able to open in the intact insulin-secreting cell when all the K^+ channels can be closed in inside-out patches and open cells by the application of 2 mmol/l ATP to the inside of the membrane and the intracellular concentration of ATP is between 4 and 6 mmol/l (Petersen and Findlay 1987)? The simplest explanation for this discrepancy is that in the intact cell, additional modulators of channel gating exist that are able to influence the sensitivity of channels to ATP. One effective modulator is ADP, which has been shown to open ATP-inhibited channels even in the presence of a greater than 20:1 excess of ATP to ADP (Dunne et al. 1988 b). As well as ADP, AMP (Dunne 1988) and the pyridine nucleotides (Dunne et al. 1988 a) have also been shown to reduce the sensitivity of K^+ channels to ATP, though to a much lesser extent.

It has been estimated that because of the high sensitivity of the K_{ATP} channel to ATP, with a K_i of approximately 15 μmol/l (Cook and Hales 1984; Rorsman and Trube 1985), between 90%–99% of the channels in the normal resting cell will be permanently inhibited. Cook and his collaborators (1988) argue that this confers a number of important metabolic advantages on the functioning β cell. Having a large number of 'spare channels' may mean that the cell has maximal sensitivity to its environment. Working close to its inactive state provides the cell with the ability to respond with the largest relative change in signal for the smallest relative change in the external stimulus. Furthermore, having the majority of channels closed is the least expensive in terms of energy, and the summation of the activities of many channels working at low levels of open probability provides the cell with a greater degree of stability, in comparison with a few channels generating the same surrent by opening for longer periods of time.

It must be stressed that the closure of ATP-sensitive K^+ channels by themselves would *not* provide the cell with a membrane depolarisation; this can only be explained if the cell maintains an inward current during stimulation. Such an inward current may be carried by either Na^+ or Cl^- ions, or indeed both. So far only single- and whole-cell Na^+ currents have been described in insulin-secreting cells, and these appear to be inactive at physiological membrane potentials. Studies of radiolabelled Cl^- fluxes have recently suggested the existence of voltage-dependent Cl^- channels in these cells (Sehlin 1987), and if Cl^- were to be accumulated by a $Na^+-K^+-2Cl^-$ co-transport mechanism (Petersen 1988a), then the opening of Cl^- channels would provide the required inward current (Petersen 1988b).

Inhibition of Insulin Secretion by the Actions of Hormones and Neurotransmitters

The actions of inhibitory hormones and neurotransmitters on insulin secretion have so far failed to hold the attention of β-cell patch-clamp electrophysiologists, except for the hyperglycemia-inducing neuropeptide galanin. In a manner similar to that with which the initiation of carbohydrate-induced membrane depolarisations can be explained by the closure of ATP-sensitive K^+ channels, inhibition of insulin-secretion, mediated by a membrane hyperpolarisation, could be brought about by the specific activation of these channels. Such a mechanism appears to underlie the inhibitory effects of galanin. The 29 amino acid polypeptide has for a number of years been known to abolish the secretion of insulin under a number of experimental conditions both in vivo and in the isolated perfused pancreas (Ahren et al. 1987).

The first electrophysiological investigations of galanin were caried out by Lazdunski and his collaborators (DeWeille et al. 1988). In this study it was demonstrated that the polypeptide is able to hyperpolarise the cell membrane and thereby reduce the spontaneous electrical activity of the cell through the specific activation of ATP-sensitive K^+ channels. Dunne et al. (1989) demonstrated directly that galanin was able to open K^+ channels. Using outside-out membrane patches, with GTP, ATP and ADP on the cytosolic surface of the membrane, galanin was found to provoke a pronounced and fully reversible activation of K^+ channels. Furthermore, since the inhibitory action of the neuropeptide on carbohydrate-induced insulin secretion and its hyperpolarizing effect were abolished in cells that had been pretreated with *pertussis* toxin for a number of hours, it was concluded that the effects of galanin were mediated by the activation of a *pertussis* toxin-sensitive G protein (Dunne et al. 1989).

Conclusions and Perspectives

There is now firm evidence that the three types of ion channel presented in Fig. 2 do exist in the insulin-secreting cell preparation, but a number of questions remain unanswered.

1. Although there can now be little doubt that the closure of K_{ATP} channels initiates the membrane depolarisation in response to carbohydrate stimulation, the mechanism by which channel closure is brought about is

far from proven. Several current hypotheses have been reviewed, and although possible, indeed plausible, their role in stimulus-secretion coupling is by no means certain. Alternative mechanisms to explain the various channel closures and openings will doubtless be put forward, and the ideas presented in this article re-evaluated. To this end, it is significant that the internal second messenger system in exocrine cells is currently undergoing redefinition in view of the novel experiments undertaken by Morris et al. (1987), using whole-cell internal perfusion of inositolpoly-phosphates. A similar approach is required for the insulin-secreting cells.

2. The advancement of current technology to detect changes in internal molecule concentrations at a high resolution would either prove or dismiss the role(s) of the various nucleotides in stimulus-secretion coupling.

3. It must also be remembered that the majority of patch-clamp investigations of insulin-secreting cells conducted so far have addressed themselves to the events that mediate the initial depolarisation of the membrane. Under steady-state conditions of carbohydrate stimulation, membrane potential fluctuations are complex, consisting of oscillatory waves of depolarisation and repolarisation generating plateau potentials upon which are superimposed Ca^{2+} spike potentials. The cellular mechanisms that mediate these changes in potential along with the ionic events responsible for them have so far remained unaddressed and therefore unanswered.

4. Finally, since the ion channels identified to date appear to be very similar in a number of different insulin-secreting cell preparations, investigations of ion channels in diabetic systems, including animal and human tissues, are of obvious importance. It would not be surprising if defects in the regulatory processes of channel gating prevail in tissues expressing the disease.

References

Ashcroft FM (1988) Adenosine 5'-triphosphate-sensitive potassium channels. Annu Rev Neurosci 11: 97–118

Ashcroft FM, Harrison DE, Ashcroft SJH (1984) Glucose induces closure of single potassium channels in isolated rat pancreatic B-cells. Nature 312: 446–448

Ashcroft FM, Kakei M, Kelly R, Sutton R (1987) ATP-sensitive K^+ channels in isolated human pancreatic B-cells. FEBS Lett 215: 9–12

Ashcroft FM, Ashcroft SJH, Berggren P-O, Botholz C, Rorsman P, Trube G, Welsh M (1988) Expression of K^+ channels in Xenopus laevis oocytes injected with poly(A^+) mRNA from the insulin-secreting B-cell line HIT T15. FEBS Lett 239: 185–189

Ahren B, Rorsman P, Berggren P-O (1988) Galanin and the endocrine pancreas. FEBS Lett 229: 233–237

Bigay J, Deterre P, Pfister C, Chabre M (1987) Fluoride complexes of aluminium or beryllium act on G proteins as reversibly bound analogues of the γ-phosphate of GTP. EMBO J 6: 2907–2913

Cachelin AB, De Payer JE, Kokobun S, Reuter H (1983) Calcium channel modulation by 8 bromo-cyclic AMP in cultures heart cells. Nature 304: 462–464

Cook DL, Hales CN (1984) Intracellular ATP directly blocks K^+ channels in pancreatic B-cells. Nature 311: 271–273

Cook DL, Ikeuchi M, Fujimoto WY (1984) Lowering of pH_i inhibits Ca^{2+}-activated K^+ channels in pancreatic B-cells. Nature 311: 269–271

Cook DL, Satin LS, Ashford MLJ, Hales CN (1988) ATP-sensitive K^+ channels in pancreatic B-cells. Spare-channel hypothesis. Diabetes 37: 495–498

Dean PM, Matthews EK (1968) Electrical activity in pancreatic islet cells. Nature 219: 389–390

De Weille J, Schmid-Antomarchi H, Fosset M, Lazdunski M (1988) ATP-sensitive K^+ channels that are blocked by hypoglycemia-inducing sulphonylureas in insulin-secreting cells are activated by galanin, a hyperglycemia-inducing hormone. Proc Natl Acad Sci USA 83: 517–521

Dunne MJ (1988) Ion channels in insulin-secreting cells. PhD thesis, Liverpool University, England

Dunne MJ, Petersen OH (1986a) Intracellular ADP activates K^+ channels that are inhibited by ATP in an insulin-secreting cell line. FEBS Lett 208: 59–62

Dunne MJ, Petersen OH (1986b) GTP and GDP activation of K^+ channels that can be inhibited by ATP. Pflügers Arch 407: 564–565

Dunne MJ, Findlay I, Petersen OH, Wollheim CB (1986) ATP-sensitive K^+ channels in an insulin-secreting cell-line are inhibited by D-glyceraldehyde and activated by membrane permeabilization. J Membr Biol 93: 271–279

Dunne MJ, Ilott MC, Petersen OH (1987) Interactions of diazoxide, tolbutamide and ATP^{4-} on nucleotide-dependent K^+ channels in an insulin-secreting cell line. J Membr Biol 99: 215–224

Dunne MJ, Findlay I, Petersen OH (1988a) The effects of pyridine nucleotides on the gating of ATP-sensitive K^+ channels in insulin-secreting cells. J Membr Biol 102: 205–216

Dunne MJ, West-Jordan J, Abraham RJ, Edwards RTH, Petersen OH (1988b) The gating of nucleotide dependent K^+ channels in insulin-secreting cells can be modulated by changes in the ratio ATP^{4-}/ADP^{3-} and by nonhydrolyzable analogues of ATP and ADP. J Membr Biol 104: 165–177

Dunne MJ, Bullett MJ, Li G, Wollheim CB, Petersen OH (1989) Galanin activates nucleotide-dependent K^+ channels via a pertussis toxin-sensitive G-protein. EMBO J 8: 412–420

Findlay I (1987) The effects of magnesium upon the ATP-sensitive K^+ channel in an insulin-secreting cell line. J Physiol (Lond) 391: 611–629

Findlay I, Dunne MJ (1985) Voltage-activated Ca^{2+} currents in insulin-secreting cells. FEBS Lett 189: 281–285

Findlay I, Dunne MJ (1986) ATP maintains ATP-inhibited K^+ channels in an operational state. Pflügers Arch 407: 238–240

Findlay I, Dunne MJ, Petersen OH (1985a) High conductance K^+ channel in pancreatic islet cells can be activated and inactivated by internal calcium. J Membr Biol 83: 169–175

Findlay I, Dunne MJ, Petersen OH (1985b) ATP-sensitive inward rectifier and voltage- and calcium-activated K^+ channels in cultured pancreatic islet cells. J Membr Biol 88: 165–172

Grapengiesser E, Gylfe E, Hellman B (1988) Glucose-induced oscillations of cytoplasmic Ca^{2+} in the pancreatic B-cell. Biochem Biophys Res Commun 151: 1299–1304

Hamill OP, Marty A, Neher E, Sakmann B, Sigworth FJ (1981) Improved patch-clamp techniques for high resolution current recordings from cells and cell-free membrane patches. Pflügers Arch 391: 85–100

Hedeskov CJ (1980) Mechanism of glucose-induced insulin secretion. Physiol Rev 60: 442–509

Kakei M, Kelly RP, Ashcroft SJH, Ashcroft FM (1986) The ATP-sensitivity of K^+ channels in rat pancreatic B-cells is modulated by ADP. FEBS Lett 208: 63–66

Lacerda AE, Rampe D, Brown AM (1988) Effects of protein kinase C activators on cardiac Ca^{2+} channels. Nature 335: 249–251

Matthews EK, Sakamoto Y (1975) Electrical characteristics of pancreatic islet cells. J Physiol (Lond) 246: 421–437

Morris AP, Gallacher DV, Irvine RF, Petersen OH (1987) Synergism of inositol trisphosphate and tetrakisphosphate in activating Ca^{2+}-dependent K^+ channels. Nature 330: 653–655

Ohno-Shosaku T, Zunkler BJ, Trube G (1987) Dual effects of ATP on K^+ currents in mouse pancreatic B-cells. Pflügers Arch 408: 133–138

Partridge LD, Swandulla D (1988) Calcium activated non-specific cation channels. Trends Neurosci 11: 69–72

Petersen OH (1988a) The control of ion channels and pumps in exocrine acinar cells. Comp Biochem Physiol 4: 717–720

Petersen OH (1988b) Control of potassium channels in insulin-secreting cells. ISI Atlas of Science: Biochemistry 1: 144–149

Petersen OH, Dunne MJ (1988) Regulation of insulin-secreting cells by control of potassium ion channels. In: Thorn NA, Treiman M, Petersen OH (eds) Molecular mechanisms in secretion (25th Alfred Benzon symposium 1987). Munksgaard, Copenhagen, pp 30–41

Petersen OH, Findlay I (1987) Electrophysiology of the pancreas. Physiol Rev 67: 1054–1116

Petersen OH, Maruyama Y (1984) Calcium-activated potassium channels and their role in secretion. Nature 307: 693–396

Plant TD (1988a) Properties and calcium-dependent inactivation of calcium currents in cultured mouse pancreatic B-cells. J Physiol (Lond) 404: 731–747

Plant TD (1988b) Na^+ currents in cultured mouse pancreatic B-cells. Pflügers Arch 411: 429–435

Prentki M, Matschinski FM (1987) Ca^{2+}, cAMP and phospholipid-derived messengers in coupling mechanisms of insulin secretion. Physiol Rev 67: 1185–1248

Reuter H (1983) Calcium channel modulation by neurotransmitters, enzymes and drugs. Nature 301: 569–574

Ribalet B, Eddlestone GT, Ciani S (1988) Metabolic regulation of the K(ATP) and a maxi-K(V) channel in the insulin-secreting RINm5F cell. J Gen Physiol 92: 219–237

Rorsman P, Trube G (1985) Glucose-dependent K^+ channels in pancreatic B-cells are regulated by intracellular ATP. Pflügers Arch 405: 305–309

Rorsman P, Trube G (1986) Calcium and delayed potassium currents in mouse pancreatic B-cells under voltage-clamp conditions. J Physiol (Lond) 374: 531–550

Rorsman P, Arkhammar P, Berggren P-O (1986) Voltage-activated Na^+ currents and their suppression by phorbol ester in clonal insulin-producing RINm5F cells. Am J Physiol 251: C912–C919

Rorsman P, Ashcroft FM, Trube G (1988) Single channel Ca^{2+} currents in mouse pancreatic B-cells. Pflügers Arch 412: 597–603

Sakmann B, Neher E (1983) Single-channel current recording. Plenum, New York

Satin LS, Cook DL (1985) Voltage-gated Ca^{2+} current in pancreatic B-cells. Pflügers Arch 404: 385–387

Satin LS, Cook DL (1988) Evidence for two calcium currents in insulin secreting cells. Pflügers Arch 411: 401–409

Sehlin J, Taljedal I-B (1975) Glucose-induced decrease in Rb^+ permeability in pancreatic B-cells. Nature 253: 635–636

Sehlin J (1987) Evidence for voltage-dependent Cl^- permeability in mouse pancreatic B-cells. Biosci Rep 7: 67–72

Sturgess NC, Ashford MLJ, Cook DL, Hales CN (1985) The sulphonylurea receptor may be an ATP-sensitive potassium channel. Lancet 8453: 474–475

Sturgess NC, Hales CN, Ashford MLJ (1986) Inhibition of calcium-activated, non-selective cation channel in a rat insulinoma cell line, by adenine derivatives. FEBS Lett 208: 397–400

Trube G, Rorsman P, Ohno-Shosaku T (1986) Opposite effects of tolbutamide and diazoxide on the ATP-dependent K^+ channel in mouse pancreatic B-cells. Pflügers Arch 407: 493–499

Velasco JM, Petersen JUH, Petersen OH (1988) Single-channel Ba^{2+} currents in insulin-secreting cells are activated by glyceraldehyde stimulation. FEBS Lett 231: 366–370

Wollheim CB, Biden TJ (1987) Signal transduction in insulin secretion: comparison between fuel and receptor agonist. Ann NY Acad Sci 488: 317–333

Wollheim CB, Ullrich S, Pozzan T (1984) Glyceraldehyde but not cyclic AMP-stimulated insulin release in preceeded by a rise in cytosolic free calcium. FEBS Lett 177: 17–22

Wollheim CB, Dunne MJ, Peter-Riesch B, Bruzzone R, Pozzan T, Petersen OH (1988) Activators of protein kinase C depolarise insulin-secreting cells by closing K^+ channels. EMBO J 7: 2443–2449

Zunkler BJ, Lenzen S, Manner K, Panten U, Trube G (1988a) Concentration-dependent effects of tolbutamide, meglitinide, glipizide, glibenclamide and diazoxide on ATP-regulated K^+ currents in pancreatic B-cells. Naunyn Schmiedebergs Arch Pharmacol 337: 225–230

Zunkler BJ, Lins S, Trube G, Panten U (1988b) Concentration-dependent effects of tolbutamide, meglitinide, glipizide, glibenclamide and diazoxide on ATP-regulated K^+ currents in pancreatic B-cells. Pflügers Arch 411: 613–619

5 Gastric Mucosa

Electrophysiological Aspects of Gastric Ion Transport

E. Frömter, S. Curci, and A. H. Gitter

Introduction

In comparison to nerve, muscle, and numerous epithelial organs such as intestine, kidney, and exocrine glands, electrophysiological studies on gastric epithelia have been less successful in the past. The reason for this is twofold: (1) In contrast, for example, to intestine, it is quite difficult to obtain viable in vitro preparations of mammalian gastric mucosa because cessation of blood circulation apparently leads to oxygen deficiency or catabolic poisoning and tends to render the tissue unresponsive to secretory stimuli. (2) In contrast to other epithelia, gastric mucosa has a very complex architecture. Fundus mucosa consists of a layer of surface epithelial cells (SEC) that is perforated by the openings of numerous gastric glands that are densely packed underneath the SEC layer and are composed of different cell types: enzyme and HCl secreting oxyntic cells (OC) in amphibia, and separate enzyme secreting chief cells (CC) and HCl secreting parietal cells (PC) in mammals, together with mucous neck cells (MC) and endocrine cells (EC). Since virtually only SEC could be punctured in the past, a detailed analysis of the major transport events was not possible.

To resolve this complex analysis problem, besides electrophysiology, different experimental approaches have been taken. Individual glands of rabbit stomach (Berglindh and Öbrink 1976), individual cells of mammalian and amphibian stomach (Soll 1978; Ayalon et al. 1982; Blum et al. 1971), as well as more or less purified membrane vesicle preparations of individual cell surface membranes (Forte et al. 1967; Lee et al. 1974; Sachs et al. 1976) have been developed and have been used for uptake studies based on fluorescence or tracer techniques. These studies have established that the central active mechanism in HCl secretion is an electroneutral ATP-driven K^+-H^+ exchange pump (Sachs et al. 1976; Forte and Lee 1977). It resides in the luminal cell membrane of PC or, respectively, OC and operates in parallel with passive K^+ and Cl^- conductances (Wolosin and Forte 1984;

Young · Wong, Epithelial Secretion of Water and Electrolytes
© Springer-Verlag Berlin · Heidelberg 1990

Cuppoletti and Sachs 1984) which allow K^+ ions to recirculate for continued pumping and Cl^- ions to follow the secreted H^+ ions towards the gland lumen. In addition, direct evidence has been obtained for $Cl^- - HCO_3^-$ exchange which facilitates Cl^- entry and HCO_3^- exit across the basolateral cell membrane of PC (Muallem et al. 1985; Paradiso et al. 1986).

In order to characterize the ionic transport mechanisms of individual cell membranes more completely, however, electrophysiological studies are indispensable. Thus, microelectrode experiments have recently also been performed on isolated gastric glands and attempts have been undertaken to isolate individual cell types and to grow them in monolayer culture for separate investigation in Ussing chambers. In addition, recently, techniques have been developed that allow individual OC of intact frog or *Necturus* gastric mucosa to be reliably investigated with microelectrodes. Taken together, these and other new approaches have not only opened up the field for future successful investigation with electrophysiological techniques, but have already helped to clarify some previous controversies and have provided new insight into the transport properties of gastric cells. In this review we intend to summarize the knowledge that the new approaches have provided. For reason of space, however, no attempt will be made to cover the older literature completely (for review see Durbin 1967; Sachs et al. 1978; Forte et al. 1980).

Electrophysiological Approaches to Study Gastric Ion Transport

Transepithelial Potential and Resistance Measurements

As mentioned above the proper interpretation of transepithelial studies of open circuit potentials (V_t), resistances (R_t), and short circuit current (I_{sc}) is hampered by the complex nature of gastric mucosal architecture. Generally, it has been found that resting stomachs filled with bicarbonate Ringer solution or isolated mucosae bathed on either surface with identical Ringer solutions generate a lumen-negative V_t that varies between -10 and -60 mV depending on the species investigated (Durbin 1967). This potential difference reflects the sum of all active cation and anion fluxes that can be determined when the tissue is short-circuited. In the resting state I_{sc} is usually well accounted for by the sum of net active Na^+ absorption (not present in all species) and net active Cl^- secretion (Hogben 1955), while net K^+ and H^+ fluxes are negligibly small. Upon stimulation with histamine, V_t, I_{ss}, and R_t decrease, while H^+ secretion and Cl^- secretion increase in virtually all species studied: frog (Hogben 1955), rat and guinea pig (Sernka and Hogben 1969), piglet (Forte and Machen 1975), and dog (Kuo and Shanbour 1979).

Much effort has been made in the past to identify whether or not H^+ and Cl^- secretion are independent rheogenic processes. Since frog gastric fundus mucosa bathed in Cl^--free SO_4^{2-}-Ringer-solution was found to generate a reversed (lumen-positive) I_{sc}, and since the rate of H^+ secretion could be altered by applied voltages (Rehm 1956; Rehm and Lefevre 1965; Shoemaker and Sachs 1972), it was concluded that H^+ secretion was an independent rheogenic active transport. The same conclusion was also reached for active Cl^- secretion (Hogben 1955; Starlinger et al. 1986) for which two different mechanisms were postulated: (1) nonacidic active Cl^- secretion (observed in the resting state when active H^+ secretion was negligible) and (2) acidic active Cl^- secretion (observed after stimulation). In an attempt to define single cell membrane transport mechanisms, V_t and R_t measurements have been performed under conditions of unilateral ion substitution or during application of more or less specific inhibitors. These studies have identified Na^+ and K^+ conductances on the apical surface of gastric mucosa of several species without being able, however, to clarify whether the observed conductances were located in SEC or OC (or, respectively, PC or CC). Moreover, corresponding studies have provided evidence for a K^+ permeability and for a Na^+-K^+ pump on the basolateral surface of gastric mucosa. These data shall not be presented and discussed in detail here (see, for example, Harris and Edelman 1964). We want to mention, however, that recently more or less direct evidence was published for a basolateral bicarbonate conductance (Schwartz et al. 1985), a $Na^+-HCO_3^-$ cotransporter (Klemperer et al. 1983), and a rheogenic $Na^+-(Cl^-)_n$ cotransporter with $n>1$ (Carrasquer et al. 1982). These data, however, were only in part convincing, and the cellular localization of the postulated transport mechanisms remained unidentified.

Usually, more direct insight into an ion transport mechanism can be obtained if instead of macroscopic I_{sc} or V_t the frequency and amplitude of the microscopic fluctuations ("noise") of I_{sc} or V_t are analyzed, which reflect molecular properties of the underlying transport mechanism. Such studies have been very fruitful in the analysis of ion transport across frog skin (van Driessche and Zeiske 1985). To our knowledge, however, thus far only one such study has been performed on gastric mucosa, from which the authors have concluded that the current fluctuations observed in the presence and absence of inhibitors (e.g., Ba^{2+}) support the existence of apical K^+ channels and Cl^- channels in stimulated frog gastric mucosa (Zeiske et al. 1983).

Cell Potential Measurements

Surface Epithelial Cells

Since the first experiments by Villegas in 1962, a considerable number of microelectrode experiments has been undertaken on SEC of various species of frog and on *Necturus*. When mucosae were bathed on either surface in identical NaCl Ringer solution, the membrane potential of SEC, referred to the serosal surface, was usually estimated to be around -50 mV (cytoplasm negative, see, for example, Villegas 1962; Shoemaker and Sachs 1972; Shoemaker 1978). Recently, however, higher values have been obtained which range up to -70 mV (Curci and Schettino 1984) and are more likely to be correct.

As in transepithelial measurements, attemps have been made to determine ionic cell membrane permeabilities by suddenly changing apical or basolateral ion concentrations or by applying selective inhibitors (e.g., Ba^{2+}). Such experiments have provided evidence for a small apical K^+ conductance (Shoemaker and Sachs 1972) and for an amiloride-inhibitable apical Na^+ conductance in *Necturus* SEC (Demarest et al. 1986), but the results for Cl^- were conflicting. While Shoemaker and Sachs (1972) and Machen and Zeuthen (1982) postulated the presence of a significant Cl^- conductance, other investigators could not confirm these data, neither in frog nor in *Necturus* (Curci and Schettino 1984; Schettino and Curci 1985; Demarest et al. 1986). Using the same approaches, the basolateral cell membrane of SEC was found to have both a large K^+ and a significant Cl^- conductance (Shoemaker and Sachs 1972; Spenney et al. 1974; Curci and Schettino 1984).

Oxyntic Cells

The first attempts to puncture oxyntic cells were made by advancing microelectrodes from the luminal surface deep into the mucosa with or without later histological identification of the puncture site. Using this approach, Villegas (1962) and Shoemaker (1978) obtained serosal membrane potentials of between -14 and -20 mV, which, as many experts felt, were not convincing. Consequently it was thought that OC, which are covered at the serosal surface with a thick layer of muscle fibers and connective tissues, might not be amenable to micropuncture. Recently, however, two laboratories succeeded in dissecting off the connective tissue layer and puncturing OC directly (Demarest and Machen 1985; Curci et al. 1987). These experiments yielded serosal cell membrane potentials of around -40 to -50 mV or, respectively, -60 to -70 mV (cytoplasm negative) which could be kept stable for hours and clearly show that the older measurements were artifacts. By performing serosal ion substitution experiments, it was also possible to investigate ionic conductances of the serosal cell membrane. Thus

———————————————————————————————➤

Fig. 1. Response of basolateral cell membrane potential (V_s) of frog oxyntic cell to reduction of serosal HCO_3^- and/or Na^+ concentration. Trace record of V_s (*lower line, left ordinate*) and of transepithelial potential difference (V_t, *upper line, right ordinate*) during reduction of serosal HCO_3^- from 17.8 to 6 mmol/l or during replacement of serosal Na^+ by N-methyl-D-glucamine. Note net anionic charge efflux in both cases and lack of response to HCO_3^- in Na^+-free conditions, indicating the presence of rheogenic $Na^+-(HCO_3^-)_n$ cotransport with $n \geq 1$ (from Curci et al. 1987)

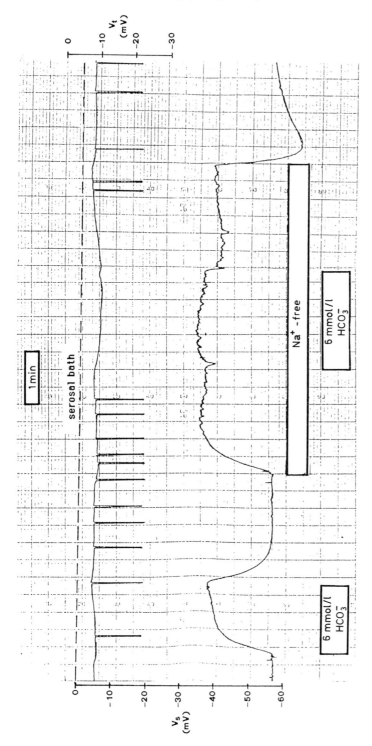

a barium-inhibitable K^+ conductance was observed, but no evidence was obtained for a significant Cl^- conductance (S. Curci and collaborators, unpublished). Instead, when changing serosal HCO_3^- and serosal Na^+ concentration, a rheogenic $Na^+-(HCO_3^-)_n$ cotransport mechanism was detected (Fig. 1) that could be inhibited by the disulfonic stilbene, 4-acetamino-4'-isothiocyanatostilbene-2,2'-disulfonic acid (SITS). It resembles closely the renal $Na^+-(HCO_3^-)_3$ cotransporter that has recently been described (Boron and Boulpaep 1983; Yoshitomi et al. 1985). It may explain the anomalous dependence of V_t on Na^+ and its dependence on HCO_3^- that led Rehm and collaborators to postulate rheogenic $Na^+-(Cl^-)_n$ cotransport and/or a HCO_3^- conductance (see above). In contrast to the renal cotransporter, however, the stoichiometry of the gastric cotransporter, which may also be present in antrum (Flemström and Sachs 1975), is not yet known.

Thus far, only preliminary observations are available on whether, and if so, how these basolateral ionic permeabilities of OC change during stimulation by histamine or cyclic AMP. They indicate that the K^+ conductance increases slightly, both in *Necturus* (Demarest et al. 1986) and frog (S. Curci and collaborators, unpublished), while $Na^+-(HCO_3^-)_n$ permeability appears to decrease (Curci et al. 1988).

Parietal Cells and Chief Cells

As compared to amphibian tissue, much less progress has been made in mammalian tissue. Regarding SEC properties there is only one report on microelectrode experiments in intact mammalian gastric mucosa (Canosa and Rehm 1968), and recent attempts to grow isolated SEC in monolayer cultures are not yet far advanced (Ayalon et al. 1982; Rutten et al. 1985). Recently, some attempts have also been made to puncture PC and non-PC of isolated gastric tubules and of gastric cell cultures of newborn rats. However, the results were not fully convincing. Kafoglis et al. (1984) reported membrane potentials of ca. $-7\,mV$ (obtained on isolated rabbit glands) while Okada and Ueda (1984) and Schettino et al. (1985) reported values between -20 and $-40\,mV$ (on cultured cells or on microdissected rabbit glands). Attempts to identify ionic conductances have confirmed the presence of a K^+ conductance and the absence of a significant Cl^- conductance in the basolateral membrane of rabbit PC. In one study, however, it was observed that Cl^- substitution led to a gradual progressive hyperpolarization of the cells towards values of -70 to $-80\,mV$ (Schettino et al. 1985) for which no equivalent observation on frog oxyntic cells is available. This finding might reflect an increased K^+ conductance after cellular HCO_3^- uptake in exchange for Cl^-. Unpublished observations from of Köhler and Frömter point to the presence of conductive HCO_3^- transport also in rabbit PC.

Other Electrophysiological Measurements

Cellular Ionic Activity Measurements

Thus far, only a few attempts have been made to determine intracellular ion concentrations in gastric cells with microelectrodes. These have been restricted to SEC of *Necturus* and frog gastric mucosa and to PC of isolated gastric tubules of rabbit. In frog SEC, a cytoplasmic K^+ activity of 99 mmol/l was observed (Schettino and Curci 1980) which indicates that K^+ has accumulated in the cytoplasm above electrochemical equilibrium with respect to the serosal fluid. This accumulation appears to reflect the operation of an active Na^+-K^+ pump in the serosal cell membrane. In addition, intracellular Cl^- concentration was determined in the SEC of frog and *Necturus* by Machen and Zeuthen (1982), by Curci and Schettino (1984), and Curci et al. (1986) who all showed that also Cl^- had accumulated above equilibrium with respect to serosal fluid to values of 15 to 29 mmol/l; these values may be slight overestimates, however, because of some interference problems with the microelectrodes. The transport mechanism(s) responsible for the accumulation have not yet been identified. Studies on isolated gastric tubules that attempted to measure the intracellular H^+ and K^+ concentrations of parietal cells (Kafoglis et al. 1984) did not achieve reliable results.

Patch-Clamp Experiments

Thus far, only a few attempts have been made to investigate gastric cells with patch-clamp techniques. After little-rewarding trials on isolated PC of rabbit (Loo et al. 1985), one laboratory succeeded in identifying single K^+ conductance channels on isolated cells and on the basolateral surface of gastric glands of *Necturus* which had been isolated with the help of collagenase and pronase (Ueda et al. 1987). Two types of K^+ channels with linear current–voltage relations and conductances of 67 or 33 pS in symmetrical (100 mmol/l) KCl solutions were observed. The open probability of the larger conductance channel, which occurred less frequently, increased with membrane depolarization and with increasing intracellular Ca^{2+} concentration. The smaller conductance channel was activated by the cAMP pathway. Although the stimulation-dependent opening of K^+ channels observed in these patch-clamp experiments seems to agree with the hyperpolarization of the OC observed by Demarest and Machen (1985) under histamine stimulation, it should be noticed that this hyperpolarization was not associated with a significant increase of the potential response to K^+ concentration steps. Since it cannot be excluded that cell isolation resulted in redistribution of single channels, it cannot be excluded either that possibly the small K^+ channel might have actually originated from the apical cell membrane. An equivalent of the larger, less frequent K^+ channel was also observed in our laboratory on the basolateral membrane from identified PC of isolated rabbit gastric tubules (see Fig. 2).

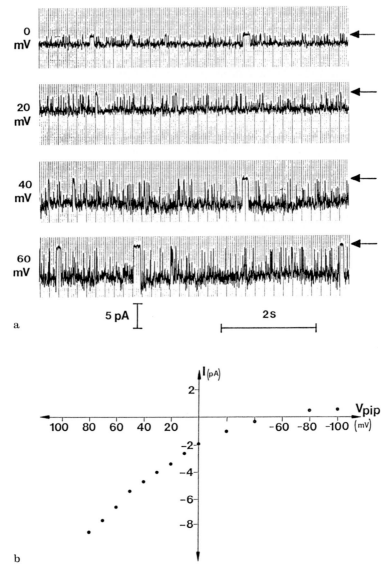

Fig. 2a, b. Single K^+ channel of basolateral cell membrane from parietal cell of collagenase-isolated rabbit gastric gland. Cell-attached measuring configuration. **a** Current traces at different pipette voltages as indicated. *Arrows* indicate closed state. Note high, voltage-independent open probability, probably reflecting high intracellular Ca^{2+} concentration. **b** Current voltage relation. *Abscissa*, pipette voltage; *ordinate*, single channel current. In four similar channels zero-voltage conductance was $57\,pS \pm 6$ S.D. Note Goldman-rectification reflecting 150 mmol/l KCl as pipette-filling solution and low cytoplasmic K^+ concentration following the isolation procedure and long-time incubation of the gland in HCO_3^--Ringer solution at 22 °C. The PC were identified as described by Köhler and Frömter (1985). The observations suggest that the $60\,pS$ K^+ channel of *Necturus* OC is also present in basolateral membrane of rabbit PC

Equivalent Circuit Analysis to Identify Routes of Transepithelial Ion Flow and Their Relative Importance

While two-dimensional intraepithelial current spread analysis and combined transepithelial and intraepithelial impedance analysis have been successfully applied to determine individual cell membrane resistances and junctional shunt resistances in flat-sheet epithelia (Frömter 1972; Kottra and Frömter 1985), in contrast to *Necturus* antrum mucosa (Ashley et al. 1985), measurements on gastric fundus mucosa have not been very successful thus far. This reflects again the tremendous problems in investigating a tissue which forms fluid-filled pits and glands and in addition consists of different cell types that may or may not be coupled by gap junctions and might possibly develop different types of tight junctions between different cells.

Spenney et al. (1974) analyzed horizontal current spread in *Necturus* fundus and concluded that the resistance of the paracellular shunt was only 3.8 times higher than the resistance of the cells. This value appears surprisingly low in view of the enormous H^+ gradients that the tight junctions have to resist in protecting the mucosa from damage. On the other hand, it remains doubtful whether the data are quantitatively reliable since they were obtained by applying simple 2D-cable equations to the highly complex mucosal structure: the fact that the calculated space constant was reported to be 400 µm while the distance between individual crypts was only 150 µm would forbid this analysis if the authors' assumption that SEC and OC are highly coupled were correct.

Further attempts to identify equivalent circuit parameters of bullfrog gastric mucosa have been made by Clausen et al. (1983) with the help of transepithelial impedance measurements. Data obtained under progressive stimulation with histamine could be fitted to a one-cell type model (representing OC, but neglecting SEC) with "distributed" effects. Those effects ought to arise from cable-like intraepithelial structures (glands, lateral spaces, microvilli) which were not identified, however. The authors interpreted their results as indicating that the transepithelial electrical properties were largely determined by the OC, that the glandular fluid space did not represent a major resistance to current flow, and that the fall in transepithelial resistance upon stimulation was mainly reflecting the increasing apical surface area of OC.

Although the experimental basis for these conclusions is not convincing – because more detailed information would have been necessary to justify the neglect of SEC, of cell-to-cell coupling, and of paracellular shunt conductances – the predominance of the OC in determining the overall electrical properties of *Necturus* gastric mucosa has recently been confirmed by vibrating probe measurements. Using a vibrating point electrode to scan current densities above the crypts and above the surrounding surface epithelium, Demarest et al. (1986) have demonstrated that in amiloride-treated *Necturus* stomach virtually all short-circuit current originates from the crypts (see Fig. 3) and that in the absence of amiloride the surrounding

SEC contribute only a minor component of Na^+ current, but no Cl^- current to I_{sc}. Moreover, the authors showed that apical application of amiloride decreased V_t and increased R_t only slightly, although it greatly increased the cell membrane potential and the ratio of apical to basal cell membrane resistance of SEC, but not of OC. This result clearly demonstrates a preponderance of the OC in determining the overall electrical properties of *Necturus* stomach epithelium in agreement with conclusions reached by Rehm and collaborators from less direct electrophysiological experiments on frog stomach based on the use of various inhibitors (O'Callaghan et al. 1974; Rehm et al. 1983; Rehm et al. 1986).

On the other hand, opposing views have also been reached from electrophysiological (Shoemaker and Sachs 1972) and other experiments (McGreevy 1984). In the latter experiments either the apical or the basolateral surface of rabbit fundic mucosa was exposed to anoxic conditions, and it was observed that V_t and R_t decreased in the first case, but did not change in the latter although the glands showed all signs of histological damage. More direct evidence for an important contribution of SEC to overall electrical properties of frog gastric mucosa (*Rana esculenta*) was recently obtained by S. Curci and collaborators (unpublished) who compared changes of V_t with membrane potential changes of SEC and OC in response to basolateral K^+ concentration steps before and after histamine and found that V_t changed in parallel with the basolateral membrane potential (V_s) of SEC, while V_s of OC remained constant.

Summarizing this discussion, we conclude that the relative importance of SEC and OC in determining overall electrical properties of gastric mucosa may differ in different animal species and/or in different functional states. The quantitative determination of this relation, however, is important and remains a challenge for all future transport investigations on gastric mucosa.

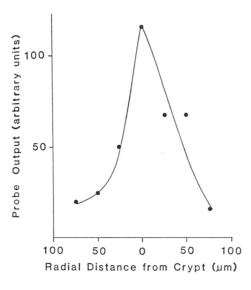

Fig. 3. Current-density profile above a crypt opening of *Necturus* gastric mucosa in the presence of amiloride (10^{-6} mmol/l). *Abscissa*, radial distance from crypt opening, in μm; *ordinate*, observed current density in arbitrary units. A vibrating probe was moved across a crypt opening 30 μm above the mucosal surface while current density was continously measured. Average current density above crypts was 505 and above SEC 4.4 μA/cm² (from Demarest et al. 1986)

Other important questions, e.g., whether SEC and OC are electrically coupled or whether the tight junctions between the different cells are tight or not, cannot be answered today.

Gastric Ion Transport Mechanisms

Active H^+ Secretion

In experiments on membrane vesicles it has been convincingly demonstrated that active H^+ secretion arises from the operation of an electroneutral K^+-, H^+-ATPase (Sachs et al. 1976; Forte and Lee 1977). Upon stimulation with histamine, elaborate structural alterations occur in the apical cell membrane of PC (OC in amphibia; Ito and Schofield 1974; Forte et al. 1977; Gibert and Hersey 1982) which result in exposure of the ATPase towards the glandular lumen. The controversial observations of the microscopic electro-neutrality and the macroscopic electrogenicity of the H^+ pump (see also Hersey et al. 1985) can be largely reconciled today when considering the role of a K^+ conductance which has also been identified in the apical cell membrane in vesicle studies (Wolosin and Forte 1984; Gunther et al. 1987). Since the electroneutral pump absorbs one K^+ ion in exchange for each H^+ ion secreted, the continuous operation of the pump requires the continuous recirculation of K^+ from cytosol to gland lumen. If this flux proceeds as an independent ion flux across a conductance pathway, it will generate a lumen-positive electrical current that matches the rate of active H^+ secretion. Indeed, when inhibiting the H^+ pump by omeprazole, Reenstra et al. (1986) observed active K^+ secretion, as the model would predict. However, the fact that active K^+ secretion reached only less than 2% of the preexisting active H^+ secretion is difficult to explain. The authors invoked diffusional restraints from the collapsing glandular lumen, which seem unlikely, however, in view of the unimpaired rate of Cl^- secretion and of almost identical diffusional properties of K^+ and Cl^- in aqueous solutions. Insufficient basolateral K^+ uptake can also be excluded because the continued active Cl^- secretion seen under these conditions probably results from a stimulation of the Na^+-K^+ pump (see also below). Alternatively, it might be that the apical K^+ conductance shuts down when luminal pH rises or cell pH falls after cessation of H^+ secretion or that the electrical driving force across the apical cell membrane changes under omeprazole so as to prevent K^+ efflux, but not Cl^+ efflux.

As a consequence of H^+ secretion by the apical H^+-ATPase, OH^- accumulates in the cell and in the presence of carbonic anhydrase near the pump site (Vega et al. 1985) is immediately converted to HCO_3^- and leaves the basolateral cell surface via an electroneutral $Cl^--HCO_3^-$ exchanger. This transport mechanism was postulated long ago by Rehm and Sanders (1975), but its operation was convincingly demonstrated only recently in cell pH studies on isolated gastric glands with the help of fluorescence techniques (Muallem et al. 1985; Paradiso et al. 1986, 1987). Whether $Na^+ - (HCO_3^-)_n$ cotransport (Curci et al. 1987) contributes significantly to HCO_3^- exit is unknown at present. The observed decrease of HCO_3^--dependent potential changes during stimulation of gastric secretion rather points against an involvement of $Na^+ - (HCO_3^-)_n$ cotransport in active H^+ secretion (Curci et al. 1988).

Active Cl⁻ Secretion

For many years it has been known that resting stomach mucosa actively secretes Cl^- ions (nonacidic Cl^- secretion) and that following stimulation by histamine, Cl^- secretion increases in conjunction with, but independent of H^+ secretion (acidic Cl^- secretion). While the latter was always thought to originate from OC or PC, for some time it was thought that the non-acidic Cl^- secretion arises from SEC (Machen and Zeuthen 1982). Electrophysiological evidence discussed above, however, has indicated that SEC are not capable of performing the postulated secondary active Cl^- transport, neither in frog nor in *Necturus* (Curci and Schettino 1984; Schettino and Curci 1985). Thus it appears that *all* active Cl^- secretion originates from OC, both in the resting state and after stimulation (see also Demarest et al. 1986).

Since in contrast to the H^+-, K^+-ATPase, no Cl^--ATPase has been convincingly demonstrated, it is generally held that Cl^- secretion occurs via secondary active transport in coupling with active Na^+ pumping (in the resting state) and/or in coupling with HCO_3^- backflux, and hence essentially active H^+ secretion (in the stimulated state). The model concept is depicted in Fig. 4. It has great similarities with the model of secondary active chloride secretion in shark rectal gland (De Silva et al. 1977; Greger and Schlatter 1984) which has also been confirmed for many other tissues such as intestine, respiratory epithelia, and exocrine glands. It consists of a serial arrangement of two functionally different membranes. (1) The basolateral cell membrane, across which Cl^- ions are accumulated inside the cell against their electrochemical gradient. This uptake is coupled to Na^+ uptake and energized by the Na^+ gradient which in turn is generated by the $Na^+ - K^+$ pump; and (2) the apical cell membrane, which is permeable to Cl^- ions and allows Cl^- to proceed passively into the lumen following its electrochemical ion gradient. The gastric model of Cl^- secretion equals that of other epithelia insofar as the apical cell membrane is concerned. Here a stimulable Cl^- conductance is required which has already been identified in studies on membrane vesicles (Wolosin and Forte 1984; Cuppoletti and Sachs 1984; Takeguchi and Yamazaki 1986) but it differs from the other models with regard to the basolateral cell membrane. Here, instead of $Na^+ - K^+ - 2Cl^-$ cotransport, a pair of antiporters for $Cl^- - HCO_3^-$ exchange and $Na^+ - H^+$ exchange is necessary, which has also been identified recently in the basolateral cell membrane of PC (Muallem et al. 1985; Paradiso et al. 1986,

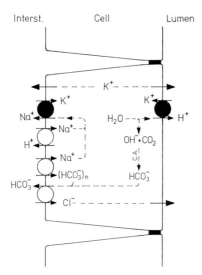

Fig. 4. Transport model for frog oxyntic cell. *Solid circles*, ATP-dependent ion pumps; *open circles*, co- and countertransporters; *arrows*, ionic conductances; *C.A.*, carbonic anhydrase

1987). The advantage of this arrangement is that in the stimulated state, Cl^- can be taken up in exchange for HCO_3^- (which is generated in the cell during H^+ secretion) without involving Na^+-H^+ exchange and, hence, without requiring extra energy as it does in the resting state.

The essential features of the model (Na^+ dependence, inhibition by ouabain, independence of omeprazole) have recently been tested and confirmed by Reenstra et al. (1987) in I_{sc} and tracer-flux measurements on frog stomach mucosa. The fact that specific inhibition of the H^+ pump by omeprazole does not significantly decrease Cl^- secretion (see also Starlinger et al. 1986; Bunce and Spraggs 1988) implies that either Na^+-H^+ exchange is stimulated (Muallem et al. 1988) or $Na^+-(HCO_3^-)_n$ cotransport is activated to bring enough HCO_3^- into the cell for continued exchange against Cl^-. The postulated stimulation might be a consequence of a relative intracellular acidosis that might possibly develop after cessation of H^+ secretion.

Active Na^+ Absorption

The gastric mucosa of most species (with the exception of the frog) is capable of actively absorbing Na^+ ions. The varying amount of Na^+ absorption adds an electrical current of equal sign onto the current from active Cl^- secretion and may be largely responsible for the observed variations in open circuit V_t (Durbin 1967). As clearly demonstrated by Demarest et al. (1986), active Na^+ absorption is a property of SEC. It appears to obey the Ussing model of Na^+ absorption in frog skin (Koefoed-Johnsen and Ussing 1958), with an amiloride-inhibitable Na^+ conductance in the apical cell membrane and an active Na^+-K^+ pump in the basolateral cell membrane.

K^+ Secretion/Absorption

Most studies of transepithelial K^+ transport across gastric mucosa have demonstrated net K^+ secretion (Hogben 1955; Makhlouf 1974; Sen et al. 1980) without being able to identify the cellular origin of this flux. In principle both cell types, SEC and OC, could be involved since both are thought to contain a Na^+-, K^+-ATPase on the basolateral cell surface and K^+ conductance pathways at the apical cell surface. On the other hand, in the stimulated state it may be expected that the (K^+-resorptive) H^+ pump comes into play and, hence, that K^+ may be actively absorbed. This has indeed been observed in the study cited above by Reenstra et al. (1986). To further prove the mechanism of K^+ absorption, the latter authors observed that inhibition of the H^+-, K^+-ATPase by omeprazole inverted the direction of K^+ transport, leading to net secretion. Although the involvement of a H^+-, K^+-ATPase shall not be questioned, it might be worth mentioning that the significance of small active net fluxes as determined from unidirectional tracer fluxes on short-circuited preparations is difficult to assess. The reason is again the complex microarchitecture of gastric musoca which presents two major problems: (1) during continued secretion, the fluid in the gland lumen cannot effectively be replaced by the mucosal bath fluid, as would be necessary for defined flux measurements, and (2) the longitudinal resistance of the cable-like glands does not allow V_t to be brought exactly to zero across all SEC and all OC simultaneously. These problems have been thoroughly discussed by Rehm (1968, 1975) who concluded that the latter effect was irrelevant because ion concentration gradients would develop along the glands that would exactly compensate for possible potential gradients. This, however, would require that the cell membranes be impermeable to water, which is not true. In view of these problems, one should be reluctant to put too much emphasis on the absolute magnitude of transepithelial net fluxes determined under short-circuit conditions.

Active HCO_3^- Secretion

During inhibition of acid secretion by histamine (H_2) receptor antagonists, or SNC^-, the gastric fundus mucosa of frog and *Necturus* was found to secrete alkali actively (OH^-, HCO_3^-; Flemström 1977; Takeuchi et al. 1982). The net rate of this secretion amounts at best to $\sim 5\%$–10% of the rate of stimulated H^+ secretion. Since alkalinization is not only restricted to fundic mucosa but occurs also in antrum (Flemström and Sachs 1975), it was thought to originate from SEC. The mechanism of HCO_3^- secretion has not yet been identified. From ion substitution studies, however, it may be concluded that alkali secretion depends on the presence of Na^+, HCO_3^-, and possibly Cl^- in the basolateral solution and that it can be inhibited by basolateral application of the disulfonic stilbene DIDS. This points to the involvement of $Na^+ - HCO_3^-$ cotransport or of the coupled $Na^+ - H^+$ and

$Cl^- - HCO_3^-$ exchanges for HCO_3^- uptake into the cell. The mechanism of HCO_3^- or OH^- exit across the apical cell membrane is completely unknown.

Conclusions

As it may have become evident from the foregoing discussion, electrophysiological experiments have contributed only little to the present model concepts of gastric ion transport. This may change in the future, however, when new techniques such as noise analysis and patch-clamp analysis are applied more frequently to determine molecular details of transport mechanisms. In addition, the membrane properties of identified cells could and should be investigated further with microelectrodes, including ion-selective microelectrodes and shielded microelectrodes for impedance measurements. The quantitative interpretation of potential and/or resistance changes in response to ion substitutions, stimulants, or inhibitors, however, is still hampered by the lack of decent information on equivalent circuit parameters of gastric epithelium. It is of paramount importance, therefore, that the relative conductances of SEC and OC, the resistance of the glandular fluid columns, and the resistances of the tight junctions be determined to allow the electrical measurements to be analyzed quantitatively.

Unfortunately, gastric mocusa presents additional problems here, in that the circuit parameters are not constant, but may be expected to differ from species to species and from functional state to functional state. This adds another degree of complexity to the well-known histological complexity of this epithelium.

Acknowledgement. The secretarial assistance of Mrs I. Harward is gratefully acknowledged.

References

Ashley SW, Soybel DI, De L, Cheung LY (1985) Microelectrode studies of Necturus antral mucosa. II. Equivalent circuit analysis. Am J Physiol 248: G574–G579

Ayalon A, Sanders MJ, Thomas LP, Amirian DA, Soll AH (1982) Electrical effects of histamine on monolayers formed in culture from enriched canine gastric chief cells. Proc Natl Acad Sci USA 79: 7009–7013

Berglindh T, Öbrink KJ (1976) A method for preparing isolated glands from the rabbit gastric mucosa. Acta Physiol Scand 96: 150–159

Blum AL, Shah GT, Wiebelhaus VD, Brennan FT, Helander HF, Ceballos R, Sachs G (1971) Pronase method for isolation of viable cells from *Necturus* gastric mucosa. Gastroenterology 61: 189–200

Boron WF, Boulpaep EL (1983) Intracellular pH regulation in the renal proximal tubule of the salamander. Basolateral $NaHCO_3$ transport. J Gen Physiol 81: 53–94

Bunce KT, Spraggs CF (1988) Stimulation of electrogenic chloride secretion by prostaglandin E_2 in guinea-pig isolated gastric mucosa. J Physiol (Lond) 400: 381–394

Canosa CA, Rehm WS (1968) Microelectrode studies of dog's gastric mucosa. Biophys J 8: 415–430

Carrasquer G, Chu TC, Rehm WS, Schwartz M (1982) Evidence for electrogenic Na – Cl symport in the in vitro frog stomach. Am J Physiol 242: G620–G627

Clausen C, Machen TE, Diamond JM (1983) Use of AC impedance analysis to study membrane changes related to acid secretion in amphibian gastric mucosa. Biophys J 41: 167–178

Cuppoletti J, Sachs G (1984) Regulation of gastric acid secretion via modulation of a chloride conductance. J Biol Chem 259: 14952–14959

Curci S, Schettino T (1984) Effect of external sodium on intracellular chloride activity in the surface cells of frog gastric mucosa. Pflügers Arch 401: 152–159

Curci S, Schettino T, Frömter E (1986) Histamine reduces Cl^- activity in surface epithelial cells of frog gastric mucosa. Pflügers Arch 406: 204–211

Curci S, Debellis L, Frömter E (1987) Evidence for rheogenic sodium bicarbonate cotransport in the basolateral membrane of oxyntic cells of frog gastric fundus. Pflügers Arch 408: 497–504

Curci S, Debellis L, Frömter E (1988) Effect of stimulation on the sodium bicarbonate cotransport in frog stomach oxyntic cells. In: Wong PYD, Young JA (eds) Exocrine secretion. Hong Kong University Press, Hong Kong, p 55

Demarest JR, Machen TE (1985) Microelectrode measurements from oxyntic cells in intact Necturus gastric mucosa. Am J Physiol 249: C535–C540

Demarest JR, Scheffey C, Machen TE (1986) Segregation of gastric Na and Cl transport: a vibrating probe and microelectrode study. Am J Physiol 251: C643–C648

De Silva P, Stoff J, Field M, Fine L, Forrest JN, Epstein FH (1977) Mechanism of active chloride secretion by shark rectal gland: role of Na^+-, K^+-ATPase in chloride transport. Am J Physiol 233: F298–F306

Durbin RP (1967) Eletrical potential differences of the gastric mucosa. In: Code CF (ed) Alimentary canal. American Physiological Society, Washington, pp 879–888 (Handbook of physiology, section 6, vol II)

Flemström G (1977) Active alkalinization by amphibian gastric fundic mucosa in vitro. Am J Physiol 233: E1–E12

Flemström G, Sachs G (1975) Ion transport by amphibian antrum in vitro. I. General characteristics. Am J Physiol 228: 1188–1198

Forte JG, Lee HC (1977) Gastric adenosine triphosphatases: a review of their possible role in HCl secretion. Gastroenterology 73: 921–926

Forte JG, Machen TE (1975) Transport and electrical phenomena in resting and secreting piglet gastric mucosa. J Physiol (Lond) 244: 33–51

Forte JG, Forte TM, Saltman P (1967) K^+-stimulated phosphatase of microsomes from gastric mucosa. J Cell Physiol 69: 293–304

Forte JG, Machen TE, Öbrink KJ (1980) Mechanisms of gastric H^+ and Cl^- transport. Annu Rev Physiol 42: 111–126

Forte TM, Machen TE, Forte JG (1977) Ultrastructural changes in oxyntic cells associated with secretory function: a membrane recycling hypothesis. Gastroenterology 73: 941–955

Frömter E (1972) The route of passive ion movement through the epithelium of Necturus gallbladder. J Membr Biol 8: 259–301

Gibert AJ, Hersey (1982) Morphometric analysis of parietal cell membrane transformations in isolated gastric glands. J Membr Biol 67: 113–124

Greger R, Schlatter E (1984) Mechanism of NaCl secretion in the rectal gland of spiny dog fish (Squalus acanthias). I. Experiments in isolated in vitro perfused rectal gland tubulus. Pflügers Arch 402: 63–75

Gunther RD, Bassilian S, Rabon EC (1987) Cation transport in vesicles from secreting rabbit stomach. J Biol Chem 262: 13966–13972

Harris JD, Edelman IS (1964) Chemical concentration gradients and electrical properties of gastric mucosa. Am J Physiol 206: 769–782

Hersey SJ, Sachs G, Kasbekar DK (1985) Acid secretion by frog gastric mucosa is electroneutral. Am J Physiol 248: G246–G250

Hogben CAM (1955) Active transport of chloride by isolated frog gastric epithelium. Origin of gastric mucosal potential. Am J Physiol 180: 641–649

Ito S, Schofield GG (1974) Studies on the depletion and accumulation of microvilli and changes in the tubulovesicular compartment of mouse parietal cells in relation to gastric acid secretion. J Cell Biol 63: 364–382

Kafoglis K, Hersey SJ, White JF (1984) Microelectrode measurements of K^+ and pH in rabbit gastric glands: effect of histamine. Am J Physiol 246: G433–G444

Klemperer G, Lelchuk S, Caplan SR (1983) Na^+-coupled Cl^- transport in the gastric mucosa of the guinea pig. J Bioenerg Biomembr 15: 121–134

Koefoed-Johnsen V, Ussing HH (1958) The nature of the frog skin potential. Acta Physiol Scand 42: 298–308

Köhler M, Frömter E (1985) Identification of mitchondria-rich cells in unstained vital preparations of epithelia by autofluorescence. Pflügers Arch 403: 47–49

Kottra G, Frömter E (1984) Rapid determination of intraepithelial resistance barriers by alternating current spectroscopy. II. Test of model circuits and quantification of results. Pflügers Arch 402: 421–432

Kuo YJ, Shanbour LL (1979) Chloride, sodium, potassium and hydrogen ion transport in isolated canine gastric mucosa. J Physiol (Lond) 291: 367–380

Lee J, Simpson G, Scholes P (1974) An ATPase from dog gastric mucosa; changes of outer pH in supensions of membrane vesicles accompanying ATP hydrolysis. Biochem Biophys Res Commun 60: 825–832

Loo DDG, Mendlein JD, Berglindh T, Soll AH, Sachs G, Wright EM (1985) Single channel and whole cell currents in unstimulated isolated parietal cells. Fed Proc 44: 463

Machen TE, Zeuthen T (1982) Cl^- transport by gastric mucosa: cellular Cl^- activity and membrane permeability. Philos Trans R Soc Lond [Biol] 299: 559–573

Makhlouf GM (1974) A model for passive transport of potassium by the stomach: evidence from in vitro studies. Am J Physiol 227: 1285–1288

McGreevy JM (1984) Gastric surface cell function: potential difference and mucosal barrier. Am J Physiol 247: G79–G87

Muallem S, Burnham C, Blissard D, Berglindh T, Sachs G (1985) Electrolyte transport across the basolateral membrane of the parietal cells. J Biol Chem 260: 6641–6653

Muallem S, Blissard D, Cragoe EJ, Sachs J (1988) Activation of the Na^+/H^+ and Cl^-/HCO_3^- exchange by stimulation of acid secretion in the parietal cell. J Biol Chem 263: 14703–14711

O'Callaghan J, Sanders SS, Shoemaker RL, Rehm WS (1974) Barium and K^+ on surface and tubular cell resistances of frog stomach with microelectrodes. J Physiol (Lond) 227: 273–288

Okada Y, Ueda S (1984) Electrical membrane responses to secretagogues in parietal cells of the rat gastric mucosa in culture. J Physiol (Lond) 354: 109–119

Paradiso AM, Negulescu PA, Machen TE (1986) Na^+-H^+ and $Cl^--OH^-(HCO_3^-)$ exchange in gastric glands. Am J Physiol 250: G524–G534

Paradiso AM, Tsien RY, Machen TE (1987) Digital image processing of intracellular pH in gastric oxyntic and chief cells. Nature 325: 447–450

Reenstra WW, Bettencourt JD, Forte JG (1986) Active K^+ absorption by the gastric mucosa: inhibition by omeprazole. Am J Physiol 250: G455–G460

Reenstra WW, Bettencourt JD, Forte JG (1987) Mechanisms of active Cl^- secretion by frog gastric mucosa. Am J Physiol 252: G543–G547

Rehm WS (1956) Effect of electrical current on gastric hydrogen ion and chloride ion secretion. Am J Physiol 185: 325-331

Rehm WS (1968) An analysis of the short-circuiting technique applied to in vivo tissues. J Theor Biol 20: 341–354

Rehm WS (1975) Ion transport and short-circuit technique. Curr Top Membr Transport 7: 217–270

Rehm WS, Lefevre ME (1965) Effect of dinitrophenol on potential, resistance and H^+ rate of frog stomach. Am J Physiol 208: 922–930

Rehm WS, Sanders SS (1975) Implications of the neutral carrier Cl^-/HCO_3^- exchange mechanism in gastric mucosa. Ann NY Acad Sci 264: 442–455

Rehm WS, Chu TC, Schwartz M, Carrasquer G (1983) Mechanisms responsible for SCN increase in resistance of frog gastric mucosa. Am J Physiol 245: G143–G156

Rehm WS, Carrasquer G, Schwartz M (1986) Sites of resistance changes with inhibition of acid secretion in frog stomach. Am J Physiol 250: G639–G647

Rutten M, Rattner D, Silen W (1985) Transepithelial transport of guinea pig gastric mucous cell monolayers. Am J Physiol 249: C503–C513

Sachs, G, Chang H, Rabon E, Schackmann R, Lewin M, Saccomani G (1976) A non-electrogenic H^+ pump in plasma membrane of hog stomach. J Biol Chem 251: 7690–7698

Sachs G, Spenney JG, Lewin M (1978) H^+ transport: regulation and mechanism in gastric mucosa and membrane vesicles. Physiol Rev 58: 106–173

Schettino T, Curci S (1980) Intracellular potassium activity in epithelial cells of frog fundic gastric mucosa. Pflügers Arch 383: 99–103

Schettino T, Curci S (1985) On the luminal membrane permeability to Cl^- of *Necturus* gastric surface cells. Pflügers Arch 403: 331–333

Schettino T, Köhler M, Frömter E (1985) Membrane potentials of individual cells of isolated gastric glands of rabbit. Pflügers Arch 405: 58–65

Schwartz M, Carrasquer G, Rehm WS (1985) Evidence for HCO_3^- conductance pathways in nutrient membrane of resting frog fundus. Biochem Biophys Acta 819: 187–194

Sen PC, Tague LL, Ray TK (1980) Secretion of H^+ and K^+ by bullfrog gastric mucosa: characterization of K^+ transport pathways. Am J Physiol 239: G485–G492

Sernka TJ, Hogben CAM (1969) Active ion transport by isolated gastric mucosae of rat and guinea pig. Am J Physiol 217: 1419–1424

Shoemaker RL (1978) Micropuncture studies using the amphibian fundic gastric mucosa, in vitro. Acta Physiol Scand [Special Suppl], p 173–180

Shoemaker RL, Sachs G (1972) Microelectrode studies of *Necturus* gastric mucosa. In: Sachs G, Heinz E, Ullrich KJ (eds) Gastric secretion, Academic Press New York, New York, p 147–164

Soll AH (1978) The actions of secretagogues on oxygen uptake by isolated mammalian parietal cells. J Clin Invest 61: 370–380

Spenney JG, Shoemaker RL, Sachs G (1974) Microelectrode studies of fundic gastric mucosa: cellular coupling and shunt conductance. J Membrane Biol 19: 105–128

Starlinger MJ, Hollands MJ, Rowe PH, Mathiews JB, Silen W (1986) Chloride transport of frog gastric fundus: effects of omeprazole. Am J Physiol 250: G118–G126

Takeguchi N, Yamazaki Y (1986) Disulfide cross-linking of H,K-ATPase opens Cl^- conductance, triggering proton uptake in gastric vesicles. J Biol Chem 261: 2560–2566

Takeuchi K, Merhav A, Silen W (1982) Mechanism of luminal alkalinization by bullfrog fundic mucosa. Am J Physiol 243: G377–G388

Ueda S, Loo DDF, Sachs G (1987) Regulation of K^+ channels in the basolateral membrane of *Necturus* oxyntic cells. J Membrane Biol 97: 31–41

Van Driessche W, Zeiske W (1985) Ionic channels in epithelial cell membranes. Physiol Rev 65: 833–903

Vega FV, Olaisson H, Mårdh S (1985) Distribution of carbonic anhydrase in cells and membranes isolated from pig gastric mucosa. Acta Physiol Scand 124: 573–579

Villegas L (1962) Cellular location of the electrical potential difference in frog gastric mucosa. Biochim Biophys Acta 64: 359–367

Wolosin JM, Forte JG (1984) Stimulation of the oxyntic cell triggers K^+ and Cl^- conductances in apical H^+-, K^+-ATPase membrane. Am J Physiol 246: C537–C545

Yoshitomi K, Burckhardt BC, Frömter E (1985) Rheogenic sodium-bicarbonate cotransport in the peritubular cell membrane of rat renal proximal tubule. Pflügers Arch 405: 360–366

Zeiske W, Machen TE, Van Driessche W (1983) Cl^-- and K^+-related fluctuations of ionic current through oxyntic cells in frog gastric mucosa. Am J Physiol 245: G797–G807

6 Liver

Hepatic Electrolyte Transport and Bile Formation

J. Graf*

Introduction

According to the osmotic theory of bile formation proposed by Sperber (1959), bile solutes are transported across the hepatobiliary epithelium against a concentration gradient. Their luminal accumulation promotes transepithelial water flow.

Fluid transport by hepatocytes and bile ductular epithelial cells produces canalicular and ductular secretion, respectively. Ductular bile formation appears to result from active bicarbonate secretion and is subject to hormonal stimulation (Tavoloni 1987). Canalicular bile formation is measured by the clearance of substances that readily permeate hepatocytes, but not duct cells (e.g. erythritol). Since active secretion of bile acids accounts for a fraction of the canalicular bile flow, and since many exogenous compounds are also actively excreted into the canalicular lumen, they thus promote fluid secretion. The mechanism of canalicular fluid secretion in the absence of bile acids and of exogenous compounds continues to be a matter for speculation, and both active secretion of endogenous organic compounds and active transport of inorganic ions have been invoked as responsible (for references see Van Dyke et al. 1982; Boyer 1983; Graf 1983; Anwer and Hegner 1983; Scharschmidt and Van Dyke 1983; Moseley and Boyer 1985; Arias 1986; Boyer 1986; Coleman 1987; Erlinger 1988; Frimmer and Ziegler 1988). This article summarizes present concepts of the role of inorganic electrolyte transport in canalicular bile formation.

---

* Dedicated to my year long mentor, Professor Dr. Adolf Lindner, at the occasion of his 75th birthday

Young · Wong, Epithelial Secretion of Water and Electrolytes
© Springer-Verlag Berlin · Heidelberg 1990

Approaches to Study Hepatobiliary Electrolyte Transport

Hepatic transport of electrolytes has been studied in a number of preparations including the intact animal, the isolated perfused liver (Claret and Mazet 1972; Graf 1983; Anwer and Hegner 1983; Fritz and Scharschmidt 1987 a, b), isolated hepatocytes (Berthon et al. 1980, 1983, 1985; Scharschmidt and Stephens 1981; Van Dyke and Scharschmidt 1983; Field and Jenkinson 1985; Gebhardt 1986), isolated cell membrane vesicles prepared from the basolateral (blood sinusoidal) and apical (luminal) surface domain of the hepatocyte (Sips et al. 1980; Ruifrok and Meijer 1982; Boyer et al. 1983; Duffy et al. 1983; Inoue et al. 1983 a; Blitzer and Donovan 1984; Meier et al. 1984 b) and, more recently, in hepatocyte couplets (Graf et al. 1984, 1987; Gautam et al. 1987). This last preparation is unique. It is an in vitro gland composed of a pair of contiguous liver cells that develop a secretory lumen between one another. The luminal wall is composed of two half shells of apical cell membrane united by a circular tight junctional belt that separates the lumen from the extracellular bathing media. This luminal space expands in tissue culture by acquisition of additional luminal membrane and by secretion of bile. In this preparation the luminal spaces can be punctured with microelectrodes so that classical methods of epithelial electrophysiology can be applied.

Does Electrolyte Transport into Bile Promote Canalicular Bile-Salt-Independent Bile Formation?

Paracellular Electrolyte Transport

Concepts of bile canalicular electrolyte secretion have been previously reviewed (Van Dyke et al. 1982; Anwer and Hegner 1983; Graf 1983; Graf et al. 1987) and are only briefly summarized here. In pulse-chase experiments performed in the isolated perfused rat liver, the rate constants ($k\ min^{-1}$) of isotopic ion exchange ($^{24}Na^+$, $^{42}K^+$, $^{36}Cl^-$) between the blood sinusoidal compartment and hepatocytes and their intracellular ion concentrations (mmol/l) have been determined: $k_{Na}=0.17$; $k_K=0.014$; $k_{Cl}=0.077$; $[Na]_i=16.4$; $[K]_i=113$; $[Cl]_i=25.5$ (Claret and Mazet 1972). It was then shown that equilibration of specific radioactivities between bile and the sinusoidal compartment proceeds at a faster rate ($k_{Na}=1.01$; $k_K=0.61$; $k_{Cl}=0.50$; Graf and Peterlik 1975; Graf 1983), corroborating an earlier suggestion that a large fraction of biliary ion secretion bypasses the liver cells (Leong et al. 1957). It was also shown that biliary ion concentrations very rapidly follow concentration changes applied to the perfusion medium (Graf 1983). Conforming to their morphological appearance in freeze-etch preparations (Lagarde et al. 1981), leaky tight junctions between hepatocytes were considered to allow for the rapid transepithelial permeation of electrolytes across a paracellular pathway. This suggestion was substantiated by the electrophysiological observation in isolated hepatocyte couplets that the conductance of the tight junctions (g_T) is considerably higher than the conductances of the apical-canalicular (g_C) and basolateral-sinusoidal (g_S) liver cell membranes ($g_T = 40.5$ nS; $g_C = 1.3$ nS; $g_S = 6.5$ nS; Graf et al. 1987). It has been proposed that tight junctions may possess an adequate degree of permeability under physiological conditions (Reichen and Simon 1988). Thus, tight junctions should be leaky enough to allow ready permeation of electrolytes into the lumen, but tight enough to prevent backleak of those biliary solutes that are actively secreted by the hepatocytes into bile and thereby sustain water flow. This suggestion is supported by studies in the perfused rat liver showing that replacement of Na^+ or Cl^- in the perfusion medium by Li^+ or NO_3^- has little effect on bile flow rate, whereas replacement by bulkier organic ions such as choline, acetate or isethionate reduces bile flow rate (Van Dyke et al. 1982; Anwer and Hegner 1983; Graf 1983).

Gradual reduction of extracellular Ca^{2+} concentration first increases bile flow rate, but cholestasis ensues when $[Ca^{2+}]_0$ is reduced below 0.1 mmol/l (Graf 1976b; Reichen et al. 1985; Reichen and Simon 1988). This finding may be interpreted as being due to a gradual increase in tight junction permeability. Cholestasis could thus be produced by both too high or too low a paracellular permeability.

Two other observations indicate passive paracellular permeation of NaCl: (1) bile-to-perfusate concentration gradients of NaCl are less potent in inducing osmotic water flow than equivalent concentration gradients of sucrose, indicating that the reflection coefficient of NaCl is less than unity (Graf 1983), and (2) the decrease of the luminal volume of isolated cell couplets in bathing media made hypertonic by addition of sucrose or raffinose exceeds the magnitude of volume changes that would occur if only water left the lumen to readjust isotonicity, indicating that permeant solutes, most probably NaCl, also leave the lumen (Graf et al. 1984). In similar experiments it was also noted that cell shrinking in hypertonic media precedes the reduction of the luminal volume, suggesting that transepithelial water flux takes a transcellular rather than a paracellular route (Graf et al. 1989; Fig. 1). The luminal volume of cell couplets also shrinks rapidly when Cl^- in the external medium is replaced by gluconate. The luminal volume shrinks to approximately 30% of its original size, whilst the cell volume decreases only to approximately 85%, again indicating that Cl^- (and the accompanying cation) rapidly permeates across the tight junctions and that the canalicular luminal concentration of Cl^- and the permeant cation (Na^+) is high (near the external bath concentration; L. Schild and J. Graf, preliminary observation).

Rapid transport of large molecules from blood to bile (e.g. inulin, horse radish peroxidase, dextrans) has frequently been interpreted to indicate that these molecules permeate across the paracellular shunt pathway, particularly

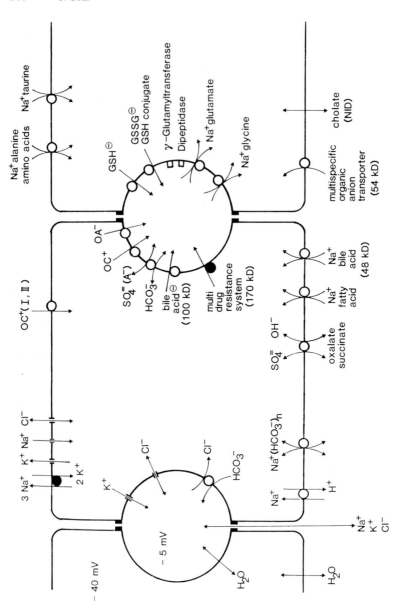

in unphysiological conditions. In contrast, transcellular vesicular transport of extracellular space markers has been demonstrated (La Russo 1985; Lake et al. 1985; Lowe et al. 1985; Coleman 1987; Reichen and Simon 1988), and recent evidence indicates that this transcytotic transport exhibits a fast temperature-sensitive component (Fuchs et al. 1988). Whether paracellular permeation of such molecules occurs to any significant extent may also be questioned in view of the fact that the tight junctions effectively prevent the backleak of much smaller bile solutes that are secreted by the hepatocytes.

The dependence of bile flow on the presence of a particular ionic species has been frequently interpreted as indicating that active cellular transport of inorganic ions is responsible for bile-salt-independent canalicular bile formation, but, as outlined above, such dependence observed in ion replacement studies in the perfused liver may merely indicate that a particular ionic species is sufficiently permeant across the epithelium, in particular the paracellular pathway, whereas the replacing ion is not (Van Dyke et al. 1982; Scharschmidt and Van Dyke 1983; Anwer and Hegner 1983; Graf 1983). This argument also applies to a study that showed that bile flow is reduced when perfusate bicarbonate is replaced by the bufferion tricine (Hardison and Wood 1978). Proof of the concept that active cellular inorganic ion transport *per se* could maintain canalicular bile-salt-independent bile formation would require the demonstration that at least one inorganic cation or anion is transported into the canalicular lumen against a transepithelial electrochemical gradient. Based on this thermodynamic consideration, bile formation was studied by impeding bile flow by liver perfusion with a medium made hypertonic by addition of sucrose. Since sucrose is only slowly transported into the canalicular lumen, the concentrations of other biliary solutes would have to rise in order to provide bile isotonic with the perfusate and to allow bile secretion to occur. It was found that biliary concentrations of Na^+ and K^+ rose, while those of Cl^- and HCO_3^- fell slightly thus increasing the biliary 'cation–anion gap' (Graf 1983). These biliary organic anions, the concentration of which rose during

---

Fig. 1. Sinusoidal and canalicular membrane transport mechanisms participating in bile formation. Two bile canalicular spaces in between three liver cells are shown. *Full circles* represent primary active transport utilizing ATP. *Open circles with arrows* represent carrier-mediated and secondary active transport driven by the trans-membrane gradients of Na^+, pH, or the electrical membrane potential (*encircled charge symbol*), *arrows on opposite sides* indicate countertransport (antiport), *arrows on the same side* indicate cotransport (symport). The molecular weight of well characterized carrier proteins is given (kD). The *left hand section* depicts mechanisms of electrolyte transport, including the sinusoidal Na^+-, K^+-ATPase, sinusoidal and luminal ion channels, paracellular ion permeation across the tight junction, the intracellular and the canalicular luminal electric potential, and carriers involved in H^+ and HCO_3^- transport. The *right hand section* depicts the transport mechanism for organic solutes. OC^+, organic cations (two sinusoidal transport systems); OA^-, organic anions; *GSH* and *GSSG*, reduced and oxidized glutathione; *boxes*, glutathione degrading enzymes; *NID*, non-ionic diffusion

hypertonic perfusion, are mostly glutamic acid conjugates probably representing transglutamylation products derived from secreted glutathione (Graf 1983; Kaplowitz et al. 1983; Inoue et al. 1983b; Jansen et al. 1987a; Ballatori et al. 1988b). It may therefore be assumed that cellular secretion of endogenous organic anions, which do not permeate the tight junctions produces an osmotic gradient, promoting bile formation, whereas inorganic. ions distribute passively between perfusate and bile, conforming to the Gibbs-Donnan equilibrium. Observation of a small lumen-negative electric potential (-5 mV) in the isolated couplet system supports this concept (Graf et al. 1987) and explains the biliary inorganic cation–anion gap.

Transcellular Electrolyte Transport

Studies with isolated canalicular cell membrane vesicles have shown that this membrane domain posesses ion channels for K^+ and Cl^- (Meier et al. 1985; Sellinger et al. 1989; Thalhammer et al. 1989). Although canalicular luminal ion concentrations have not yet been determined directly, it is conceivable that these ion channels allow for secretion of K^+ and Cl^- down an electrochemical gradient driven by the high intracellular K^+ concentration and the negative intracellular electric potential (-40 mV), respectively. In view of the high tight junctional conductance, substantial backleak of secreted ions across the paracellular pathway is likely to occur, and cellular transport of these ions may therefore be inefficient in promoting canalicular bile flow.

A carrier system for electroneutral $Cl^- - HCO_3^-$ exchange has also been identified at the luminal cell membrane (Meier et al. 1985). This transport system could serve for HCO_3^- secretion driven by an inwardly directed Cl^- concentration gradient. If effective, this mechanism should result in a high biliary bicarbonate concentration and a canalicular luminal pH above electrochemical equilibrium, but neither has been demonstrated thus far (Hardison and Wood 1978; Graf 1983; Corbic et al. 1985; Henderson et al. 1985).

High bicarbonate concentrations in final bile have been observed during hypercholeresis, a term indicating that choleresis induced by unconjugated lipophilic bile acids (e.g. ursodesoxycholic acid, UDCA) exceeds that of conjugated, less lipophilic bile acids (e.g. taurocholic acid), i.e. a larger volume of bile is produced per mole of bile acid excreted (Yoon et al. 1986; Palmer et al. 1987). Although the mechanism of this process is not understood in detail, the inhibitory effects of amiloride and acetazolamide on UDCA-induced choleresis (Garcia-Marin et al. 1985a, b; Lake et al. 1987; Renner et al. 1988) could indicate that the secreted bile acid is protonated within the biliary lumen by H^+ derived from the dissociation of carbonic acid. While HCO_3^- remains in the lumen, the undissociated lipophilic bile acid could be reabsorbed by non-ionic diffusion, driven by an alkaline intracellular pH established by $Na^+ - H^+$ exchange. Reabsorption would occur downstream in the biliary tree at a late canalicular or ductular site from where the bile acid may be brought back by the blood stream to the site of secretion. With each cycle in this 'cholehepatic circulation' one HCO_3^- ion would be secreted (Yoon et al. 1986; Palmer et al. 1987). The primary driving force for bile flow in this model is therefore the canalicular secretion of the bile acid, and part of the amount secreted is replaced by bicarbonate downstream in the biliary tree.

In summary, evidence that active secretion of any electrolyte could promote canalicular water flow is still lacking.

The Role of Hepatocellular Electrolyte Transport As an Energy Source of Hepatobiliary Transport Processes

Hepatocellular electrolyte transport plays an important role in generating the driving forces for the transport of organic solutes: transmembrane ion concentration gradients and the cell membrane potential are established by the primary action of the Na^+-, K^+-ATPase and provide the energy for coupled and electrogenic transport processes, respectively. The following paragraphs describe steady-state transmembrane ion-concentration gradients and their generation through the activity of the $Na^+ - K^+$ pump and give an account of transport mechanisms associated with the dissipation of these ion gradients.

Cellular Ion Concentration Gradients

Intracellular ion concentrations have been determined in many studies using various techniques (Claret and Mazet 1972; Scharschmidt and Stephens 1981; Graf 1983). Representative values obtained with ion-sensitive electrodes in isolated cell couplets are (mmol/l: $[K^+]_i = 117$; $[Na^+]_i = 16.3$; $[Cl^-]_i = 23.6$; $pH_i = 7.0$ (Henderson et al. 1986; Graf et al. 1987).

The high intracellular concentration of K^+ and the low concentration of Na^+ are maintained by the activity of the Na^+-, K^+-ATPase. This active transport is electrogenic (Graf and Peterson 1974; Graf et al. 1987), coupling Na^+-extrusion and K^+ uptake at an apparent ratio of 3:2. Calculated for a single cell, the pump transports K^+ at an approximate rate of 0.2–0.5 $\times 10^{-15}$ mol/s into the cell, thus imposing a considerable demand on cellular energy metabolism (Graf 1976a; Van Dyke and Scharschmidt 1983; Berthon et al. 1983; Graf et al. 1987). The pump is activated both by a rise of intracellular $[Na^+]$ and extracellular $[K^+]$ (Graf and Peterson 1974; Graf et al. 1987). Na^+ uptake through coupled transport processes (alanine and taurocholic acid uptake, $Na^+ - H^+$ exchange) thus stimulates Na^+ pumping (Van Dyke and Scharschmidt 1983; Kristensen 1986; Graf et al. 1988a). Hormonal stimulation of the pump (Berthon et al. 1983, 1985; Lynch et al.

1986) and dependence of pump activity on membrane lipid fluidity (Keeffe et al. 1979, 1980; Schachter 1984) has also been demonstranted.

According to histochemical (Blitzer and Boyer 1984), immunocytochemical (Sztul et al. 1987), membrane isolation (Boyer et al. 1983; Sellinger et al. 1988) and electropyhsiological studies (Graf et al. 1987), the pump is predominantly, if not exclusively, located in the basolateral-sinusoidal cell membrane. Due to the high conductance of this membrane (see above), inhibition of the electrogenic pump by ouabain causes only a small membrane depolarization (Graf and Peterson 1974; Graf et al. 1987) and, analogously, inhibition or activation of other electrogenic transport processes has little effect on cell membrane potential (Folke and Paloheimo 1975; Kristensen 1986; Fritz and Scharschmidt 1987a, b).

The intracellular negative membrane potential (-40 mV) is largely due to the high membrane K^+ conductance, and it is steeply dependent on transmembrane K^+ concentration gradients (Graf and Peterson 1978; Graf et al. 1987). Accordingly, facilitation of K^+ fluxes by hormones acting through inositol-1,4,5-triphosphate (IP_3) and cytosolic Ca^{2+} concentration (Burgess et al. 1981, 1984, Jenkinson et al. 1983; Cook and Haylett 1985; Field and Jenkinson 1985), or by a rise of intracellular pH (Henderson et al. 1988), or during volume regulatory decrease in hypotonic media (Berthon et al. 1980; Graf et al. 1988a) causes membrane hyperpolarization, whereas inhibition by applying of Ba^{2+}, apamin and quinine (Burgess et al. 1981; Cook and Haylett 1985; Wondegem and Castillo 1988), a decrease in temperature (Wondergem and Castillo 1986), or during volume regulatory increase (Graf et al. 1988a) causes membrane depolarization. Electrogenic transport processes (e.g. bile acid secretion, see below) may therefore be modulated through changes of K^+ concentration gradients or changes of membrane K^+ conductance.

The transmembrane Cl^- concentration gradient appears to be in electrochemical equilibrium (Claret and Mazet 1972; Lyall et al. 1987; Fritz and Scharschmidt 1987b), and it has been shown that $[Cl^-]_i$ follows variations of the membrane potential (Graf et al. 1987). It is therefore assumed that Cl^- distributes passively through conductive membrane Cl^- channels. These are subject to hormonal regulation (Field and Jenkinson 1985). As noted above a $Cl^- - HCO_3^-$ exchanger has been identified at the luminal cell membrane. The efficiency of this antiport is unknown so that possible effects of a pH (or HCO_3^-) gradient across the luminal cell membrane on intracellular Cl^- concentration remains undetermined.

Transport Processes at the Sinusoidal Cell Membrane

In contrast to channel-mediated transmembrane fluxes of K^+ and Cl^-, a large fraction of the Na^+ influx is coupled to transport of various other solutes by a common carrier molecule, and thus, the inward directed sodium concentration gradient provides the energy for these secondary active transport mechanisms (Graf et al. 1988b). Sodium-coupled transport mechanisms serve to regulate intracellular pH, intracellular calcium concentration (Schanne and Moore 1986; for primary active Ca^{2+} transport mechanisms see Grollman 1988) and the cellular uptake from the blood stream of bile acids, fatty acids and amino acids. Regulation of intracellular pH serves many vital cellular functions such as control of metabolism, proliferation and cell volume (Kashiwagura et al. 1984; Graf et al. 1988a, c).

The Na^+-H^+ antiport protects the cell from intracellular acidification. This transporter was initially identified in isolated basolateral membrane vesicles (Arias and Forgac 1984; Moseley et al. 1986b; Fuchs et al. 1986). More recently, it has been shown that Na^+-H^+ exchange is activated by intracellular acidification, reaching a maximal activity of approximately 0.9 $\times 10^{-15}$ mol/s per cell (calculated from Henderson et al. 1986), whereas pH_i under control conditions is little affected by inhibition of Na^+-H^+ exchange by amiloride. Amiloride has little effect on unstimulated bile flow, but reduces the stimulatory effects of bile acids, particularly of ursodesoxycholic acid, possibly by interfering with the cholehepatic circulation of this bile acid, as described above.

A $Na^+-(HCO_3^-)_n$ symport has also been identified in basolateral membrane vesicles and cultured hepatocytes (Renner et al. 1987; Gleeson et al. 1988; Meier et al. 1988). This transporter is electrogenic $(n>1)$ and inhibited by 4-acetamino-4'-isothiocynatostilbene-2,2'-disulphonic acid (SITS). The functional significance of this transporter is not yet established, and, depending on its stoichiometry (n is unknown) and the amount of charge transfer, it may serve both HCO_3^- uptake and intracellular alkalinization driven by the transmembrane Na^+ gradient or HCO_3^- expulsion and intracellular acidification driven by the membrane potential. The transporter could thus operate bidirectionally and set the intracellular pH at a certain level, depending on the Na^+ gradient, the external HCO_3^- concentration and the membrane potential (Fig. 1).

Transport of organic solutes in the liver has been reviewed recently (Petzinger et al. 1989). Na^+-dependent transport systems have been identified at the sinusoidal and canalicular cell membrane, some participating directly or indirectly in the biliary excretion of organic solutes. At the sinusoidal cell membrane, Na^+-dependent transport systems for several groups of amino acids exist (Kilberg 1982). As an example, alanine transport has been extensively studied. This transport is electrogenic, coupling Na^+ and alanine uptake at a ratio of 1:1 (Folke and Paloheimo 1975; Sips et al. 1980; Kristensen and Folke 1983; Fritz and Scharschmidt 1987a). It exhibits low affinity ($K_m = 4$–7 mmol/l; Kristensen 1986), but high transport capacity ($V_{max} =$ approximately 1.3×10^{-15} mol/s per cell) and is under hormonal control (Kilberg et al. 1985). A comparison to the transport rate of the Na^+-, K^+-ATPase (see above) shows that this rapid intracellular accumulation of Na^+ and alanine requires cell volume compensation, possibly involving release of KCl and stimulation of the Na^+-K^+ pump (Van Dyke and Scharschmidt 1983; for references see also Kristensen 1986 and Graf et al.

1988a). In addition, dissipation of the Na^+ gradient by alanine uptake may inhibit other Na^+-dependent transport systems such as taurocholic acid uptake (Blitzer et al. 1983). With respect to bile formation, sinusoidal uptake of amino acids such as glutamate (Sips et al. 1982; Gebhardt and Mecke 1983; Taylor and Rennie 1987), glutamine (Kilberg et al. 1980) and taurine (Bucuvalas et al. 1987) may be also required to supply substrates continuously for the intracellular synthesis of bile secretory products such as glutathione, glutathione conjugates or amino acid conjugates of bile acids and other compounds. Uptake of fatty acids into liver cells is also energized by the inwardly directed Na^+ concentration gradient and probably mediated by a 40 kDa carrier protein (Stremmel et al. 1985, 1986; Stremmel 1987).

Bile acids, returning to the liver after their intestinal reabsorption, are avidly taken up into liver cells. A Na^+-dependent uptake system with high affinity for taurocholic acid at the basolateral cell membrane has been studied extensively (for references see Frimmer and Ziegler 1988; Petzinger et al. 1989). Some of these studies indicate electrogenicity of this transporter (coupling ratio $2 Na^+$: 1 bile acid), suggesting that uptake is favoured by the Na^+ gradient and the electrical membrane potential (Edmondon et al. 1985; Fritz and Scharschmidt 1987a). The presence of Cl^- facilitates Na^+-dependent bile acid uptake (Duffy et al. 1983; Meier et al. 1984a; Petzinger and Frimmer 1984), but it is presently unknown whether cotransport of Cl^- occurs. Affinity labelling with photolabile bile acid derivatives identified presumptive transport molecules (Kramer et al. 1982; Wieland et al. 1984; Fricker et al. 1987; Ananthanarayanan et al. 1988), a 48-kDa protein being the likely candidate for Na^+-dependent bile acid transport (Von Dippe et al. 1986). This transporter apparently accepts a variety of other substrates such as steroids, cyclic oligopeptides and various drugs, including cationic compounds (Zimmerli et al. 1987; Frimmer and Ziegler 1988; Kurz et al. 1989). A second protein (54 kDa) may be responsible for Na^+-independent bile acid uptake (Wieland et al. 1984; Fricker et al. 1987; Kurz et al. 1989) and similar sized or identical molecules transport a variety of organic anions including sulfobromophthalein and bilirubin (for references see Wieland et al. 1984; Stremmel and Berk 1986; Berk et al. 1987, 1989). The driving force for concentrative uptake of these last mentioned compounds is unknown (e.g. Sottocasa et al. 1982) although it is known that transport requires the presence of Cl^- (Wolkoff et al. 1987). Requirement of inorganic anion has also been demonstrated for uptake of certain organic cations (Ruifrok 1982; Joppen et al. 1985; Meijer 1987; Meijer et al. 1989).

The pH gradient at the sinusoidal cell membrane has also been invoked to provide the energy for various transport processes. Since the transmembrane pH gradient is established by secondary active transport ($Na^+ - H^+$ exchange) these transport processes are termed 'tertiary active'. A carrier system for $OH^- - SO_4^{2-}$ exchange has been demonstrated in isolated membrane vesicles. This transporter also accepts dicarboxylic acids (oxalate, succinate) and is competitively inhibited by cholate (Hugentobler and Meier

1986). The pH-gradient-driven transport of cholate has also been demonstrated in isolated membrane vesicles (Blitzer et al. 1986), but it has been questioned whether this transport is carrier mediated since pH gradient-dependent transport occurs also in protein-free artifical lipid membranes, suggesting non-ionic diffusion of this bile acid (Caflish et al. 1987). Ambiguity also exists about the efficiency of this transport system since pH_i is less than pH_e. Energization of uptake by the pH gradient would require us to assume that pH_i is greater than pH_e in the microenvironment of the cell membrane, perhaps provided by $Na^+ - H^+$ exchange. In contrast, an outwardly directed proton concentration gradient ($pH_i < pH_o$) was suggested to drive uptake of certain low-molecular-weight organic cations by a countertransport system (Meijer 1987; Meijer et al. 1989).

Transport Processes at the Canalicular Cell Membrane

The majority of transport processes at the canalicular membrane appear to be driven by the intracellular negative electric potential, which favours the exit of anionic bile constituents from the cytosol. Carrier-mediated transport of bile acids has been demonstrated in isolated canalicular membrane vesicles (Meier et al. 1984a, 1987a; Ruetz et al. 1987). A 100-kDa bile acid-binding protein was identified by photoaffinity labelling; the protein has been purified, reconstitution of the protein into liposomes induces DIDS-sensitive, carrier-mediated bile acid transport, and antibodies against the protein inhibit transport in membrane vesicles (Fricker et al. 1987; Ruetz et al. 1987). Electrogenicity of the transport system was demonstrated in canalicular membrane vesicles and in reconstitution experiments (Meier 1984a; Ruetz et al. 1988). Recently it was also shown in isolated cell couplets that cell hyperpolarization induced by passing current through the cell membrane stimulates bile production if taurocholic acid is present in the bathing medium (Weinman et al. 1989). Analogously, in the perfused rat liver, cell depolarization or hyperpolarization by variations of the perfusate K^+ concentration results, respectively, in a reduction and an increase of bile flow. The amplitude of these changes was increased by taurocholic acid (Graf 1989). These effects indicate that both bile salt-dependent and independent bile flow are regulated by the cell membrane potential, the latter component perhaps through electrogenic secretion of endogenous biliary anions such as glutathione.

Glutathione is synthesized by the liver cells reaching high intracellular concentration (5–7 mmol/l). Most of the reduced glutathione (GSH) is delivered into the blood, but GSH is also secreted across the luminal membrane by an electrogenic transport system (Inoue et al. 1983b, 1984b; Kaplowitz et al. 1983; Sies and Graf 1985). Secreted GSH is hydrolyzed in the lumen by γ-glutamyltranspeptidase and dipeptidases, and the split products are partially reabsorbed (Ballatori et al. 1988a, b), apparently providing the substrates for sodium gradient-driven transport of glutamate and glycine, recently identified in canalicular membrane vesicles (Ballatori et al. 1986; Moseley et al. 1986a). Oxidized glutathione (GSSG) and glutathione conjugates (excretory products of various xenobiotics) are preferentially delivered into bile (Inoue et al. 1984a; Akerboom et al. 1984). Although canalicular transport of GSSG is electrogenic (Akerboom et al. 1984), the high transmembrane concentration gradient of GSSG (Akerboom et al. 1982) may require additional driving forces, perhaps hydrolysis of ATP (Nicotera et al. 1985).

A $HCO_3^- - SO_4^{2-}$ antiport system has been demonstrated in canalicular membrane vesicles. This anion exchanger appears to be driven by the inwardly directed HCO_3^- concentration gradient and would serve for the biliary secretion of SO_4^{2-} and perhaps of sulfonated or sulfate-conjugated compounds (Meier et al. 1987b).

In addition to these transport mechanisms which are driven by the membrane potential, the transmembrane Na^+ gradient, or the pH gradient, the canalicular membrane provides also for secretion of organic cations. The driving force for this process is unknown, but may involve countertransport with inorganic cations. (Meijer 1987; Meijer et al. 1989). Direct utilization of ATP may energize the biliary excretion of anti-cancer drugs such as daunomycin (Hsu et al. 1987; Arias 1989). This transport is mediated by a 170-kDa protein initially identified in drug-resistant cell lines expressing the multidrug resistance gene (Fojo et al. 1987). Current research also concentrates on the excretory mechanism of organic anions such as bilirubin and sulfobromophthalein, the canalicular secretion of which may also be driven by the negative cell potential. New insight into this transport system may be gained through studies of a mutant rat strain that exhibits impaired anion excretory capacity analogous to the defect in human Dubin-Johnson syndrome (Jansen et al. 1987a, b).

Conclusion

Despite considerable effort, no conclusive evidence has been obtained that hepatocellular electrolyte secretion *per se* is a driving force for canalicular bile formation. Biliary electrolyte secretion appears to result mainly from diffusion across the paracellular pathway. On the other hand, hepatocellular electrolyte transport appears to provide the major driving force for the biliary secretion of organic solutes, in particular for Na^+-dependent transport across the sinusoidal cell membrane and for electrogenic transport across the luminal cell membrane (Fig. 1). In view of the multiplicity of transport systems involved, it is unnecessary to say that much has to be learned about many aspects, including the question of whether the magnitude of the identified driving forces is sufficient to explain the vectorial concentrative transport of organic solutes into bile.

References

Akerboom T, Bilzer M, Sies H (1982) The relationship of biliary glutathione disulfide efflux and intracellular glutathione disulfide content in perfused rat liver. J Biol Chem 257: 4248–4252

Akerboom T, Inoue M, Sies H, Kinne R, Arias IM (1984) Biliary transport of glutathione disulfide studied with isolated rat-liver canalicular membrane vesicles. Eur J Biochem 141: 211–215

Ananthanarayanan M, von Dippe P, Levy D (1988) Identification of the hepatocyte Na^+-dependent bile acid transport protein using monoclonal antibodies. J Biol Chem 263: 8338–8343

Anwer MS, Hegner D (1983) Role of inorganic electrolytes in bile acid-independent canalicular bile formation. Am J Physiol 244: G116–G124

Arias IM (1986) Mechanisms and consequences of ion transport in the liver. In: Popper H, Schaffner F (eds) Progess in liver disease, vol VIII. Grune and Stratton, New York, pp 145–149

Arias IM (1989) ATP in and around the bile canaliculus. In: Petzinger E, Kinne RKH, Sies H (eds) Hepatic transport of organic substances. Springer, Berlin Heidelberg New York, pp 102–117

Arias IM, Forgac M (1984) The sinusoidal domain of the plasma membrane of rat hepatocytes contains an amiloride-sensitive Na^+-H^+ antiport. J Biol Chem 259: 5406–5408

Ballatori N, Moseley RH, Boyer JL (1986) Sodium gradient dependent L-glutamate transport is localized to the canalicular domain of liver plasma membranes. J Biol Chem 261: 6216–6221

Ballatori N, Jacob R, Barrett C, Boyer JL (1988a) Biliary catabolism of glutathione and differential reabsorption of its amino acid constituents. Am J Physiol 254: G1–G7

Ballatori N, Jacob R, Boyer JL (1988b) Intrabiliary glutathione hydrolysis. A source of glutamate in bile. J Biol Chem 261: 7860–7865

Berk PD, Potter BJ, Stremmel W (1987) Role of plasma membrane ligand-binding proteins in the hepatocellular uptake of albumin-bound organic anions. Hepatology 7: 165–176

Berk PD, Potter BJ, Sorrentino D, Stremmel W, Stump D, Kiang Ch-L, Zhou Sh-L (1989) Characteristics of organic anion binding protein from rat liver sinusoidal plasma membranes. In: Petzinger E, Kinne RKH, Sies H (eds) Hepatic transport of organic substances. Springer, Berlin Heidelberg New York, pp 195–210

Berthon B, Claret M, Mazet JL, Poggioli J (1980) Volume and temperature dependent permeabilities in isolated rat liver cells. J Physiol (Lond) 305: 267–277

Berthon B, Burgess BA, Capiod T, Claret M, Poggioli J (1983) Mechanisms of action of noradrenaline on the sodium potassium pump in isolated rat liver cells. J Physiol (Lond) 341: 25–40

Berthon B, Capiod T, Claret M (1985) Effect of noradrenaline, vasopressin and angiotensin on the Na–K pump in rat isolated liver cells. Br J Pharmacol 86: 151–161

Blitzer BL, Boyer JL (1984) Localization of Na^+-, K^+-ATPase on the hepatocyte plasma membrane. Gastroenterology 87: 1206–1207

Blitzer BL, Donovan CB (1984) A new method for the rapid isolation of basolateral plasma membrane vesicles from rat liver. Characterization, validation and bile acid transport studies. J Biol Chem 259: 9295–9301

Blitzer BL, Ratoosh SL, Donovan CB (1983) Amino acid inhibition of bile acid uptake by isolated rat hepatocytes: relationship to dissipation of transmembrane Na^+ gradient. Am J Physiol 245: G399–G403

Blitzer BL, Terzakis CH, Scott KA (1986) Hydroxyl/bile acid exchange. A new mechanism for the uphill transport of cholate by basolateral liver plasma membrane vesicles. J Biol Chem 261: 12042–12046

Boyer JL (1983) New concepts of mechanisms of hepatocyte bile formation. Physiol Rev 60: 303–326

Boyer JL (1986) Mechanisms of bile acid secretion and hepatic transport. In: Andreoli TE, Hoffman JF, Fanestil DD, Schultz SG (eds) Physiology of membrane disorders. Plenum, New York, pp 609–636

Boyer JL, Allen RM, NG O-C (1983) Biochemical separation of Na^+K^+-ATPase from a "purified" light density, "canalicular"-enriched plasma membrane fraction from rat liver. Hepatology 3: 18–28

Bucuvalas JC, Goodrich AL, Suchy FJ (1987) Hepatic taurine transport: a Na^+-dependent carrier on the basolateral plasma membrane. Am J Physiol 253: G351–G358

Burgess BA, Claret M, Jenkinson DH (1981) Effects of quinine and apamin on the calcium-dependent potassium permeability of mammalian hepatocytes and red cells. J Physiol (Lond) 317: 67–90

Burgess GM, Irvine RF, Berridge MJ, McKinney JS, Putney JW (1984) Actions of inositol phosphates on Ca^{++} pools in guinea-pig hepatocytes. Biochem J 224: 741–746

Caflish C, Zimmerli B, Hugentobler G, Meier PJ (1987) pH Gradient driven cholate uptake into rat liver plasma membrane vesicles represents nonionic diffusion rather than a carrier mediated process (Abstract). Gastroenterology 92: 1722

Claret M, Mazet JL (1972) Ionic fluxes and permeabilities of cell membranes in rat liver. J Physiol (Lond) 223: 279–295

Coleman R (1987) Biochemistry of bile secretion. Biochem J 5: 122–134

Cook NS, Haylett DG (1985) Effects and apamin, quinine and neuromuscular blockers on calcium-activated potassium channels in guinea-pig hepatocytes. J Physiol (Lond) 358: 373–394

Corbic M, Munoz C, Dumont M, DeConet G, Erlinger S (1985) Effect of systemic pH, pCO_2 and bicarbonate concentration on biliary bicarbonate secretion in the rat. Hepatology 5: 594–599

Duffy MC, Blitzer BL, Boyer BL (1983) Direct determination of the driving forces for taurocholate uptake into rat liver plasma membrane vesicles. J Clin Invest 72: 1470–1481

Edmonson JW, Miller BA, Lumeng L (1985) Effect of glucagon on hepatic taurocholate uptake: relationship to membrane potential. Am J Physiol 249: G427–G433

Erlinger S (1988) Bile flow. In: Arias IM, Jacoby WB, Popper H, Schachter D, Shafritz DA (eds) The liver: biology and pathobiology. Raven, New York, pp 643–661

Field AC, Jenkinson DH (1985) The influence of noradrenaline on membrane conductance of isolated guinea-pig and rabbit hepatocytes. J Physiol (Lond) 369: 106P

Fitz JG, Scharschmidt BF (1987a) Regulation of transmembrane electrical potential gradient in rat hepatocytes in situ. Am J Physiol 252: G56–G64

Fitz JG, Scharschmidt BF (1987b) Intracellular chloride activity in intact liver: relationship to membrane potential and bile flow. Am J Physiol 252: G699–G706

Fojo AT, Ueda K, Slamon DJ, Poplack DG, Gottesmann MM, Pastan I (1987) Expression of a multi-drug-resistance gene in human tumors and tissues. Proc Natl Acad Sci USA 84: 265–269

Folke M, Paloheimo M (1975) The effect of alanine on cell membrane potentials in rat liver. Acta Physiol Scand 95: 44A

Fricker G, Schneider S, Gerok W, Kurz G (1987) Identification of different transport systems for bile salts in sinusoidal and canalicular membranes of hepatocytes. Biol Chem Hoppe Seyler 368: 1143–1150

Frimmer M, Ziegler K (1988) The transport of bile acids in liver cells. Biochim Biophys Acta 947–99

Fuchs R, Thalhammer T, Peterlik M, Graf J (1986) Electrical and molecular coupling between sodium and proton fluxes in basolateral membrane vesicles of rat liver. Pflügers Arch 406: 430–342

Fuchs R, Klapper H, Peterlik M, Mellman I (1988) Characterization and isolation of rat liver endosomes destined for lysosomes and for bile. Hepatology 8: 1420

Garcia-Marin JJ, Dumont M, Corbic M, DeConet G, Erlinger S (1985a) Effect of acid-base balance and acetazolamide on ursodeoxycholate-induced biliary bicarbonate secretion. Am J Physiol 248: G20–G27

Garcia-Marin JJ, Corbic M, Dumont M, DeConet G, Erlinger S (1985b) Role of H^+ transport in ursodeoxycholate-induced biliary HCO_3^- secretion in the rat. Am J Physiol 249: G335–G341

Gautam A, NG O-C, Boyer JL (1987) Isolated rat hepatocyte couplets in short-term tissue culture: structural characteristics and plasma membrane reorganization. Hepatology 7: 216–223

Gebhardt R (1986) Use of isolated and cultured hepatocytes in studies on bile formation. In: Guillouzo A, Guguen-Guillouzo C (eds) Research in isolated and cultured hepatocytes. Libbey, London, pp 353–376

Gebhardt R, Mecke D (1983) Glutamate uptake by cultured rat hepatocytes is mediated by hormonally inducible, sodium dependent transport systems. FEBS Lett 161: 275–278

Gleeson D, Smith ND, Scaramuzza DM, Boyer JL (1988) Bicarbonate dependent and independent pH regulatory mechanisms in rat hepatocytes. Gastroenterology 94: A542

Graf J (1976a) Sodium pumping and bile secretion. In: Preisig R, Bircher J, Paumgartner G (eds) The liver: quantitative aspects of structure and function. Edito Cantor, Aulendorf, pp 370–385

Graf J (1976b) Some aspects of the role of cyclic AMP and calcium in bile formation. In: Case M, Goebell H (eds) Stimulus secretion coupling in the gastrointestinal tract. MTP, Lancester, pp 305–328

Graf J (1983) Canalicular bile salt independent bile formation: concepts and clues from electrolyte transport in rat liver. Am J Physiol 244: G233–G246

Graf J (1989) Effects of hydrostatic pressure and liver cell membrane potential on hepatic bile acid transport. In: Petzinger E, Kinne RKH, Sies H (eds) Hepatic transport of organic substances. Springer, Berlin Heidelberg New York, pp 299–300

Graf J, Peterlik M (1975) Mechanisms of transport of inorganic ions into bile. In: Taylor W (ed) The hepatobiliary system – fundamental and pathological mechanisms. Plenum, New York, pp 43–58

Graf J, Peterson OH (1974) Electrogenic sodium pump in mouse liver parenchymal cells. Proc R Soc London [Biol] 187: 363–367

Graf J, Peterson OH (1978) Cell membrane potential and resistance in liver. J Physiol (Lond) 284: 105–126

Graf J, Gautam A, Boyer L (1984) Isolated rat hepatocyte couplets: a primary secretory unit for electrophysiologic studies of bile secretory function. Proc Natl Acad Sci USA 81: 6516–6520

Graf J, Henderson RM, Krumpholz B, Boyer JL (1987) Cell membrane and transepithelial voltages and resistances in isolated rat hepatocyte couplets. J Membr Biol 95: 241–254

Graf J, Haddad P, Häussinger D, Lang F (1988a) Cell volume regulation in liver. Renal Physiol Biochem 11: 202–220

Graf J, Henderson RM, Boyer JL (1988b) Electrophysiological and energetic aspects of hepatobiliary transport in isolated rat hepatocyte couplets. In: Davison JS, Shaffer EA (eds) Gastrointestinal and hepatic secretion: mechanisms and control. University of Calgary Press, Calgary, pp 24–29

Graf J, Henderson RM, Meier PJ, Boyer JL (1988c) Regulation of intracellular pH in hepatocytes. In: Häussinger D (ed) pH Homeostasis: mechanisms and control. Academic, London, pp 43–60

Graf J, Schild L, Boyer JL, Giebisch G (1989) Osmotic water flux in a two-cell gland derived from isolated hepatocytes. FASEB J 3: A983

Grollman EF (1988) Calcium signals in liver. In: Arias IM, Jakoby WB, Popper H, Schachter D, Shafritz DA (eds) The liver: biology and pathobiology. Raven, New York, pp 777–783

Hardison WGM, Wood GA (1978) Importance of bicarbonate in bile salt independent fraction of bile flow. Am J Physiol 235: E158–E164

Henderson RM, Graf J, Boyer JL (1985) Measurement of intracellular and intracanalicular pH in isolated rat hepatocyte couplets using microelectrodes. Fed Proc 44: 1395

Henderson RM, Graf J, Boyer JL (1986) Na–H exchange regulates intracellular pH in isolated rat hepatocyte couplets. Am J Physiol 252: G109–G113

Henderson RM, Krumpholz B, Boyer JL, Graf J (1988) Effect of intracellular pH on potassium conductance in liver. Pflügers Arch 412: 334–335

Hsu J, Gatmaitan Z, Willingham M, Gottesmann MM, Pastan I, Cornwell M, Arias IM (1987) The multidrug-resistance system and anti-cancer drug transport by rat liver canalicular membrane vesicles (Abstract). Hepatology 7: 1104

Hugentobler G, Meier PJ (1986) Multispecific anion exchange in basolateral (sinusoidal) rat liver plasma membrane vesicles. Am J Physiol 251: G656–G664

Inoue M, Kinne R, Tran T, Biempica L, Arias IM (1983a) Rat liver canalicular membrane vesicles: isolation and topological characterization. J Biol Chem 258: 5183–5188

Inoue M, Kinne R, Tran T, Arias IM (1983b) The mechanism of biliary secretion of reduced glutathione analysis of transport process in isolated rat liver canalicular membrane vesicles. Eur J Biochem 134: 467–471

Inoue M, Akerboom TPM, Sies H, Kinne R, Tran T, Arias IM (1984a) Biliary transport of glutathione S-conjugate by rat liver canalicular membrane vesicles. J Biol Chem 259: 4998–5002

Inoue M, Kinne R, Tran T, Arias IM (1984b) Glutathione transport across hepatocyte plasma membranes. Analysis using isolated rat-liver sinusoidal-membrane vesicles. Eur J Biochem 138: 491–495

Jansen PLM, Groothius GMM, Peters WHM, Meier DKF (1987a) Selective hepatobiliary transport defect for organic anions and neutral steroids in mutant rats with hereditary-conjugated hyperbilirubinemia. Hepatology 7: 71–76

Jansen PLM, Peters WHM, Meijer DKF (1987b) Hepatobiliary excretion of organic anions in double-mutant rats with a combination of defective canalicular transport and uridine 5'-diphosphate-glucuronyltransferase deficiency. Gastronterology 93: 1094–1103

Jenkinson DH, Haylett DG, Cook NS (1983) Calcium-activated potassium channels in liver cells. Cell Calcium 4: 429–434

Joppen C, Petzinger E, Frimmer M (1985) Properties of iodopamide uptake by isolated hepatocytes. Naunyn Schmiedebergs Arch Pharmacol 331: 393–397

Kaplowitz N, Eberle DE, Petrini J, Touloukian J, Corvasce MC, Kuhlenkamp J (1983) Factors influencing the efflux of hepatic glutathione into bile in rats. J Pharmacol Exp Ther 224: 141–147

Kashiwagura T, Deutsch CJ, Taylor J, Erecinska M, Wilson DF (1984) Dependence of gluconeogenesis, urea synthesis, and energy metabolism of hepatocytes on intracellular pH. J Biol Chem 259: 237–243

Keeffe EB, Scharschmidt BF, Blankenship NM, Ockner RK (1979) Studies of relationships among bile flow, liver plasma membrane Na,K-ATPase, and membrane microviscosity in the rat. J Clin Invest 64: 1590–1598

Keeffe EB, Blankenship NM, Scharschmidt BF (1980) Alteration of rat liver membrane fluidity and ATPase activity by chlorpromazine hydrochloride and its metabolites. Gastroenterology 79: 222–231

Kilberg MS (1982) Amino acid transport in isolated rat hepatocytes. J Membr Biol 69: 1–12

Kilberg MS, Handlogten ME, Christensen HN (1980) Characteristics of an amino acid transport system in rat liver for glutamine, asparagine, histidine and closely related analogs. J Biol Chem 255: 4011–4019

Kilberg MS, Barber EF, Handlogten ME (1985) Characteristics and hormonal regulation of amino acid transport system A in isolated rat hepatocytes. Curr Top Cell Regul 25: 133–163

Kramer W, Bickel U, Buscher HP, Gerok W, Kurz G (1982) Bile-salt binding polypeptides in plasma membranes of hepatocytes revealed by photoaffinity labeling. Eur J Biochem 129: 13–24

Kristensen LO (1986) Associations between transports of alanine and cations across cell membrane in rat hepatocytes. Am J Physiol 251: G575–G584

Kristensen LO, Folke M (1983) Coupling ratio of electrogenic Na^+-alanine cotransport in isolated rat hepatocytes. Biochem J 210: 621–624

Kurz G, Müller M, Schramm U, Gerok W (1989) Identification and function of bile salt binding polypeptides of hepatocyte membrane. In: Petzinger E, Kinne R, Sies H (eds) Hepatic transport of organic substances. Springer, Berlin Heidelberg New York, pp 267–278

La Russo NF (1985) Proteins in bile: how they get there and what they do. Am J Physiol 247: G199–G205

Lagarde S, Elias W, Wade JB, Boyer JL (1981) Structural heterogeneity of hepatocyte "tight" junctions: a quantitative analysis. Hepatology 1: 793–798

Lake JR, Licko V, Van Dyke RW, Scharschmidt BF (1985) Biliary secretion of fluid-phase markers by the isolated perfused rat liver. Role of transcellular vesicular transport J Clin Invest 76: 676–684

Lake JR, Van Dyke RW, Scharschmidt BF (1987) Effects of Na^+ replacement and amiloride on ursodeoxycholic acid-stimulated choleresis and biliary bicarbonate secretion. Am J Physiol 252: G163–G169

Leong GF, Holloway RJ, Brauer RW (1957) Potassium transfer from plasma to bile in isolated perfused rat liver (Abstract). Fed Proc 16: 316

Lowe PJ, Kan KS, Barnwell SG, Sharma RK, Coleman R (1985) Transcytosis and paracellular movements of horseradish peroxidase across liver parenchymal tissue from blood to bile. Effects of alpha-naphthylisothiocyanate and colchicine. Biochem J 229: 529–537

Lyall V, Croxton TL, Armstrong WM (1987) Measurement of intracellular chloride activity in mouse liver slices with microelectrodes. Biochim Biophys Acta 903: 56–67

Lynch CJ, Wilson PB, Blackmore PF, Exton JH (1986) The hormone sensitive hepatic Na^+-pump; evidence for regulation by diacylglycerol and tumor promoters. J Biol Chem 261: 14551–14556

Meier P, Meier-Abt AS, Barett C, Boyer L (1984a) Mechanisms of taurocholate transport in canalicular and basolateral rat liver plasma membrane vesicles. Evidence for an electrogenic canalicular organic anion carrier. J Biol Chem 259: 10614–10622

Meier PJ, Sztul ES, Reuben A, Boyer JL (1984b) Structural and functional polarity of canalicular and basolateral plasma membrane vesicles isolated in high yield from rat liver. J Cell Biol 98: 991–1000

Meier PJ, Knickelbein R, Moseley RH, Dobbins JW, Boyer JL (1985) Evidence for carrier-mediated chloride/bicarbonate exchange in canalicular rat liver plasma membrane vesicles. J Clin Invest 1256–1263

Meier PJ, Meier-Abt ASt, Boyer JL (1987a) Properties of the canalicular bile acid transport system in rat liver. Biochem J 242: 465–469

Meier PJ, Valantinas J, Hugentobler G, Rahm I (1987b) Bicarbonate sulfate exchange in canalicular rat liver plasma membrane vesicles. Am J Physiol 253: G461–G468

Meier PJ, Renner ER, Zimmerli B, Scharschmidt BF (1988) Hepatocytes exhibit electrogenic basolateral Na^+/HCO_3^- cotransport. Clin Res 36: 559A

Meijer DKF (1987) Current concepts on hepatic transport of drugs. J Hepatol 4: 259–268

Meijer DKF, Mol W, Müller M, Kurz G (1989) Mechanism of hepatobiliary transport of cationic drugs studied with the intact organ and on the membrane level. In: Petzinger E, Kinne R K-H, Sies H (eds) Hepatic transport of organic substances. Springer, Berlin Heidelberg New York, pp 344–367

Moseley RH, Boyer JL (1985) Mechanisms of electrolyte transport in the liver and their functional significance. Semin Liver Dis 5: 122–135

Moseley RH, Ballatori N, Murphy SM (1986a) Na^+-glycine cotransport in canalicular liver plasma membrane vesicles – a potential mechanism for the reabsorption of an amino acid constituent of glutathione from bile (Abstract). Hepatology 6: 1207

Moseley RH, Meier PJ, Aronson PS, Boyer JL (1986b) $Na^+ - H^+$ exchange in rat liver basolateral but not canalicular plasma membrane vesicles. Am J Physiol 250: G35–G43

Nicotera P, Baldi C, Svenson S-A, Larsson R, Bellomo G, Orrenius S (1985) Glutathione S-conjugates stimulate ATP hydrolysis in the plasma membrane fraction of rat hepatocytes. FEBS Lett 187: 121–125

Palmer KR, Gurantz D, Hofmann AF (1987) Hypercholeresis induced by norchenodeoxycholate in biliary fistula rodent. Am J Physiol 252: G163–G169

Petzinger E, Frimmer M (1984) Driving forces in hepatocellular uptake of phalloidin and cholate. Biochim Biophys Acta 778: 539–548

Petzinger E, Kinne RKH, Sies H (eds) (1989) Hepatic transport of organic substances. Springer, Berlin Heidelberg New York

Reichen J, Simon FR (1988) Cholestasis. In: Arias IM, Jakoby WB, Popper H, Shafritz (eds) The liver: biology and pathobiology. Raven, New York, pp 1105–1124

Reichen J, Berr F, Le M, Warren GH (1985) Characterization of calcium deprivation-induced cholestasis in the perfused rat liver. Am J Physiol 249: G48–G57

Renner EL, Lake JR, Scharschmidt BF (1987) Hepatocytes express a mechanism for Na^+/HCO_3^- transport unrelated to Na^+/H^+ or Cl^-/HCO_3^- exchange (Abstract). Clin Res 35: 412

Renner EL, Lake JR, Cragoe EJ, Scharschmidt BF (1988) Ursodeoxycholic acid choleresis: relationship to biliary HCO_3^- and effects of $Na^+ - H^+$ exchange inhibitors. Am J Physiol 254: G132–G241

Ruetz St, Fricker G, Hugentobler G, Winterhalter K, Kurz G, Meier PJ (1987) Isolation and characterization of the putative canalicular bile salt transport system of rat liver. J Biol Chem 262: 11324–11330

Ruetz St, Hugentobler G, Meier PJ (1988) Functional reconstitution of the canalicular bile salt transport system of rat liver. Proc Natl Acad Sci USA 85: 6147–6151

Ruifrok PG (1982) Uptake of quaternary ammonium compounds into rat liver plasma membrane vesicles. Biochem Parmacol 31: 1431–1435

Ruifrok PG, Meijer DKF (1982) Sodium-coupled uptake of taurocholate by rat liver plasma membrane vesicles. The Liver 2: 28–34

Schachter D (1984) Fluidity and function of hepatocyte plasma membranes. Hepatology 4: 140–151

Schanne FAX, Moore L (1986) Liver plasma membrane calcium transport: evidence for a Na^+-dependent Ca^{2+}-flux. J Biol Chem 261: 9886–9889

Scharschmidt BF, Stephens JE (1981) Transport of sodium, chloride, and taurocholate by cultured rat hepatocytes. Proc Natl Acad Sci USA 78: 968–990

Scharschmidt BF, Van Dyke RW (1983) Mechanisms of hepatic electrolyte transport. Gastroenterology 85: 1199–1214

Sellinger M, Barrett C, Malle P, Gordon ER, Boyer JL (1988) Is Na^+-, K^+-ATPase present on the canalicular membrane domain? Hepatology 8: 1420

Sellinger M, Weiman SA, Henderson RM, Zweifach A, Boyer JL, Graf J (1989) Properties of an anion channel in rat liver canalicular membranes. Ann NY Acad Sci (in press)

Sies H, Graf P (1985) Hepatic thiol and glutathione efflux under the influence of vasopressin, phenylephrine and adrenaline. Biochem J 226: 545–549

Sips HJ, Van Amelsvoort JMM, Van Dam K (1980) Amino acid transport in plasma-membrane vesicles from rat liver. Characterization of L-alanine transport. Eur J Biochem 105: 271–274

Sips HJ, De Graaf PA, Van Dam K (1982) Transport of L-aspartate and L-glutamate in plasma membrane vesicles from rat liver. Eur J Biochem 122: 259–264

Sottocasa GL, Baldini G, Sandri G, Lunazzi G, Tiribelli (1982) Reconstitution in vitro of sulfobromophthalein transport by bilitranslocase. Biochim Biophys Acta 685: 123–128

Sperber I (1959) Secretion of organic anions in the formation of urine and bile. Pharmacol Rev II: 109–134

Stremmel W (1987) Translocation of fatty acids across the basolateral rat liver plasma membrane is driven by an active potential-sensitive sodium-dependent transport system. J Biol Chem 262: 6284–6289

Stremmel W, Berk PD (1986) Hepatocellular uptake of sulfobromophthalein (BSP) and bilirubin is selectively inhibited by an antibody to the liver plasma membrane BSP/bilirubin binding protein. J Clin Invest 78: 822–826

Stremmel W, Strohmeyer G, Borchard F, Kochwa S, Berk PD (1985) Isolation and partial characterization of a fatty acid binding protein in rat liver plasma membranes. Proc Natl Acad Sci USA 82: 4–8

Stremmel W, Strohmeyer G, Berk PD (1986) Hepatocellular uptake of oleate is energy dependent, sodium linked, and inhibited by an antibody to a hepatocyte plasma membrane fatty acid binding protein. Proc Natl Acad Aci USA 83: 3584–3588

Sztul ES, Biemersdorfer D, Caplan MJ, Kashgarian M, Boyer JL (1987) Localization of Na^+-, K^+-ATPase α-subunit to the sinusoidal and lateral but not canalicular membranes of rat hepatocytes. J Cell Biol 1239–1248

Tavoloni N (1987) The intrahepatic biliary epithelium: an area of growing interest in hepatology. Semin Liver Dis 7: 280–292

Taylor PM, Rennie MJ (1987) Perivenous localization of Na-dependent glutamate transport in perfused rat liver. FEBS Lett 221: 370–374

Thalhammer T, Peterlik M, Graf J (1989) Membrane potential measurement in isolated rat liver plasma membrane vesicles: effects of transmembrane ion concentration gradients. Biochim Biophys Acta 979: 371–374

Van Dyke R, Scharschmidt BF (1983) (Na,K)-ATPase-mediated cation pumping in cultured rat hepatocytes. Rapid modulation by alanine and taurocholate transport and characterization of its relationship to intracellular sodium concentration. J Biol Chem 285: 12912–12919

Van Dyke RW, Stephens JE, Scharschmidt BF (1982) Effect of ion substitution on bile acid-dependent and bile acid-independent bile formation by the isolated perfused rat liver. J Clin Invest 70: 505–517

von Dippe P, Drain P, Levy D (1983) Synthesis and transport characteristics of photoaffinity probes for the hepatocyte bile acid transport system. J Biol Chem 258: 8890–8895

von Dippe P, Anathanarayanan M, Drain P, Levy D (1986) Purification and reconstitution of the canalicular bile salt transport system from hepatocyte sinusoidal plasma membranes. Biochim Biophys Acta 862: 352–360

Weinman SA, Graf J, Boyer JL (1989) Voltage-driven, taurocholate-dependent secretion in isolated hepatocyte couplets. Am J Physiol 256: G 826–G 832

Wieland T, Nassal M, Kramer W, Fricker G, Bickel U, Kurz G (1984) Identity of hepatic membrane transport systems for bile salts, phalloidin and antamide by photoaffinity labeling. Proc Natl Acad Sci USA 81: 5232–5236

Wolkoff AW, Samuelson AC, Johansen KL, Nakata R, Withers DM, Sosiak A (1987) Influence of Cl^- on organic anion transport in short-term cultured rat hepatocytes and isolated perfused rat liver. J Clin Invest 79: 1259–1268

Wondergem R, Castillo LB (1986) Effect of temperature on the transmembrane potential of mouse liver cells. Am J Physiol 251: C603–C613

Wondergem R, Castillo LB (1988) Quinine decreases hepatocyte transmembrane potential and inhibits amino acid transport. Am J Physiol 254: G795–G801

Yoon YB, Hagey LR, Hofmann AF, Gurantz D, Michelotti EL, Steinbach JH (1986) Effect of side chain shortening on the physiologic properties of bile acids: hepatic transport and effect on biliary secretion of 23-norursodeoxycholate in rodents. Gastroenterology 90: 837–852

Zimmerli B, Valentinas J, Meier PJ (1987) Multispecificity of Na^+ depent taurocholate uptake in basolateral (sinusoidal) rat liver plasma membrane (blLPM) vesicles (Abstract). Hepatology 7: 1036

7 Epididymis

Electrolyte and Fluid Transport in the Epididymis *

P. Y. D. Wong

The Role of the Epididymis in Male Reproduction

Like other glandular systems in the body, the male reproductive system can be regarded as having two functions, an endocrine and an exocrine function. The former relates to the process of spermatogenesis and its hormonal control, while the latter is concerned with the transport of electrolytes, organic solutes, proteins, and water across the epithelium of the male reproductive tract. Approaches to regulate male fertility by interference with the endocrine system have been well described (Knuth and Nieschlag 1987). Although a lot of information about the endocrine control of reproductive functions has been obtained, to date no satisfactory and acceptable method has emerged that can effect male contraception by complete suppression of spermatogenesis.

In contrast, the other function of the male reproductive system has received much less attention. It is only during the last two decades that scientists began to realize that events taking place post-testicularly are important in the full expression of fertility. It has been shown in all mammalian species studied, including man, that spermatozoa first formed in the testis are immature, immotile, and incapable of fertilizing the ovum. It is only during their transit through the epididymis that they gradually acquire their fertilizing capacity and capacity for forward motility. Maturation is assocated with morphological and functional changes in the sperm. These changes confer on the sperm the ability to ascend the female genital tract and to penetrate the zona pellucida. The epididymis plays a crucial role in sperm maturation by creating an optimal microenvironment for the sperm. It is this indispensible role played by the epididymis in sperm maturation

---

* Work carried out in the author's laboratory was supported by the World Health Organization and the University of Hong Kong.

Young · Wong, Epithelial Secretion of Water and Electrolytes
© Springer-Verlag Berlin · Heidelberg 1990

that has given rise to the 'epididymal approach', an antifertility strategy based on intervention in sperm function at a post-testicular level (Waites 1987). Similarly, the dependence of sperm function on the epididymis has led to male infertility problems with epididymal dysfunction as the cause.

Several important functions of the epididymis have been described. These include the secretion of specific sperm-coating proteins found to be responsible for capacitation, acrosome reaction, penetration of the cumulus oophorus, and zona pellucida binding. All these changes are crucial to successful fertilization (see González Echeverria et al. 1984; Tezon et al. 1982; Blaquier 1985). The epididymis is capable of secreting carnitine, inositol, and glycerophosphorylcholine aganinst a lumen-to-blood concentration gradient (Marquis and Fritz 1965; Voglmayer and Amann 1973; Brooks et al. 1974). While there is some evidence that carnitine and inositol may affect sperm motility, their influence must be due to their contribution toward a major part of the epididymal fluid osmolarity. These molecules are therefore important through their effects on the osmotic balance and volume regulation of the sperm cells. Another function of the epididymis that has only quite recently been appreciated, and which has an enormous scope in post-testicular antifertility strategy, is the secretion (excretion) of exogenous drug molecules. It has been proposed that, by analogy to the kidney tubules, the epididymis is capable of excreting (secreting) exogenous drug molecules into the epididymal lumen (Qiu and Wong 1985). This idea has been advanced by experiments that showed that para-aminohippurate, a prototype of drugs actively secreted by the renal tubules, is transported actively into the lumen of the intact epididymis of the rat (Qiu and Wong 1985). Later studies with sulfonamides and related compounds also supported this contention. In these studies, it was shown that a number of sulfonamides are accumulated in the rat epididymis; their presence in the epididymal fluid appears to be a prerequisite for their antifertility effects (Wong et al. 1987). It is, therefore, of great interest that imidazoles given to dogs appeared in the semen 1–4 h after an oral dose, during which time spermatozoa were completely immobilized (Vickery et al. 1986).

The Exocrine Functions of the Epididymis

A major function of the epididymis is its ability to transport electrolytes and water because it is a process on which the concentrations of all important constituents in the epididymis depend. Furthermore, fluid transport has an immediate effect on the sperm because spermatozoa are bathed in a milieu created by the epithelium. The fluidity of the environment affects sperm concentration and possibly the time the sperm spend in the epididymis through an effect on sperm transport in the duct (Wong 1986). It has been argued that the the male reproductive tract shares many characteristics with other exocrine glands in that the testis secretes a primary fluid that carries the spermatozoa down the excurrent duct (epididymis). As fluid flows through the duct, it undergoes secondary modification. During this process, electrolytes and organic solutes are added to the lumen and others are absorbed from lumen to blood. In this respect, the male reproductive system conforms to the two-stage hypothesis (see Wong 1984) first proposed for the salivary gland (Thaysen et al. 1954) and now thought to be applicable to exocrine glands in general (Fig. 1). Advanced technology that has benefited the study of exocrine gland functions (see Wong and Young 1988) should also be used to illuminate epididymal physiology. It is only by understan-

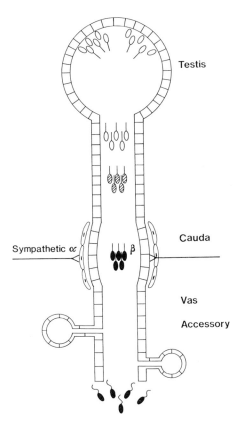

Fig. 1. The male reproductive tract can be viewed as a complex exocrine gland. A primary fluid secreted by the Sertoli's cells in the testis carries spermatozoa down the excurrent duct (epididymis). This fluid undergoes secondary modification as it flows down the duct. There is absorption of electrolytes and water and secretion of organic compounds resulting in the formation of an optimal microenvironment for sperm maturation (caput epididymis) and storage (cauda). The epididymis is innervated by sympathetic nerves. Stimulation of those nerves that supply the smooth muscle cells surrounding the duct results in ductal contraction (mediated by α-receptors), and stimulation of those leading to the epithelial cells results in fluid secretion (mediated by β-receptors). It is proposed that both ductal contraction and fluid secretion play a role in the seminal emission (Wong and Chan 1988)

ding the basic physiology of the epididymis that new methods can be devised to control male fertility or to combat infertility caused by epididymal dysfunction.

Fluid Transport in the Epididymis

Although the epididymis is normally absorptive (the epididymis reabsorbs a major part of the testicular fluid), there are large fluxes of electrolytes moving across the duct in both directions. Under basal conditions, the absorptive flux predominates over the secretory flux and this results in a net absorption of sodium and water (Wong and Yeung 1978). Under other conditions, however, when the secretory flux is increased (by secretomotor agonists) to a level exceeding the absorptive flux, net water secretion ensues. Like other secretory epithelia, active transport of anions seems to be the driving force for fluid secretion (Fig. 2).

Na^+ (Fluid) Absorption

If the lumen of the intact epididymis of the rat in vivo or that of the isolated duct of the rat cauda epididymidis in vitro is perfused with a physiological solution (Krebs-Henseleit solution), the duct reabsorbs Na^+ and water in isotonic proportions. K^+ and H^+ are secreted into the ductal lumen. This

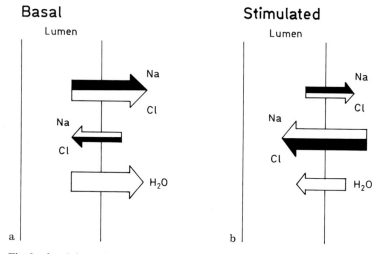

Fig. 2a, b. Schematic diagram showing electrolyte and water movements across the epididymal epithelium under **a** basal and **b** stimulated conditions. *Open arrows* and *closed arrows* indicate passive and active transport respectively

transport of Na^+ (which is linked to Cl^- absorption, H^+ secretion, and K^+ secretion) occurs in an electroneutral fashion since reabsorption is not accompanied by a detectable transepithelial potential difference (Wong et al. 1980). Like other absorbing epithelia, active Na^+ reabsorption is the driving force for fluid reabsorption, the energy being derived from the Na^+-, K^+-ATPase which has been detected histochemically in the basolateral membrane of the epididymal cells (Brandes 1974). A significant part of the fluid flowing across the epithelium appears to move through the lateral intercellular space. This is suggested by changes in the structure of the lateral intercellular spaces that accompany fluid transport (Wong et al. 1978; Cooper and Yeung 1980). Regulation of Na^+ and fluid reabsorption by the epithelium is dependent on circulating androgens (Wong and Yeung 1977) and is intimately related to the control of fluid volume homeostasis. Hence, reabsorption falls after adrenalectomy and is reversed by hormone replacement with aldosterone (Au et al. 1978). It is affected by the acid–base status of the animals (Au and Wong 1980) and is inhibited by diuretic drugs (Wong and Lee 1982; Turner and Cesarini 1983; Jenkins et al. 1983).

Anion (and Fluid) Secretion

The ability to culture epididymal cells represents a major advance in the study of epididymal function (Kierszenbaum et al. 1981; Olson et al. 1983; Byers and Dym 1986; Cuthbert and Wong 1986). Primary cultures of rat epididymal cells have been grown on permeable supports (Cuthbert and Wong 1986) and electrogenic ion secretion studied by the short-circuit current technique. It has been shown that the tissues secrete chloride and bicarbonate concurrently in response to a number of secretomotor agonists (see below). Experiments using transport inhibitors and specific channel blockers have led to the conclusion that secretion is mediated by the simultaneous activities of a $Na^+-K^+-2Cl^-$ symport, a Na^+-H^+ exchanger and a $Cl^--HCO_3^-$ exchanger in the basolateral membrane (Wong 1988a), and the opening of the anion channels in the apical membrane (Wong 1988b; Huang and Wong 1988; Fig. 3).

Secretomotor agonists stimulate secretion of anions (and fluid) by increasing intracellular cyclic AMP (see Fig. 4) which opens apical anion channels. This action of cyclic AMP has also been demonstrated by experiments involving intracellular pH (pH_i) measurement using a pH-sensitive dye, BCECF (Huang and Wong 1988). Under basal conditions, pH_i was decreased by amiloride (an inhibitor of Na^+-H^+ antiports), but increased by SITS (an inhibitor of $Cl^--HCO_3^-$ exchange) and diphenylamino-2-carboxylate (DPC), a blocker of anion channels.

Addition of β-adrenergic agonists, forskolin, and 8-Br-cyclic AMP to the cells caused the pH_i to fall to the equilibrium pH of 6.7. This agonist-induced acidosis was blocked by DPC, but was unaffected by SITS. These experi-

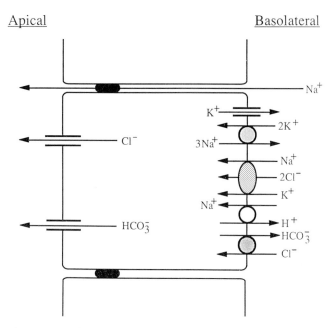

Fig. 3. Model for anion (and fluid) secretion by the epididymis. Secretion of chloride and bicarbonate drives water secretion. Secretion involves three basolateral membrane carriers, i.e., a $Na^+ - K^+ - 2Cl^-$ symport, $Na^+ - H^+$ and $Cl^- - HCO_3^-$ antiports, and apical anion channels. During secretion, the charge carried by anion efflux at the apical membrane is balanced by K^+ efflux through the basolateral K^+ channels

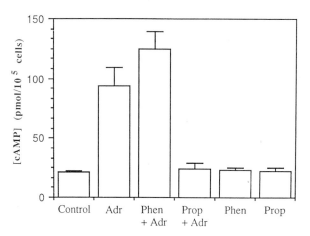

Fig. 4. Cyclic AMP concentration in monolayers of rat epididymal cells grown on millipore filters. Confluent monolayers (area $0.6\ cm^2$ were incubated in Krebs-Henseleit (K – H) solution (*control*), or K – H solution containing adrenaline (*Adr*, 1 µmol/l), or adrenaline plus phentolamine (*Phen*, 2 µmol/l), or adrenaline plus propranolol (*Prop*, 2 µmol/l), or the inhibitors alone, for 10 min before cyclic AMP was measured by radioimmunoassay. All solutions contained 1 mmol/l IBMX (3-Isobutyl-1-methyl-xanthine)

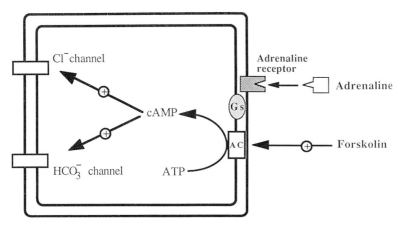

Fig. 5. Control of secretion by cyclic AMP. β-Adrenergic agonists interact with receptors leading to the formation of cyclic AMP which opens chloride and bicarbonate channels at the apical membrane and initiates secretion. Anion exit through these channels is the rate-limiting step in secretion. The activities of these channels therefore determine anion and fluid secretion and hence the fluidity of the epididymal environment. *Gs*, guanine nucleotide-regulatorybinding protein; *AC*, adenylate cyclase

ments therefore provide evidence that the paired Na^+-H^+ and $Cl^--HCO_3^-$ antiports and a HCO_3^- channel are present in the epididymal cells (Wong 1988a). These transporters are involved in the regulation of intracellular pH. β-Agonists stimulate anion secretion by stimulating the formation of cyclic AMP, which leads to the activation or insertion of anion (both Cl^- and HCO_3^-) channels in the apical membrane. Since the intracellular Cl^- and HCO_3^- activities are normally held above electrochemical equilibrium (by the symport, the $Cl^--HCO_3^-$ exchanger and the Na^+-H^+ exchanger), increasing the apical anion conductance by cyclic AMP would lead to an efflux of anions into the apical compartment (Fig. 5). This accounts for the fall in pH_i observed during stimulation. Efflux of anions at the apical membrane is rheogenic and would cause a depolarization of the basolateral membrane with subsequent activation of the K^+ channels at the basolateral side (Fig. 3). The evidence that the epididymal cells do have a basolateral K^+ conductance that plays a role in secretion came from the following experiments. Tetraethylamminium (TEA; 10 mmol/l) added to the basolateral side of the epididymal monolayer did not affect the secretory response to adrenaline (measured as a rise in short circuit current (SCC), whereas addition of Ba^{2+} (5 mmol/l) to the same side completely abolished it. These results would indicate that a basolateral K^+ channel blockable by Ba^{2+} is involved in secretion. Similar observations have been made in bicarbonate secretion in the pancreatic duct cells (Gray et al. 1988; Novak and Greger 1988). K^+ efflux is followed by K^+ reuptake via the basolateral Na^+-K^+ $-2Cl^-$ symport and the ouabain-sensitive Na^+-, K^+-ATPase. The Na^+ ions that have entered the cells by the symport and the Na^+-H^+ antiport are pumped out again by the Na^+-, K^+-ATPase. The net result of these complex ionic events is to effect a net Cl^- and HCO_3^- uptake into the cytosol through the cycling of Na^+ and K^+ across the basolateral membrane, the energy being derived from the Na^+ gradient and ultimately from the Na^+-, K^+-ATPase. The primary event in stimulus-secretion coupling, however, is the activation of an apical anion conductance by cyclic AMP (Fig. 5). The presence of a cyclic AMP-activated anion channel in the apical membrane and a voltage-dependent K^+ channel in the basolateral membrane of the epididymal cells (Fig. 3) awaits verification by patch-clamp studies.

Regulation of Anion (and Fluid) Secretion

Adrenergic agonists, autacoids, and hormones control anion secretion in the epididymal cells (Table 1). β-Adrenergic agonists have been the most extensively investigated (Wong and Chan 1988; Wong 1988a). Isoproterenol, adrenaline, noradrenaline, and phenylephrine stimulate secretion by interacting with the basolateral β-adrenergic receptors; the effect is blocked by propranolol, a β-antagonist. When β-agonists bind to their receptors, they activate adenylate cyclase, which increases intracellular cyclic AMP levels in the epididymal cells. Although the cyclic AMP level has not been measured in all cases, most of these secretomotor agonists probably involve cyclic AMP in the signal transduction mechanism (Table 1). Intracellular Ca^{2+} has been measured in epididymal cell monolayers using Fura-2. No increase in $[Ca^{2+}]_i$ was observed with these secretory agonists (Table 1). This indicates that these cyclic AMP-linked agonists do not exploit calcium as an intracellular messenger to stimulate anion secretion.

In many epithelia, signals that regulate ion transport come from the serosal surface of the cell. Table 1 shows a similar situation in the epididymal cells. Very recently we have become interested in the possibility that control

Table 1. Neurohumoral and pharmacological agents that stimulate anion secretion in primary monolayer cultures of rat epididymis

Agent	Side of action	cAMP	$[Ca^{2+}]_i$
β-Adrenergic agents	Serosal	↑	No change
Prostaglandins	Serosal	↑	No change
Adenosine triphosphate	Mucosal	↑	No change
VIP	Serosal	↑	No change
Bradykinin	Serosal > mucosal	↑	No change
ADH	Serosal > mucosal	↑	No change
Angiotensin	Serosal	↑	No change
A23187	Mucosal	Small ↑	↑

Mucosal, apical; serosal, basolateral; VIP, vasoactive intestinal peptide; ADH, antidiuretic hormone

of fluid transport in the epididymis is also exerted at the apical (mucosal) side of the epithelium. This is particularly important because normally the lumen is filled with spermatozoa. It is possible that spermatozoa can affect secretion by feedback onto the epididymal cells, and in doing so, regulate the fluidity of their own environment. Such a local control would require that some factors are released from spermatozoa. Secondly, there must be receptors for these factors in the apical membrane of the cells, and lastly, interaction of receptors with these factors leads to an alteration in fluid transport. These criteria for a local control are met by ATP which is present in spermatozoa at high concentrations (Gottlieb et al. 1987). In the rat, spermatozoa flushed out from the cauda epididymidis have been found to contain ATP in a concentration of 7.2 mmol/l of sperm cells (P.Y.D. Wong, unpublished observation).

ATP added to the apical side of the cultured monolayers of the rat epididymis stimulates short-circuit current in a dose-dependent manner (Wong and Fu 1988). The EC_{50} (concentration producing a 50% increase in

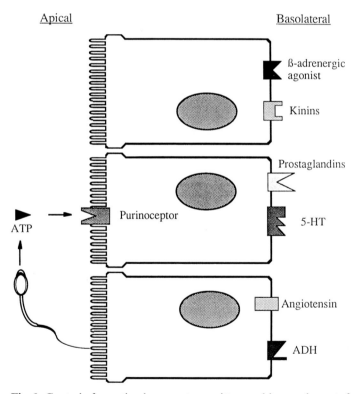

Fig. 6. Control of secretion by neurotranamitters and humoral agents from the basolateral side and by ATP from the apical side. All these controls are important in the maintenance of a normal fluid environment in the epididymis. The control of secretion by the apical purinoceptors offers a means by which spermatozoa can regulate the fluidity of their own environment

current) is 5×10^{-8} mol/l. The increase in current was not seen in Cl^--free medium, suggesting that the response was probably due to Cl^- secretion. ATP added to the lumen of the intact epididymis induced an increase in serosal-to-mucosal Cl^- flux and concomitantly reversed the net water absorption into net water secretion (Wong and Fu 1988; Wong 1988c). Our study of agonist potency showed that among the adenosine derivatives, ATP was the most potent, with adenosine the least potent in stimulating Cl^- secretion. This order of potency: ATP > ADP $\gg$ AMP = adenosine, suggests that it is the P_2-purinoceptor that mediates the secretory response to ATP. The contention was supported by the finding that 8-phenyltheophylline, a potent antagonist of P_1-purinoceptors, did not prevent the rise in SCC caused by ATP. It is possible that degenerating spermatozoa release ATP which stimulates fluid secretion locally. An increase in fluidity in the vicinity of the sperm would help resorption of the sperm fragments by the epididymal cells. This mechanism may be involved in the disposition of unejaculated aged sperm by the cauda epididymidis.

It appears that in the epididymis, various secretomotor agonists affect anion secretion by acting either from the basolateral or the apical side of the epithelium. Those that act basolaterally include the neurotransmitter, noradrenalin, blood-borne hormones, and humoral agents that are produced locally in the epididymis (prostaglandins, angiotensin, bradykinin, etc.). ATP, which is present in spermatozoa in high concentrations, may act on the purinoceptors located at the apical membrane. This local control via apical purinoceptors offers a means by which spermatozoa may control the fluidity of their own environment (Fig. 6).

Defective Fluid Secretion As a Cause of Obstructive Azoospermia

As mentioned above, the epididymis is both absorptive and secretory. Both processes are precisely controlled so that under normal conditions, there is a balance between absorption and secretion. However, if absorption and secretion are mismatched, or the secretory mechanism itself becomes defective, abnormal fluid transport across the duct will lead to an unfavourable environment which may have adverse effects on sperm function and, hence, fertility.

When rats are treated with reserpine to disrupt adrenergic influences on the epididymis (and other systems as well), sperm concentration and protein concentration in the fluid flushed out from the cauda epididymidis rise. There is also a concomitant increase in the viscosity of the fluid. These effects are secondary to a decrease in secretion leading to 'dehydration' of the epididymal lumen (Wen and Wong 1988).

The importance of the balance between absorption and secretion to spermatozoa and fertility is shown in Fig. 7. Figure 7a represents the normal

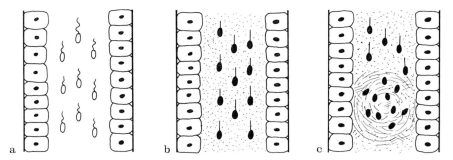

Fig. 7a — c. Schematic diagram showing how abnormal fluid transport may lead to epididymal obstruction. **a** Epididymis with normal fluid transport. **b** Defective secretion results in a rise in the viscosity of the epididymal fluid. **c** This eventually leads to the formation of a plug blocking the epididymal lumen

situation in which there is a balance between absorption and secretion. Sperm are bathed in an environment of normal fluidity. In Fig. 7b it is seen that defective anion and fluid secretion leads to a 'dehydrated' state within the lumen. The epididymal cells continuously secrete high-molecular-weight glycoproteins (Usselman and Cone 1983) that confer a high viscoelasticity on the epididymal fluid. Continuous secretion of proteins without fluid secretion would eventually lead to luminal blockage by thick mucous material (Fig. 7c), a phenomenon seen in cystic fibrosis, Young's syndrome, and some other unexplained cases of male infertility.

Epididymis and Cystic Fibrosis

Cystic fibrosis (CF) is the most common fatal genetic disease of Caucasians. The disease characteristically involves three exocrine organs: sweat glands, pancreas, and airways. In all cases, the primary disturbance is caused by defective fluid secretion leading to obstruction of the ductal part of the glands by thick inspissated material.

It is now known that these manifestations of the disease have one common cause. The secretion of chloride (and hence fluid) by the epithelium in response to β-adrenergic agonists is impaired. Electrophysiology of cultured CF airway epithelial cells has localized the defect to an apical membrane that is impermeable to Cl^- (Widdicombe et al. 1985) and suggests a defect in Cl^- channel function in CF. The patch-clamp technique has been used to study single-channel currents in CF airway epithelial cells (Frizzell et al. 1986; Welsh and Liedtke 1986). It was found that in excised patches, apical membrane Cl^- channels were present, and their conductive and kinetic properties were normal. However, when channel activities were studied in the cell-attached mode, Cl^- channels did not open normally in response to agonists that stimulate cyclic AMP production. There is no fault at the level of the signal transduction because CF cells can generate cyclic AMP in response to stimulation with secretomotor agonists. The defect must lie at a site distal to cyclic AMP generation. More recent experiments using subunit C of the cyclic AMP-dependent protein kinase on excised membrane patches of CF airway cells have further localized the defect to the regulatory protein of the apical Cl^- channels (Schoumacher et al. 1987).

The defective regulation of the Cl^- channels by cyclic AMP is not unique to the airway cells. Patch-clamp studies of the cultured nasal polyps (Kunzelmann et al. 1988) derived from CF patients have indicated that in this tissue the regulation of the chloride channels by cyclic AMP is also defective. Evidence is accumulating that a similar defect occurs in pancreatic duct cells (Gray et al. 1988). It appears that secretory epithelia that utilize cyclic AMP as the second messenger in stimulus-secretion coupling are the targets of the disease. We propose that the epididymis with secretory mechanisms so similar to these epithelia falls into the catagory of CF epithelia. The arguments to support this contention are as follows:

1. Men with CF who have survived to adulthood are infertile because of obstructive azoospermia (Di Sant'Agnese 1968; Seale et al. 1985). (Sometimes the epididymis is absent and this morphological change may be sesondary to defective secretion). Obstruction is caused by thick inspissated material blocking the lumen, a situition very similar to that seen in the airway and pancreatic ducts of CF patients.
2. The epididymis utilizes cyclic AMP as a second messenger in stimulus-secretion coupling. It is now known that CF predominately affects cyclic AMP-dependent epithelia. It is the cyclic AMP-dependent activation of Cl^- channels at the apical membrane that fails.
3. Short-circuit current measurement in cultured epididymal epithelium has indicated the presence of an apical Cl^- channel that is blocked selectively by Cl^- channel blockers, namely, diphenylamine-2-carboxylate (DPC) and 5-nitro-2-(3-phenylpropylamino)-benzoate (NPPB) (Wong 1988b). Chloride channels with the same characteristics are found in the airway cells.
4. The profiles of neurohumoral control of secretion in the epididymis and the airway are very similar (see Table 1 and Welsh 1987). This prompts one to speculate that the two tissues have similar properties with respect to their physiology and pathology.

Area for Future Research

In view of the possibility that the epididymis may fall into the class of CF epithelia, there is a need to identify the ion channels in the epididymal cells using the patch-clamp technique. CF is not the only example in which defective secretory functions are linked to male infertility. Obstructive azoospermia seen in patients with Young's syndrome (sinopulmonary disease; Handelsman et al. 1984) may also have a similar pathophysiological basis. Similarly, a number of unexplained cases of male infertility may well be the result of abnormal fluid transport.

If secretion occurs by the mechanism shown in Fig. 3, there must be a Cl^- (and HCO_3^-) channel at the apical membrane and a K^+ channel at the basolateral membrane. During secretion, Cl^- and HCO_3^- exit through the apical anion channel driven by their electrochemical gradients. K^+ enters cells through the $Na^+ - K^+ - 2Cl^-$ symport and the Na^+-, K^+-ATPase. For secretion to continue, the excess K^+ ions that have accumulated intracellularly would have to leave the cells. The regulated K^+ channel at the basolateral membrane therefore provides a pathway for K^+ efflux. These ion channels play an integral role in anion and fluid secretion and determine the fluidity of the environment in which spermatozoa are bathed. An understanding of the secretory mechanism at the level of the ion channel is therefore important to the future development of post-testicular male fertility-regulating agents as well as to the understanding of male infertility caused by epididymal dysfunction.

References

Au CL, Wong PYD (1980) Luminal acidification by the perfused rat cauda epididymidis. J Physiol (Lond) 309: 419–428

Au CL, Ngai HK, Yeung CH, Wong PYD (1978) Effect of adrenalectomy and hormone replacement on sodium and water transport in the perfused rat cauda epididymis. J Endocrinol 77: 265–266

Blaquier JA, Cameo MS, deLarminat MA, Pineiro L, Tezon J, Vasquez M (1985) Some studies on the physiology of the human epididymis. Abstract, Proceedings of the 3rd International congress of andrology, Boston, 27 April–2 May 1985

Brandes D (1974) Fine structure and cytochemistry of male sex accessory organs. In: Brandes D (ed) Male accessory sex organs. Structure and function in mammals. Academic, New York, pp 17–113

Brooks DE, Hamilton DW, Mallek AH (1974) Carnitine and glycerylphosphorylcholine in the reproductive tract of the rat. J Reprod Fertil 36: 141–146

Byers SW, Dym M (1986) Growth and characterization of polaized monolayers of epididymal epithelial cells and Sertoli cells in dual environment culture chambers. J Androl 7: 59–68

Cooper TG, Yeung CH (1980) Epithelial structure of the rat cauda epididymidis after luminal perfusion. Int J Androl 3: 361–374

Cuthbert AW, Wong PYD (1986) Electrogenic anion secretion in cultured rat epididymal epithelium. J Physiol (Lond) 378: 335–346

Di Sant'Agnese PA (1968) Fertility and the young adult with cystic fibrosis. N Engl J Med 279: 103–103

Frizzell RA, Rechkemmer G, Shoemaker RL (1986) Altered regulation of airway epithelial cell chloride channels in cystic fibrosis. Science 233: 558–560

González Echeverria FM, Cuasnicú PS, Piazza A, Pineiro L, Blaquier JA (1984) Addition of an androgen-free epididymal protein extract increases the ability of immature hamster spermatozoa to fertilize in vivo and in vitro. J Reprod Fertil 71: 433–437

Gottlieb C, Svanborg K, Eneroth P, Bygdeman M (1987) Adenosine triphosphate in human seman: a study on conditions for a bioluminescence assay. Fertil Steril 47: 992–999

Grey MA, Greenwell JR, Argent BE (1988) Ion channels on pancreatic duct cells and their role in bicarbonate secretion. In: Wong PYD, Young JA (eds) Exocrine secretion. Hong Kong University Press, Hong Kong, pp 11–15

Handelsman DJ, Conway AJ, Boylan LM, Turtle JR (1984) Young's syndrome. Obstructive azoospermia and chronic sinopulmonary infections. N Engl J Med 310: 3–9

Huang SJ, Wong PYD (1988) Intracellular acidosis induced by secretomotor agonists in cultured epididymal epithelium of the rat. In: Wong PYD, Young JA (eds) Exocrine secretion. Hong Kong University Press, Hong Kong, pp 87–88

Jenkins AD, Lechene CP, Howards SS (1983) Effect of spironolactone on the elemental composition of the intraluminal fluids of the seminiferous tubules, rete testis and epididymis of rat. J Urol 129: 851–854

Kierszenbaum AL, Lea O, Petrusz P, French F, Tres LL (1981) Isolation, culture, and immunocytochemical characterization of epididymal epithelial cells from pubertal and adult rats. Proc Natl Acad Sci USA 78: 1675–1679

Knuth UA, Nieschlag E (1987) Endocrine approaches to male fertility control. In: Burger HG (ed) Bailliere's clinical endocrinology and metabolism, vol 1, no 1. Bailliere Tindall, London, pp 113–131

Kunzelmann K, Ünal Ö, Beck C, Emmrich P, Arndt H, Greger R (1988) Ion channels of cultured respiratory epithelial cells of patients with cystic fibrosis. Pflügers Arch 411: R68 (Abstract)

Marquis NR, Fritz IB (1965) Effect of testosterone on the distribution of carnitine, acetylcarnitine, and carnitine acetyltransferase in tissues of the reproductive system of male rats. In: Wolf G (ed) Recent research on carnitine. Its relation to lipid metabolism. MIT Press, Cambridge, MA, pp 31–34

Novak I, Greger R (1988) Electrophysiological study of transport systems in isolated perfused pancreatic ducts: properties of the basolateral membrane. Pflügers Arch 411: 58–68

Olson GE, Jonas-Davies J, Hoffman LH, Orgebin-Crist MC (1983) Structural features of cultured epithelial cells from the adult rat epididymis. J Androl 4: 347–360

Qiu JP, Wong PYD (1985) Secretion of para-aminohippurate by the rat epididymis. J Physiol (Lond) 364: 241–248

Schoumacher RA, Shoemaker RL, Halm DR, Tallant EA, Wallace RW, Frizzell RA (1987) Phosphorylation fails to activate chloride channels from cystic fibrosis airway cells. Nature 330: 752–753

Seale TW, Flux M, Rennert OM (1985) Reproductive defects in patients of both sexes with cystic fibrosis: a review. Ann Clin Lab Sci 15: 152–158

Tezon JG, Cuasnicú PS, Scorticoti C, Blaquier JA (1982) Development and characterization of a model system for the study of epididymal physiology in man. In: De Nicola A, Blaquier JA, Soto RJ (eds) Physiopathology of hypophysial disturbances and diseases of reproduction. Alan Liss, New York, pp 251

Thaysen JH, Thorn NA, Schwartz IL (1954) Excretion of sodium, potassium, chloride and carbon dioxide in human parotid saliva. Am J Physiol 178: 155–159

Turner TT, Cesarini DM (1983) The ability of the rat epididymis to concentrate spermatozoa. Responsiveness to aldosterone. J Androl 4: 197–202

Usselman C, Cone RA (1983) Rat sperm are mechanically immobilized in the caudal epididymis by 'immobulin', a high molecular weight glycoprotein. Biol Reprod 29: 1241–1253

Vickery BH, Grigg MB, Goodpasture JC, Bergström KK, Walker KAM (1986) Toward same-day, orally administered male contraceptive. In: Zatuchni GI, Goldsmith JM, Spieler JM, Sciarra JJ (eds) Male contraception, advances and future prospect. Harper and Row, Philadelphia, pp 227–236

Voglmayr JK, Amann RP (1973) The distribution of free myo-inositol in fluid, spermatozoa, and tissues of the bull genital tract and observations on its uptake by the rabbit epididymis. Biol Reprod 8: 504–573

Waites GMH (1987) Post-testicular antifertility methods. In: Diczfalusy E, Bygdeman M (eds) Fertility regulation for today and tomorrow. Raven, New York, pp 247–263

Welsh MJ (1987) Electrolyte transport by airway epithelia. Physiol Rev 67: 1143–1184

Welsh MJ, Liedtke CM (1986) Chloride and potassium channels in cystic fibrosis airway epithelia. Nature 322: 467–470

Wen RQ, Wong PYD (1988) Reserpine treatment increases viscosity of fluid in the epididymis of rats. Biol Reprod 38: 969–974

Widdicombe JH, Welsh MJ, Finkbeiner WE (1985) Cystic fibrosis decreases the apical membrane chloride permeability of monolayers cultured from cells of tracheal epithelium. Proc Natl Acad Sci USA 82: 6167–6171

Wong PYD (1984) The exocrine functions of the epididymis. In: Case RM, Lingard JM, Young JA (eds) Secretion, mechanisms and control. Manchaster University Press, Manchester, pp 143–147

Wong PYD (1986) Fluid transport and sperm maturation in the epididymis. Biomed Res 7 [Suppl 2]: 233–240

Wong PYD (1988a) Mechanism of adrenergic stimulation of anion secretion in cultured rat epididymal epithelium. Am J Physiol 254: F121–F133

Wong PYD (1988b) Inhibition by chloride channel blockers of anion secretion in cultured epididymal epithelium and intact epididymis of rats. Br J Pharmacol 94: 155–163

Wong PYD (1988c) Control of anion and fluid secretion by apical P_2-purinoceptors in the rat epididymis. Br J Pharmacol 95: 1315–1321

Wong PYD, Chan TPT (1988) Adrenergic control of electrogenic anion secretion in primary cultures of rat epididymal cells. In: Davison JS, Shaffer EA (eds) Gastrointestinal and hepatic secretion. University of Calgary Press, Calgary, pp 216–219

Wong PYD, Fu WO (1988) Apical purinoceptor controls anion aund fluid secretion by the rat epididymis. In: Wong PYD, Young JA (eds) Exocrine secretion. Hong Kong University Press, Hong Kong, pp 215–218

Wong PYD, Lee WM (1982) Effects of spironolactone (aldosterone antagonist) on electrolyte and water content of the cauda epididymidis and fertility of male rats. Biol Reprod 27: 771–777

Wong PYD, Yeung CH (1977) Hormonal regulation of fluid resorption in isolated rat cauda epididymidis. Endocrinology 101: 1391–1397

Wong PYD, Yeung CH (1978) Absorptive and secretory functions of the perfused rat cauda epididymidis. J Physiol (Lond) 275: 13–26

Wong PYD, Young JA (eds) (1988) Exocrine secretion. Hong Kong University Press, Hong Kong

Wong YC, Wong PYD, Yeung CH (1978) Ultrastructural correlation of water resorption in isolated cauda epididymidis. Experientia 34: 485–487

Wong PYD, Au CL, Ngai HK (1980) The isolated duct of the rat cauda epididymidis as a model for isosmotic transport studies. Jpn J Physiol 30: 1–15

Wong PYD, Lau HK, Fu WO (1987) Antifertility effects of some sulfonamide and related compounds and their accumulation in the rat epididymis. J Reprod Fertil 81: 259–267

8 Salt Glands

Ultrastructure and X-Ray Microanalysis of Vertebrate Salt Glands

A.T. Marshall

Introduction

The functional significance of salt glands in vertebrates was discovered by Schmidt-Nielsen and his colleagues some 30 years ago (e.g. Schmidt-Nielsen et al. 1957). All of these glands secrete sodium chloride, usually at a higher concentration than is present in the blood, and in some cases, high concentrations of potassium and bicarbonate are also secreted.

There has been a considerable volume of research on the structure, role in osmotic and ionic regulation and the cellular mechanisms of secretion of the glands (Minnich 1979; Van Lennep and Young 1979; Holmes and Phillips 1985). The secretory mechanism at the cellular level has been largely elucidated in the elasmobranch rectal gland. A simple model has been developed that incorporates features common to a variety of vertebrate transporting epithelia. It depends on the secondary active transport of chloride coupled to sodium and potassium transport via a common carrier. The driving force for the movement of sodium via the common carrier is the gradient maintained by basolaterally distributed Na^+-, K^+-ATPase. Chloride diffuses passively across the apical membrane, and sodium and water follow via a paracellular route (Epstein and Silva 1981).

There are a number of structural similarities in salt glands. They all appear to be tubular glands, usually, having a main duct which branches into secondary ducts which in turn may branch into ducts termed central canals into which the secretory tubules drain. The secretory tubules are composed of principal cells as a major component with other cell types present as minor components. It is generally considered that the principal cells are the sites of active ion transport into the lumen.

Young · Wong, Epithelial Secretion of Water and Electrolytes
© Springer-Verlag Berlin · Heidelberg 1990

Ultrastructure

The ultrastructure of the avian salt gland has been extensively investigated (e.g. Komnick 1963). The salt glands of various groups of reptiles have been described at the ultrastructural level, e.g. marine and estuarine turtles (Abel and Ellis 1966; Cowan 1971), lizards (e.g. Van Lennep and Komnick 1970), sea snakes (Dunson and Dunson 1974) and saltwater crocodiles (Taplin and Grigg 1981). In elasmobranchs salt gland ultrastructure has also been described (e.g. Bulger 1963, 1965).

Principal Cells

The principal cells of all salt glands have some features in common and others which, superficially, appear to be major differences. In both reptiles and elasmobranchs the principal cells have highly amplified lateral cell membranes (Fig. 1), whereas in birds there is also amplificiation of the basal membranes (Fig. 2). The lateral amplificiations are in the form of plications or leaflets. In reptilian (Ellis and Goertemiller 1976) and avian (Ellis et al. 1977) cells the plications run in a base-to-apex direction (Fig. 3) on all lateral cell surfaces. It seems probable that this is the case also in elasmobranchs. The functional significance of the different emphasis on basal and lateral folding of the cell membranes in birds, reptiles and elasmobranchs remains obscure. Suggestions that this difference is related to a much higher secretion rate in birds than in reptiles and elasmobranchs do not seem tenable since Marshall and Cooper (1988) have shown that secretion rates from turtle lacrimal salt glands can be very high when appropriately stimulated. Estimates of the ratio of basolateral to apical membrane surface areas have been made in a bird and a lizard (see Van Lennep and Komnick 1970). The ratios 1000:1 and 1400:1 are similar.

In all salt glands so far investigated, cytochemically detected Na^+-, K^+-ATPase is found associated with the basolateral cell borders (Fig. 4). This

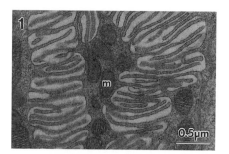

Fig. 1. Interdigitating plications of lateral cell membranes in principal cells of sea turtle lacrimal salt gland. *m*, mitochondria

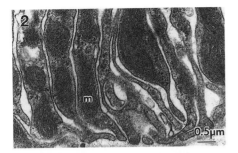

Fig. 2. Infoldings of basal cell membrane in principal cells of duck nasal salt gland. *m*, mitochondria

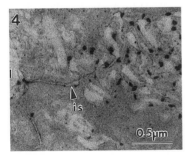

Fig. 3. Plications on lateral cell surface of principal cells of sea turtle lacrimal salt gland. *l*, lumen

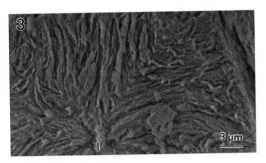

Fig. 4. Reaction sites of cytochemically detected Na^+-, K^+-ATPase on lateral cell membranes of principal cells of duck nasal salt gland. *l*, lumen; *is*, intracellular space

has been demonstrated in birds (e.g. Ernst 1972), turtles and lizards (Ellis and Goertemiller 1976) and elasmobranchs (Eveloff et al. 1979). Carbonic anhydrase has been shown to have a distribution parallel to Na^+-, K^+-ATPase in the elasmobranch rectal gland (Lacy 1983) with the reaction product deposited on the extracellular side of the basolateral membranes.

Glycosaminoglycans or glycoproteins have been revealed cytochemically to be associated with the basolateral membranes in birds (Martin and Philpott 1974), turtles (Ellis and Able 1964) and elasmobranchs (Bulger 1963; Van Lennep 1968). The cytochemical evidence suggests the presence of a non-sulphated polyanionic compound. Martin and Philpott (1974) demonstrated that the probable identity of this compound in birds is sialic acid.

At the apical ends of the intracellular spaces the adjacent cell membranes come together to form a series of junctional elements (Fig. 5). Much interest has centred on the nature of the zonulae occludentes or tight junctions, and these have been investigated in birds (e.g. Ellis et al. 1977) and elasmobranchs (e.g. Forrest et al. 1982). In all of these studies it has been shown that the zonulae occludentes consist of a small number of parallel sealing strands, typically two to three, and that although the apical surface area of the cells is very small, the apical junctions are highly convoluted because the cells interdigitate. This gives a very high junctional length per square centimetre of luminal surface area, measured in elasmobranchs to be some 100 m/cm^2. Although the junctions between sea turtle principal cells have not been studied by freeze fracture, scanning electron microscopy (A. T. Marshall and S. Saddlier, unpublished data) suggests that these cells do not interdigitate extensively.

Certain speculations arise from the forgoing. The enormous basolateral membrane amplificiation is related to the apparent requirement for Na^+-, K^+-ATPase as has been convincingly demonstrated by the correlation of increasing membrane surface area with the Na^+-, K^+-ATPase content during salt adaptation in ducks (Merchant et al. 1985). If the $Na^+ - K^+ - 2Cl^-$ co-transporter is similarly distributed, permitting the transport into the cell of $2Cl^-$ ions for every Na^+ ion transported out by the Na^+-, K^+-ATPase (Epstein and Silva 1981), then, with a basolateral to apical surface area ratio of 1000, the Cl^- flux across the apical membrane must be very high indeed. Marshall et al. (1987) have calculated the Na^+ flux across the luminal surface of the secretory tubules in the duck nasal gland to be 0.02–0.21 $\times 10^{-8} \text{ μmol μm}^{-2} \text{ s}^{-1}$, depending on the concentration of the tubule fluid. The Cl^- flux across the apical membrane would have to be slightly higher than this. Using the values of Merchant et al. (1985) for basolateral surface

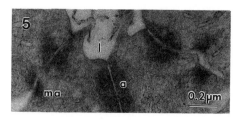

Fig. 5. Junctional complexes in principal cells of sea turtle salt gland. *l*, lumen; *a*, zonula adherens; *ma*, macula adherens

area ($10\,000\,\mu m^2$), and the number of Na^+-, K^+-ATPase molecules per μm^2 (4000), and assuming a corresponding distribution of the $Na^+ - K^+ - 2Cl^-$ co-transporter, then the transport rate of Cl^- by the co-transporter would be approximately $3-30\,Cl^-$ ions per transport complex per second.

The flow of water across the luminal surface has been calculated by Marshall et al. (1987) to be between 0.33×10^{-8} and $0.22 \times 10^{-7}\,\mu l\,\mu m^{-2}\,s^{-1}$ depending on whether post-tubular water reabsorption occurs or not. If Na^+ and water transport are considered to be paracellular and it is assumed that the junctional length per unit surface area of the lumen is similar to that of elasmobranchs (Ernst et al. 1981; Forrest et al. 1982), i.e. about $100\,m/cm^2$, then the Na^+ flux in terms of junctional length would be $2 \times 10^{-4} - 21 \times 10^{-4}\,\mu mol\,m^{-1}\,s^{-1}$ and water flow would be $3.5 - 220\,\mu l\,m^{-1}\,s^{-1}$.

The presence in birds of a highly charged polyanionic polysaccharide or glycoprotein in the intercellular spaces, associated with the basal infoldings, seems to have received little attention or comment since its role was considered by Martin and Philpott (1974). Compounds such as this must exert an influence on the distribution of cations immediately adjacent to the membranes. A possible role may be to promote recycling of Na^+ and K^+ across the cell membrane by accumulation of cations and Donnan exclusion of anions or to trap divalent cations originating from the interstitial fluid, thereby reducing their effective concentration in the intercellular spaces. It is interesting that Lacy (1983) states that the reaction product for the cytochemical localisation of carbonic anhydrase is deposited in regions of high pH and that in the case of the elasmobranch rectal gland, deposition occurs within the intercellular spaces, thereby implying that the intercellular space has a high pH. The intercellular polysaccharide would presumably be maximally dissociated under these conditions. Senson and Maren (1984) have proposed that carbonic anhydrase facilitates CO_2 transfer from sites of metabolism to capillary blood by its conversion to HCO_3^-. Thus the intercellular space must accumulate HCO_3^- during secretion.

A vexed question that has occupied several investigators is whether the intercellular spaces are dilated during secretion. The ultrastructural appearance could be ascribed to the physiological state of the cells or to the osmotic effects of fixation (e.g. Cowan 1986). Frozen-hydrated and freeze-substituted preparations of turtle salt glands (A. T. Marshall, unpublished data) clearly show that the spaces are indeed dilated in active glands, which perhaps implies that water transport is paracellular. It seems possible that a flow of water restricted to the apical junctions would be more likely to result in dilation of the intercellular space than would trancellular transport with water entering the cell over the total basolateral cell surface.

Duct System

The duct system of salt glands has been relatively neglected. It has been described in the elasmobranch rectal gland (Bulger 1965) and in the avian nasal gland (Marshall et al. 1987). Marshall et al. (1985, 1987) have proposed that the duct system in the duck plays a role in modifying the primary secretion. In the duck, the main ducts consist of large columnar cells with a layer of cuboidal basal cells. Between the cells are complex intercellular spaces, and the columnar cells resemble the cells of rabbit gall bladder. The duct system of the elasmobranch rectal gland (Bulger 1965) resembles the amphibian bladder. In the turtle, the distal part of the duct system (central canals) consists of columnar cells, but proximally is formed from a stratified or pseudostratified epithelium, similar to that of the rectal gland, and is rich in mucocytes (Marshall and Saddlier 1989). In both the rectal gland and the turtle lacrimal gland the duct system is characterised by cells with complex intercellular spaces. The zonulae occludentes in the rectal gland duct have the morphological characteristics of tight junctions (Ernst et al. 1981), and the junctional length per unit surface area of lumen is much less than in the secretory tubules. In the duck, Na^+-, K^+-ATPase has been cytochemically located along the lateral membranes of the columnar cells of the duct (Marshall et al. 1987), and carbonic anhydrase is associated with the lateral cell membranes of the cells in the rectal gland duct (Lacy 1983). Whilst the proximal regions of the duct systems in turtles and elasmobranchs are well endowed with mucocytes, it seems probable that the columnar duct cells in the duck also have the capacity, although more limited, to secrete mucus since extensive Golgi bodies and apical vesicles are commonly seen in these cells (Marshall et al. 1987). The duct systems in birds, elasmobranchs and turtles are all highly vascularised.

The morphology and cytochemistry of the duct systems suggest that the ducts may be more than just simple conduits and that they may have a role in modifying the secretion.

X-Ray Microanalysis

Two X-ray microanalytical investigations of the duck nasal salt gland have been carried out (Andrews et al. 1983; Marshall et al. 1985). Both of these investigations found high chloride concentrations (approximately 50 mmol/l) in the principal cells. This is higher than could reasonably be expected from a passive electrochemical equilibrium. Analysis of the principal cells of the sea turtle lacrimal salt gland (Marshall 1988a, b) reveals that the Cl^- concentration in the principal cells is also very high and that Na^+ is higher in secreting glands than non-secreting glands. These findings support the notion of active chloride uptake (presumably via the $Na^+ - K^+ - 2Cl^-$ co-transporter). Intracellular values in principal cells are given in Table 1.

Table 1. X-ray microanalysis of secretory tubule principal cells

	H_2O %	Na^+ (mmol/l)	K^+	Cl^-	Mg^{2+} (mmol/kg)	Ca^{2+}
Duck	77					
NS (N = 3, n = 15)		37 ± 4	112 ± 3	52 ± 3	17 ± 2	9 ± 1
S (N = 5, n = 80)		44 ± 4	116 ± 4	55 ± 3	16 ± 3	7 ± 2
Turtle	88					
NS (N = 3, n = 94)		13 ± 1	174 ± 2	81 ± 2	10 ± 1	4 ± 0
S (N = 5, n = 149)		$34 \pm 1*$	160 ± 3	81 ± 2	$13 \pm 1*$	3 ± 0

NS, not secreting; S, secreting
Mean $\pm$ SEM; N, number of animals; n, number of analyses, $* P < 0.05$

The analyses of Marshal et al. (1985) were carried out on frozen hydrated specimens (Fig. 6) and it was thus possible to analyse a number of lumina, both in the secretory tubules and in the duct system. The results of these analyses are shown in Fig. 7. They indicate that the initial secretion of the principal cells is not hyperosmotic to the blood. Indeed, the analyses suggest that it is slightly hypo-osmotic to the blood and that it is concentrated in the duct system. It may further be deduced that K^+ is secreted by the principal cells and that it is reabsorbed in the secondary ducts.

As in the duck, analyses of the lumina of sea turtle secretory tubules showed that the secreted fluid is also slightly hypo-osmotic to the blood and has a high K^+ concentration (Table 2; Marshall 1988a, b). If the luminal fluids in both the duck and turtle secretory tubules are truely hypo-osmotic this would pose a problem in explaining how secretion took place. It may be that the small osmotic deficiency is attributable to undetected small-

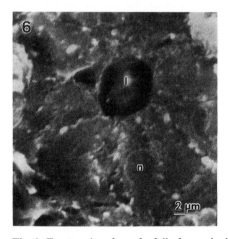

Fig. 6. Fractured surface of a fully frozen-hydrated bulk sample of secretory tubule of duck nasal gland. *l*, lumen; *n*, nucleus

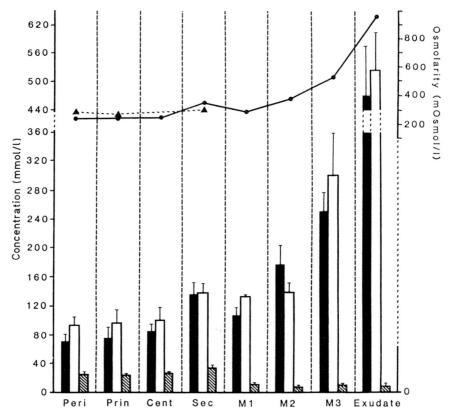

Fig. 7. Comparison of elemental concentrations in lumina of secretory tubules at position of peripheral (*Peri*) and principal (*Prin*) cells, central (*Cent*) canals of the lobules, secondary (*Sec*) ducts of the gland and different positions (*M*) along the main duct, and exudate in secreting nasal salt glands of ducks. Calculated osmolalities for cells (*dotted line*) and lumina (*solid line*) are also shown. *Solid bars*, Na; *open bars*, Cl; *hatched bars*, K

Table 2. Composition of luminal fluids in turtle salt gland

	Na^+	Cl^-	K^+ mmol/l	Mg^{2+}	Ca^{2+}
Secretory tubules					
NS (n = 4)	114 ± 13	174 ± 16	44 ± 12	6 ± 2	2 ± 2
S (n = 5)	122 ± 16	167 ± 30	38 ± 5	10 ± 2	5 ± 2
Central canals					
NS (n = 1)	178	215	11	10	–
S (n = 1)	101	126	15	11	7

NS, not secreting; S, secreting; n, number of analyses
Mean $\pm$ SEM

molecular-weight organic compounds. It should be noted, however, that hypo-osmotic secretion is not unknown since it apparently occurs in *Carausius* malpighian tubules (Taylor 1974).

The secondary duct cells in both ducks and turtles contain high concentrations of Cl^-, approximately 56 mmol/l in ducks and 86 mmol/l in turtles (Marshall et al. 1985; A.T. Marshall, unpublished data). This is perhaps further evidence of an active role for the duct cells.

The finding of K^+ in the secretory tubule lumen requires consideration in the light of the failure of Greger et al. (1987) to find K^+ channels on the luminal membrane of the principal cells of the rectal gland. This seems to indicate that either K^+ is not present in high concentration in the fluid secreted by the secretory tubules in the rectal gland or that if it is, as in the duck and turtle, it enters via the paracellular route.

The results of these X-ray microanalytical analyses are interesting to compare with those obtained from other secretory epithelia. There is only slender evidence of an increase in Na^+ concentration in duck nasal salt gland during secretion, but somewhat stronger evidence in the turtle lacrimal salt gland. This increase is consistent with X-ray microanalytical observations on the cells of the secretory coil of sweat glands and in parotid salivary gland cells (see Wilson et al. 1988). The failure to detect a fall in K^+ concentration during activity in salt glands is contrary to observations on sweat glands and parotid salivary glands. An increase in Cl^- concentration has been observed in active sweat glands and in mandibular salivary glands (Sasaki et al. 1983), but not in avian and turtle salt glands nor in parotid salivary glands.

Measurements of intracellular ion concentrations in stimulated and unstimulated rectal gland secretory tubule cells are contradictory. An increase in Na^+ activity from 11 to 30 mmol/l and a small decrease in Cl^- activity with K^+ remaining constant have been reported by Greger and Schlatter (1985), whereas Welsh et al. (1983) found Cl^- to remain unchanged, and Epstein et al. (1981) report a fall in both Na^+ and Cl^- and an increase in K^+.

Post-Tubular Modification

The finding of an almost iso-osmotic fluid in tubule lumina of salt glands that were actively secreting prior to removal and freezing must mean that either a large osmotic and ionic gradient across the epithelium has dissipated in the short time between excision and freezing or that modification of the fluid occurs in the duct system. For osmotic re-equilibration to occur, secretion of Na^+ and Cl^- would have to cease rapidly whilst the epithelium continued to be permeable to water. Perhaps arguing against a rapid osmotic re-equilibration are the findings of Shuttleworth and Thomson (1986) that in the perfused rectal gland, Na^+ concentration in the secreted

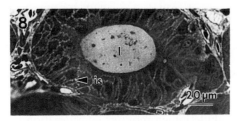

Fig. 8. Light micrograph of freeze-substituted sea turtle lacrimal salt gland showing dilated intercellular spaces in central canal/secondary duct. *l*, lumen; *is*, intercellular space

fluid remains constant over a wide range of perfusion rates. They also showed that secretion occurred in the unstimulated gland with a similar Na^+ concentration in the secreted fluid and that the relation between secretion and perfusion rate was unaffected by a reduction in oxygen availability of 80%.

Marshall et al. (1987) have measured the surface area of the duct system in ducks raised on fresh water and ducks raised on saline. The increase in secretory tubule tissue in the saline-raised birds was paralleled by an increase in the duct system, suggesting a functional relation between the two. The values for surface area were used to calculate values for Na^+ flux or water flux across the duct epithelium, assuming either Na^+ secretion or water reabsorption. These values are high, being for salt-adapted ducks 0.85×10^{-8} μmol Na^+ μm^{-2} s^{-1} and 0.88×10^{-7} μl H_2O μm^{-2} s^{-1}, but are not greatly different from the values given previously which are calculated for fluxes across the luminal surface of the secretory tubules. In the context of water reabsorption, the intercellular spaces in the duct epithelia of ducks and turtles are dilated in freeze-substituted sections (A. T. Marshall, unpublished data; Fig. 8), which suggests that they may well be filled with fluid when glands are in the secreting state.

Possible mechanisms facilitating water reabsorption might involve ion recycling in the basal cell layers and the development of hyperosmotic interspaces. In turtles and elasmobranchs the mucous layer on the luminal surface of the duct might result in ion gradients between lumen and cell surfaces with a consequent reduction in the effective osmotic gradient across the epithelium. Such a phenomenon has been proposed for the fish oesophagus (Shephard 1982).

References

Abel JH, Ellis RA (1966) Histochemical and electron microscopic observations on the salt secreting lacrymal glands of marine turtles. Am J Anat 118: 337–358

Andrews SB, Mazurkiewicz JE, Kirk RG (1983) The distribution of intracellular ions in the avian salt gland. J Cell Biol 96: 1389–1399

Bulger RE (1963) Fine structure of the rectal (salt-secreting) gland of the spiny dogfish *Squalus acanthias*. Anat Rec 147: 95–127

Bulger RE (1965) Electron microscopy of the stratified epithelium lining the secretory canal of the dogfish rectal gland. Anat Rec 151: 589–608

Cowan FBM (1971) The ultrastructure of the lachrymal "salt" gland and the Harderian gland in the euryhaline *Malaclemys* and some closely related stenohaline emydines. Can J Zool 49: 691–697

Cowan FNM (1986) A stereological analysis of the effect of buffer osmolarity on a salt secreting epithelium, under variable physiological conditions. J Microsc 142: 87–94

Dunson WA, Dunson MK (1974) Interspecific differences in fluid concentration and secretion rate of sea snake salt glands. Am J Physiol 227: 420–438

Ellis RA, Abel JH (1964) Intercellular channels in the salt-secreting glands of marine turtles. Science 144: 1340–1343

Ellis RA, Goertemiller CC (1976) Scanning electron microscopy of intercellular channels and the localization of ouabain sensitive p-nitrophenyl phosphatase activity in the salt-secreting lacrymal glands of the marine turtle *Chelonia mydas*. Cytobiologie 13: 1–12

Ellis RA, Goertemiller CC, Stetson DL (1977) Significance of extensive 'leaky' cell junctions in the avian salt gland. Nature 268: 555–556

Epstein FH, Silva P (1981) Na–K–Cl cotransport in chloride-transporting epithelia. Ann NY Acad Sci 372: 187–197

Epstein FH, Stoff JS, Silva P (1981) Hormonal control of secretion in shark rectal gland. Ann NY Acad Sci 372: 613–625

Ernst SA (1972) Transport adenosine triphosphatase cytochemistry. II. Cytochemical localization of ouabain-sensitive, potassium dependent phosphatase activity in the secretory epithelium of the avian salt gland. J Histochem Cytochem 20: 23–38

Ernst SA, Hootman SR, Schreiber JH, Riddle CV (1981) Freeze-fracture and morphometric analysis of occluding junctions in rectal glands of the elasmobranch fish. J Membrane Biol 58: 101–114

Eveloff J, Karnaky KJ, Silva P, Epstein FH, Kinter WB (1979) Elasmobranch rectal gland cell. Autoradiographic localization of [3H] onabain-sensitive Na-K-ATPase in rectal gland of dogfish, *Squalus acanthias*. J Cell Biol 83: 16–32

Forrest JN, Boyer JL, Ardito TA, Murdaugh HV, Wade JB (1982) Structure of tight junctions during Cl secretion in the perfused rectal gland of the dogfish shark. Am J Physiol 242: C388–C392

Greger R, Schlatter E (1985) cAMP increases the apical Cl⁻ conductance in the rectal gland of *Squalus acanthias*. In: Gilles R, Gilles-Baillien M (eds) Transport processes, ion-, and osmoregulation. Springer, Berlin Heidelberg New York

Greger R, Gögelein H, Schlatter E (1987) Potassium channels in the basolateral membrane of the rectal gland of the dogfish (*Squalus acanthias*) Pflügers Arch 409: 100–106

Holmes WN, Phillips JG (1985) The avian salt gland. Biol Rev Cambridge Philosophic Soc 60: 213–256

Komnick H (1963) Elektronenmikroskopische Untersuchungen zur funktionellen Morphologie des Ionentransportes in der Salzdrüse von *Larus argentatus*. 1. Ban und Feinstruktur der Salzdrüse. Protoplasma 56: 274–314

Lacy ER (1983) Carbonic anhydrase localization in the elasmobranch rectal gland. J Exp Zool 226: 163–169

Marshall AT (1988a) A comparison of the salt glands of birds and sea turtles. In: Wong PYD, Young JA (eds) Exocrine secretion. Hong Kong University Press, Hong Kong, pp 107–110

Marshall AT (1988b) Intracellular and luminal ion concentrations in sea turtle salt glands: X-ray microanalysis of frozen-hydrated bulk samples. Inst Phys Conf Ser 93 (3): 559–560

Marshall AT, Cooper PD (1988) Secretory capacity of the lachrymal salt gland of hatchling sea turtles, *Chelonia mydas*. J Comp Physiol 157: 821–827

Marshall AT, Saddlier S (1989) The duct system of the lachrymal salt gland of the green sea turtle, *Chelonia mydas*. Cell Tissue Res (in press)

Marshall AT, Hyatt AD, Phillips JG, Condron RJ (1985) Isosmotic secretion in the avian nasal salt gland: X-ray microanalysis of luminal and intracellular ion distributions. J Comp Physiol 156: 213–227

Marshall AT, King P, Condron RJ, Phillips JG (1987) The duct system of the avian salt gland as a transporting epithelium: structure and morphometry in the duck *Ana platyrhynchos*. Cell Tissue Res 248: 179–188

Martin BJ, Phillpot CW (1974) The biochemical nature of the cell periphery of the salt gland secretory cells of fresh and salt water adapted ducks. Cell Tissue Res 150: 193–211

Merchant JL, Papermasters DS, Barrnett RJ (1985) Correlation of Na^+-, K^+-ATPase content and plasma membrane surface area in adapted and de-adapted salt glands of ducklings. J Cell Sci 78: 233–246

Minnich JE (1979) Reptiles. In: Maloiy GMO (ed) Comparative physiology of osmoregulation in animals, vol 1. Academic, London, pp 391–641

Sasaki S, Nakagaki I, Mori H, Imai Y (1983) Intracellular calcium store and transport of elements in acinar cells of the salivary gland determined by electron probe X-ray microanalysis. Jpn J Physiol 209: 484–488

Schmidt-Nielsen K, Jorgensen CB, Osaki H (1957) Secretion of hypertonic solutions in marine birds. Fed Proc 16: 113–114

Shephard KL (1982) The influence of mucus on the diffusion of ions across the esophagus of fish. Physiol Zool 55: 23–24

Shuttleworth TJ, Thompson JL (1986) Perfusion-secretion relationships in the isolated elasmobranch rectal gland. J Exp Biol 125: 373–384

Swenson ER, Maren TH (1984) Effects of acidosis and carbonic anhydrase inhibition in the elasmobranch rectal gland. Am J Physiol 247: F86–F92

Taplin LE, Grigg GC (1981) Salt glands in the tongue of the estuarine crocodile *Crocodylus porosus*. Science 212: 1045–1047

Taylor HH (1974) The osmolarity of fluid secreted by the malpighian tubules of *Carausius morosus*. Comp Biochem Physiol A47: 1129–1134

Van Lennep EW (1968) Electron microscopic histochemical studies on salt-excreting glands in elasmobranchs and marine catfish. J Ultrastruct Res 25: 94–108

Van Lennep EW, Komnick H (1970) Fine structure of the nasal salt gland in the desert lizard *Uromastyx acanthinurus*. Cytobiologie 2: 47–67

Van Lennep EW, Young JA (1979) Salt glands. In: Giebisch G (ed) Transport organs. Springer, Berlin Heidelberg New York, pp 675–692 (Membrane transport in biology, vol 4 B)

Welsh MJ, Smith PL, Frizzell RA (1983) Intracellular chloride activities in the isolated perfused shark rectal gland. Am J Physiol 245: F640–F644

Wilson SM, Elder HY, Jenkinson D, McWilliams SA (1988) The effects of thermally induced activity in vivo upon the levels of sodium, chloride and potassium in the epithelia of the equine sweat gland. J Exp Biol 136: 489–494

9 Cystic Fibrotic Epithelia

Ion Transport Regulation in Cystic Fibrosis Epithelia

J. Bijman, A. M. Hoogeveen, B. J. Scholte, M. Kansen, A. W. M. van der Kamp, and H. R. de Jonge

Cystic fibrosis (CF) is an autosomal recessive inherited disease that is manifest predominantly among Caucasians. In the Netherlands the average age of survival is 21 years. The clinical symptoms of CF are meconium ileus, pancreatic insufficiency, and/or obstruction of the deeper regions of the airways. In 99% of patients, salt wasting in the sweat is apparent. A single locus appears to be involved in CF, and the defective gene has been located on chromosome 7 (Wainwright et al. 1985).

CF is characterized by abnormalities in the transport of salt in the epithelial cells of the organs with exocrine function, e.g., respiratory tissue, digestive tract, pancreas, and sweat gland. In the apical membrane of the epithelial cells of these organs, channel-forming proteins are embedded that selectively allow passage of chloride ions across the lipid bilayer. For example, in the distal part of the sweat gland (sweat duct), NaCl is reabsorbed from the primary sweat through sodium- and chloride-selective channels in the duct epithelial cells. This NaCl uptake process is electroconductive, i.e., it can be monitored by electrophysiological methods. Voltage and resistance measurements of the sweat duct led to the hypothesis of decreased chloride conductance in the CF sweat duct (Quinton 1983; Quinton and Bijman 1983; Bijman and Quinton 1984; Bijman and Frömter 1987). Subsequently, investigation of the chloride transport function of the sweat gland coil (Sato and Sato 1984), airway epithelium (Knowless et al. 1983), and intestine (De Jonge et al. 1987; Berschneider et al. 1988; Taylor et al. 1988) in normal subjects and patients with CF have confirmed the hypothesis that decreased chloride conductance is the common denominator of impaired salt transport in the organs affected in CF.

The chloride conductance of the (chloride-reabsorbing) sweat duct in normal and CF subjects is apparently not under neurohormonal control (J. Bijman, unpublished observations). In contrast, in the organs that secrete chloride, the chloride channel activity is regulated by a variety of hormones and neurotransmitters. Furthermore, the sensitivity of the chloride-secreting mechanism varies among the different cell types. In epithelial tissues, at least

Young · Wong, Epithelial Secretion of Water and Electrolytes
© Springer-Verlag Berlin · Heidelberg 1990

four types of intracellular messengers that are capable of activating chloride channel activity are known at present, namely, calcium (Ca^{2+}), cyclic AMP, cyclic GMP, and diacylglycerol (DAG). For example, the normal sweat gland coil and normal tracheal cells secrete chloride in response to cholinergic and β-adrenergic agonists, which utilize intracellular Ca^{2+} and cyclic AMP as second messengers, respectively. In CF cells of these tissues, cyclic AMP accumulation is normal, but chloride secretion fails when the cells are stimulated with β-adrenergic agonists (Sato and Sato 1984; Welsh and Liedtke 1986). Evidence for a defect in phosphorylation of a regulatory domain or subunit of the chloride channel has been obtained recently by exposing excised membrane patches of cultured tracheal cells from normal and CF subjects to cyclic AMP-dependent protein kinase (PK-A) and ATP (Schoumacher et al. 1987; Li et al. 1988). Under these experimental conditions and holding the membrane patch at physiological electrical potential, it was found that protein phosphorylation provoked the opening of normal, but not of CF chloride channels. In contrast, both normal and CF chloride channels were activated if the membrane patch was exposed to depolarizing membrane holding potentials, a phenomenon referred to as voltage activation of the channel. In our laboratory we recently measured chloride secretion in normal and CF intestinal epithelia in vitro and found that the secretory response towards Ca^{2+}, cyclic GMP, and cyclic AMP-related agonists is totally absent in CF intestine (de Jonge et al. 1987). The experiments also demonstrated that in the enterocyte, the CF defect is at a site distal to (a) cyclic GMP-dependent protein kinase activation (PK-G), (b) Ca^{2+} mobilization by Ca^{2+}-linked secretomotor agonists, and (c) PK-A activation by cyclic AMP.

The aforementioned results indicate that CF is a disease of decreased chloride permeability. However, heterogeneity with respect to cyclic nucleotide or Ca^{2+} regulation of the chloride conductance exists among the different epithelia. Yet other differences are found: for example, in the apical membrane of CF airway and CF intestinal epithelial cells, an increased sodium or potassium conductance is measured, respectively (Knowles et al. 1983, 1983; Boucher et al. 1986; de Jonge et al. 1987). Moreover, patch-clamp experiments in our laboratory suggest that CF chloride channels in excised patches have a delayed onset of activity when voltage activated, in contrast to chloride channels of normal cells. In this article a summary will be presented of our latest data on the analysis of the CF defect by means of electrophysiological and biochemical techniques.

Immortalization of Human Nasal CF Polyp Cells

The limited availability of suitable cell material is a serious obstacle in CF research. Nasal polyp and sweat gland epithelial cells are relatively easy to obtain, although only in small quantities; moreover, these cell populations have a limited proliferative capacity in culture and are often heterogeneous. We therefore felt the need to develop a continuously growing epithelial cell line retaining the CF genotype and phenotype. As spontaneously transformed epithelial cell lines from CF patients were not available, we chose to use a protocol developed recently for immortalization of human epithelial cells using a hybrid SV40/Adenol2 virus (Rhim et al. 1984). Epithelial cells were scraped off nasal polyps obtained from surgery after pronase treatment (1 h 37°C, 2.5 mg/ml pronase in RPMI medium plus 1% fetal calf serum). The cells were seeded on feeder cells (3T3 J2), irradiated with 30 Gy. The medium used was a mixture of DMEM and Ham's F 12 (1:1) supplemented with 1% (V/V) fetal calf serum, epidermal growth factor 10 ng/ml, hydrocortisone 0.1 μg/ml, insulin 10 μg/ml, transferrin 10 μg/ml, Na_2SeO_3 50 nmol/l, glutamine 2.4 nmol/l, penicillin 100 I.E. units/ml, and streptomycin 100 mg/l. Under these conditions the cells could be maintained for four to five passages (1:4), after which proliferation stopped. Approximately 5 million epithelial cells, passage three, from a CF patient were infected with a SV40/Adenol2 hybrid virus at a multiplicity of 1:100. Following infection the cells were passaged on fresh feeder twice more until the growth of primary cells stopped. After several weeks, clones of rapidly growing cells with epithelial morphology appeared. One of these subclones was cultured for 16 passages, after which a growth crisis typical for SV40-transformed cells occurred. A subclone with epithelial characteristics that survived the crisis (NCF3A) was characterized. Both the pre- and postcrisis CF cell lines that we isolated seem to have the phenotypic properties expected. They express large T antigen (Rhim et al. 1984), have epithelial morphology (Fig. 1), and the production of cytokeratins is indicative of their epithelial nature. Ussing chamber experiments can be performed with pre-crisis cells, i.e., they form cell layers with sufficient electrical resistance. A sustained increase of the short-circuit current is observed after addition of calcium ionophore A23187 in the presence of amiloride. This effect is reversed by the chloride channel blocker 51B. This can be interpreted as an increase of chloride transport caused by high intracellular calcium as was also observed in normal and CF nasal epithelial cells (Widdicombe 1986; Bijman et al. 1987). Isoproterenol, forskolin, and dibutyryl-cyclic AMP did not elicit an electrical response in the presence of amiloride, while cyclic AMP levels are increased dramatically in response to isoproterenol and forskolin. This indicates that the cyclic AMP-dependent signal transduction pathway involved in the opening of chloride channels does not operate in these cells. The postcrisis cell line NCF3A was not suitable for Ussing chamber measurements as it was apparently unable to form tight junctions. It could be shown by patch-clamp analysis that both pre- and postcrisis cells contained chloride channels of primary CF epithelial cells. Activation of the chloride channels by an increase of intracellular cyclic AMP was observed in NCF3A cells ($n=12$). Moreover, all chloride channels observed were activated during prolonged off-cell depolarization ($n=12$). This delayed onset of activation was a characteristic feature of chloride channels from CF

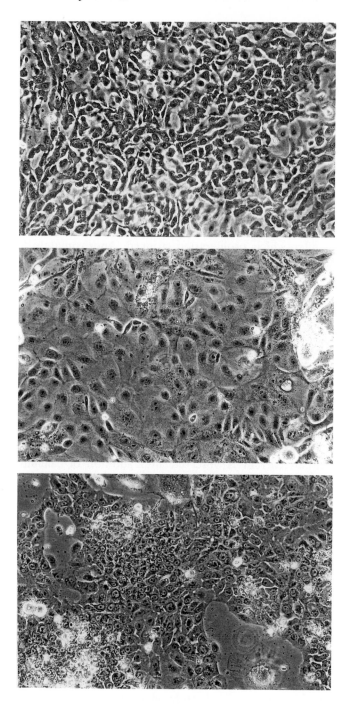

Fig. 1a – c. Light microscope images of **a** primary CF nasal polyp cells, **b** precrisis cells, and **c** immortalized cells

cells. Chloride channels of normal epithelium are activated generally within 2 min, whereas channels of CF cells are activated after 6.0 ± 2.5 min (see below). We conclude, therefore, that the behavior of the chloride channels in NCF3A is in line with the current definition of the CF phenotype: no spontaneous activity and absence of activation by increased intracellular cyclic AMP.

Patch-Clamp Analysis of Normal and CF Cells

Patch-clamp analysis of chloride channels of epithelial cells provides a useful tool to examine the CF defect at the level of the channel itself or its regulatory components in the membrane. Primary outgrowths of normal and CF sweat ducts are incubated in hydroxyethylpiperazine ethanesulfonic acid (HEPES, 5 mmol/l) buffered Ringer's solution. In excised cell membrane patches, chloride channels were present in approximately 1 in 15 successful seals of CF and normal cells. The characteristics of the chloride channel (Fig. 2) were similar to the chloride channel in cultured CF tracheal cells

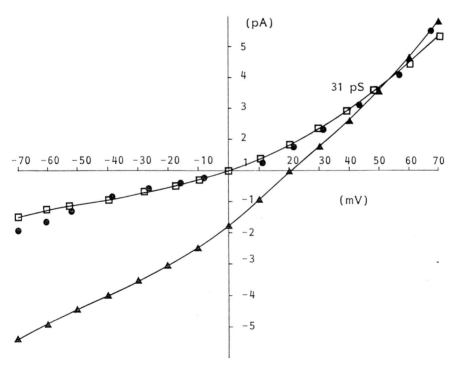

Fig. 2. Chloride channel in excised patch of cultured primary duct cell. The patch pipette was filled with 150 mmol/l NaCl; the bathing solution contained 150 mmol/l NaCl (*squares*), 420 mmol/l NaCl (*triangles*), or 140 mmol/l KCl (*dots*)

(Schoumacher et al. 1987; Li et al. 1988). The channel is rectifying for outward currents, and the conductance of the channel is 31.4 $\pm$ 3.2 pS ($n=9$). No active chloride channels are found in on-cell patches of normal unstimulated cells, which contrasts to the unstimulated chloride conductance of the sweat duct in vivo and in vitro (Bijman and Frömter 1986). This observation suggests that either the principal chloride conductance of the sweat duct resides in the paracellular junctions (Bijman and Quinton 1987) or the apparent latency of the chloride channel is due to a dedifferentiated state of the duct epithelial cells, possibly due to the cell culturing conditions. Cultured cells of normal duct exhibit chloride secretion when challenged with β-adrenergic agonists (Pedersen and Larsen 1986), but our attempts to activate the channel by catecholamine stimulation in on-cell patches have so far been unsuccesful. The chloride channel in excised patches of most normal and CF epithelial cells are activated by depolarizing the membrane potential which seems to be a characteristic property of the channel (Schoumacher et al. 1987; Li et al. 1988). Upon excision of the patch and depolarization of the membrane to 70 mV, we found that normal channels became activated almost instantaneously (1.4 $\pm$ 2.1 min, $n=16$) while CF channels opened after a lag period (7.1 $\pm$ 4.9 min, $n=12$). Whether the delayed onset of activation observed also with chloride channels of CF keratinocytes and coil cells is an intrinsic property of the CF chloride channel or is due to to the release of an inhibitory factor is at present under study.

Regulation of Chloride Secretion in Intestinal Epithelium

The possible manifestation of a chloride channel defect in intestinal epithelium from CF patients was investigated by Ussing chamber measurements of the short circuit current (I_{sc}) of stripped ileal mucosa from patients ($n=5$) undergoing resection for atresia or enterocolitis and CF patients ($n=5$) undergoing stoma surgery following meconium impaction. Endogeneous prostaglandin release was inhibited by serosal (s) and mucosal (m) indomethacin (10^{-5} mol/l). The I_{sc} response to glucose, agonists acting through Ca^{2+} (carbachol, histamine, bradykinin), through cyclic AMP (8-bromo-cyclic AMP, cholera toxin), and through cyclic GMP (8-bromo-cyclic GMP) is shown in Table 1. The negative I_{sc} response in CF observed with all agonists (except 8-bromo-cyclic GMP) was inhibited by barium (5×10^{-3} mol/l, m), bumetanide (10^{-5} mol/l, s), DIDS (10^{-5} mol/l, s) and chloride-free conditions and presumably reflects the opening of apical potassium and basolateral chloride channels by cyclic AMP and Ca^{2+}. On the basis of these results it is concluded that: (a) sodium-coupled uptake of glucose is normal in CF, (b) apical chloride channels are insensitive to the activating signals (Ca^{2+}, cyclic AMP and cyclic GMP), (c) CF enterocytes contain Ca^{2+} and cyclic AMP, but not cyclic GMP-sensitive apical potassium channels and basolateral chloride channels that are absent (or

Table 1. Transient increase of short circuit (I_{sc}) in response to agonists measured in stripped ileal mucosa from normal ($n = 5$) and CF patients ($n = 5$) mounted in an Ussing chamber

Agonist	mol/l	m, s	I_{sc} (uA/cm^2)^a	
			N	CF
Glucose	10^{-3}	m	32 ± 11	36 ± 12
Carbachol	10^{-4}	s	52 ± 18	-24 ± 5
Histamine	5×10^{-5}	s	19 ± 9	-9 ± 5
Bradykinin	10^{-6}	s	16 ± 6	-6 ± 2
8-bromo-cGMP	10^{-4}	s	23 ± 7	0 ± 0
8-bromo-cAMP	10^{-4}	s	62 ± 20	-12 ± 5
Cholera toxin	$10 \, \mu g/ml$	m	34 ± 12	-1 ± 1

m, mucosa;, s, serosa; N, normal; CF, cystic fibrosis
^{a} mean value $\pm$ sem

latent) in control tissue, and (d) the chloride channel defect in CF intestine may offer protection against secretory diarrhoea (e.g., cholera), a disease characterized by hyperactivity of chloride channels in the intestinal crypt cells.

The abnormal I_{sc} response of CF patients to both cyclic nucleotides and Ca^{2+} and the observation that the level and activation characteristics of PK-A and PK-G is normal (de Jonge, unpublished results) suggest that in CF the defect is localized distal to the PK-A and PK-G activating step. For example, the defect could be at the level of the chloride channel itself or at the level of a substrate protein shared by both kinases, a candidate being a 25-kDa proteolipid recently detected in the brush border membrane (de Jonge 1984; de Jonge and Lohmann 1985). Furthermore, our measurements seem to establish a difference in the regulatory properties and the manifestation of the CF defect at the level of the chloride channel between CF ileum and CF sweat coil and trachea since (a) the number of chloride channels in normal CF trachea and CF coil is identical (Frizzell et al. 1987), (b) the Ca^{2+} activation of the chloride channel in CF coil and trachea is normal (Welsh and Liedtke 1986; Frizzell et al. 1986), and (c) the cyclic GMP-regulated activation of the chloride channel is a unique property of intestinal cells.

Discussion

The data obtained with the immortalized nasal CF polyp cells lead us to believe that the isolated cell lines provide a useful model system for the study of cystic fibrosis. The availability of considerable amounts of well-characterized CF cell material that can be manipulated at will can be very helpful in the biochemical analysis of the disease.

When we combine the electrophysiological data of trachea (Schoumacher et al. 1987; Li et al. 1988), sweat gland, and intestinal mucosa (de Jonge et al. 1987; Berschneider et al. 1988; Taylor et al. 1988) presented in this and other studies there is evidence for: (a) a defect in cyclic GMP activation distal to PK-G in the enterocyte, (b) a defect in cyclic AMP activation of the channel at a site distal to PK-A in all tissues, (c) a defect in Ca^{2+} activation of the channel in the sweat gland duct and the enterocyte, but not in trachea and sweat coil, (d) a defect in phorbol ester activation of the channel distal to PK-C in trachea, and (e) a delay in chloride-channel activation upon excision of the patch at depolarizing holding potential, at least in nasal and sweat duct epithelial cells. These combined data suggest that the regulatory defect of the chloride channel is not cyclic nucleotide specific. The heterogeneous response to Ca^{2+} with respect to chloride-channel activation that is unmasked by the CF condition needs to be explored further. Furthermore, there is evidence that, in addition to the chloride transport defect, sodium transport in nasal airway epithelium (Knowles et al. 1983; Boucher et al. 1986) and potassium transport in intestinal epithelium (de Jonge et al. 1987; this study) become hyperactivated by the CF defect. The question remains unsettled as to whether these changes in other chloride transport processes occur in parallel with or as a consequence of the defect in chloride-channel regulation. Further research is clearly needed to establish whether the chloride-channel defect is the primary lesion or results from the deficiency (overexpression, respectively) of an activating (inhibitory, respectively) factor playing an additional role in the regulation of cation-channel activity in the apical membrane of the epithelial cells.

References

Berschneider HM, Knowles MR, Azizkhan RG, Boucher RC, Tobey NA, Orlando RC, Powell DW (1988) Altered intestinal chloride transport in cystic fibrosis. FASEB J 2: 2625–2629

Bijman J, Frömter E (1986) Direct demonstration of high transepitheleal chloride-conductance in normal human sweat duct which is absent in cystic fibrosis. Pflügers Arch 407: S123–S127

Bijman J, Quinton PM (1984) Influence of abnormal Cl$^-$ impermeability on sweating in cyctic fibrosis. Am J Physiol 247: C3–C9

Bijman J, Quinton P (1987) Lactate and bicarbonate uptake in the sweat duct of cystic fibrosis and normal subjects. Pflügers Arch 408 (5): 505–510

Bijman J, Scholte B, de Jonge HR, Hoogeveen AT, Kansen MT, Sinaasappel M, van der Kamp AWM (1987) Chloride transport in CF; chloride channel regulation in cultured sweat duct and cultured nasal polyp epithelia. In: Mastella G, Quinton PM (eds) Cellular and molecular basis of cystic fibrosis. San Francisco Press, San Francisco, pp 133–140

Boucher RC, Stutts MJ, Knowles MR, Cantley L, Gatzy JT (1986) Na$^+$ transport in cystic fibrosis respiratory epithelia. Abnormal basal rate and response to adenylate cyclase activation. J Clin Invest 78: 1245–1252

Frizzell RA, Schoumacher RA, Shoemaker RL, Halm DR (1987) Chloride channel regulation in secretory epithelial cells. Pediatr Pulmonol [Suppl] 1: 24–25

de Jonge HR (1984) The mechanisms of action of *Escherichia coli* toxin. Biochem Soc Trans 12: 180–184

de Jonge HR, Lohmann SM (1985) Mechanisms by which cyclic nucleotides and other intracellular mediators regulate secretion. Ciba Found Symp 112: 116–138

de Jonge HR, Bijman J, Sinaasappel M (1987) Relation of regulatory enzyme levels to chloride transport in intestinal epithelial cells. Pediatr Pulmonol [Suppl] 1: 54–57

Frizzell RA, Rechkemmer G, Shoemaker (1986) Altered regulation of airway epithelial cell chloride channels in cystic fibrosis. Science 233: 558–560

Knowles MJ, Gatzy J, Boucher R (1983) Relative ion permeability of normal and cystic fibrosis nasal epithelium. J Clin Invest 71: 1410–1417

Li M, McCann JD, Liedtke CM, Nairn AC, Greengard P, Welsh MJ (1988) Cyclic AMP-dependent protein kinase opens chloride channels in normal but not cystic fibrosis airway epithelium. Nature 331: 358–360

Pedersen PS, Larsen EH (1986) Effect of isoproterenol on ion transport in cell culture epithelial membranes derived from human sweat gland ducts. IRSC Med Sci 14: 108–110

Quinton PM (1983) Chloride impermeability in cystic fibrosis. Nature 301: 421–422

Quinton PM, Bijman J (1983) Higher bio-electric potentials due to decreased chloride absorption in the sweat glands of patients with cystic fibrosis. N Engl J Med 308: 1185–1189

Rhim JS, Jay G, Arnstein P, Price FM, Sanford KK, Aaronson SA (1984) Neoplastic transformation of human epidermal keratinocytes by AD12-SV40 and Kirsten sarcoma virus. Science 227: 1250–1252

Sato K, Sato F (1984) Defective beta adrenergic response of cystic fibrosis sweat glands in vivo and in vitro. J Clin Invest 73: 1763–1771

Schoumacher RA, Shoemaker RL, Halm DR, Tallant EA, Wallace RW, Frizzell RA (1987) Phosphorylation fails to activate chloride channels from cystic fibrosis airway cells. Nature 330: 752–754

Taylor CJ, Baxter PS, Hardcastle J, Hardcastle PT (1988) Failure to induce secretion in jejunum biopsies from children with cystic fibrosis. Gut 529: 957–962

Wainwright BJ, Scambler PJ, Schmidtke J, Watson EA, Law HY, Farral M, Cooke HJ, Eiberg H, Williamson A (1985) Localization of cystic fibrosis locus to human chromosome 7cen–q22. Nature 318: 384–385

Welsh MJ, Liedtke CM (1986) Chloride and potassium channels in cystic fibrosis airway epithelia. Nature 322: 476–470

Widdicombe (1986) Cystic fibrosis and β-adrenergic response of airway epithelial cell cultures. Am J Physiol 251: R818–R812

Subject Index